Bioactive Components, Diet and Medical Treatment in Cancer Prevention

Mostafa I. Waly · Mohammad Shafiur Rahman
Editors

Bioactive Components, Diet and Medical Treatment in Cancer Prevention

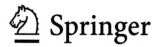 Springer

Editors
Mostafa I. Waly
Department of Food Science and Nutrition
College of Agricultural and Marine
Sciences
Sultan Qaboos University
Muscat, Oman

Mohammad Shafiur Rahman
Department of Food Science and Nutrition
College of Agricultural and Marine Sciences
Sultan Qaboos University
Muscat, Oman

ISBN 978-3-030-09300-6   ISBN 978-3-319-75693-6   (eBook)
https://doi.org/10.1007/978-3-319-75693-6

Printed on acid-free paper

This Springer imprint is published by the registered company Springer International Publishing AG
part of Springer Nature.
The registered company address is: Gewerbestrasse 11, 6330 Cham, Switzerland

..... Cancer is not cured with surgical instruments, but with a vegetarian diet and medicinal herbs...

Hippocrates

Preface

Cancer is a major public health concern not only in the Western countries but also in other parts of the world. Although modern advancements and techniques play a significant role in the treatment of cancer, cancer morbidity and mortality is still on the rise. Current research supports the notion that the primary intervention for cancer relies mainly on combating etiological and risk factors associated with cancer incidence. This approach might be succeeded through lifestyle modifications and adopting dietary intervention strategies including increase in consumption of bioactive components and functional foods that have anticancer therapeutic effects by stimulating DNA repair mechanism, promoting production of protective antioxidant enzymes, inhibiting cancer-activating enzymes and hormones, and inducing cellular antioxidant capacity.

The book includes 16 chapters that cover a broad range of methodological and theoretical approaches of functional foods, bioactive components, and natural therapeutic agents in cancer prevention. In addition to addressing the multifactorial (i.e., medical and lifestyle) aspects in the development of different types of cancers, we aimed to cover in a single volume the potential therapeutic aspects of natural antioxidants in the foods, the basic understanding of cancer risk factors, preventive measures, and possible treatments currently available.

The contributing authors to this book were selected considering their expertise in their respective fields. Individually each chapter represents a unique perspective into the biochemical and clinical basis of cancer. The chapters summarize current research findings and present novel ideas and possible mechanisms that may be of potential importance in cancer prevention. The book is structurally formatted into two sections: Bioactive Components and Cancer covers antioxidants in foods including plants and components of the diet; and Lifestyle, Medicine, and Cancer covers the risk factors and medical aspects of cancer.

We are confident that the scientific community and researchers will find in this book methods of effective treatment or at least improvements in cancer prevention. Nevertheless, the materials in this book provide a framework for further in-depth studies in order to devise new therapeutic strategies.

Muscat, Oman   Mostafa I. Waly
Muscat, Oman   Mohammad Shafiur Rahman

Contents

About the Editors

Shafiur Rahman is the author/coauthor of over 300 technical articles including more than 140 journal papers and 12 books. He is the author of the internationally acclaimed and award-wining *Food Properties Handbook*, and editor of the popular *Handbook of Food Preservation* published by CRC Press, Florida. First editions received the bestseller recognition and the third edition will be released soon. The first edition was also translated into Spanish. He has initiated the *International Journal of Food Properties* and has been serving as the founding editor-in-chief for more than 20 years, and serving in the editorial boards of ten international journals and book series. In 1998 he has been invited and continued to serve as a Food Science Adviser for the International Foundation for Science, Sweden. He was invited as a keynote/plenary speaker for more than ten international conferences in the food science and engineering area. In 2014, he has initiated and served as the Founding Chair of the International Conference on Food Properties (iCFP) and initiated the ICFP Mentoring Program for the young scientists and academics. He received the HortResearch Chairman's Award, BRAP Award, CAMS Outstanding Researcher Award 2003, and SQU Distinction in Research Award 2008. In 2008, Professor Rahman has ranked among the top five Leading Scientists and Engineers of 57 OIC Member Countries in the Agroscience Discipline. Professor Rahman is an eminent scientist and academic in the area of food processing. He is recognized for his significant contribution to the basic and applied knowledge of food properties related to food structure, engineering properties, and food stability. His total Google Scholar citation is more than 20,000 (h-index: 61) (16 November 2017), indicating high impact of his research in the international scientific community.

Mostafa I. Waly received his Ph.D. in 2003 from the Northeastern University (Boston, USA), in the field of health sciences. He is currently an associate professor in the Department of Food Science and Nutrition at the College of Agricultural and Marine Sciences, Sultan Qaboos University (Muscat, Oman). He has been working in the area of nutritional biochemistry for the past 15 years, and his research focuses on understanding the protective effect of dietary bioactive agents against oxidative stress-mediated human chronic diseases, including cancer. His laboratory studies are being used in vitro and in vivo experimental models to identify the metabolic aspects and mechanisms underlie the therapeutic effects of specific nutrients. His research work has resulted in over 90 publications in international peer-reviewed journals and acquired high ranking citations in scientific metrics such as Scopus, Researchgate, PubMed, and Google Scholar. He is the editor-in-chief and founder of the *Canadian Journal of Clinical Nutrition* and serving in the editorial boards of another eight international journals. He is an active member in the American Society for Biochemistry and Molecular Biology, American Society for Nutrition, International Society of Antioxidants in Nutrition and Health, and Society of Experimental Biology and Medicine.

Contributors

Hajar Ibrahim Salim Al-Ajmi Department of Food Science and Nutrition, College of Agricultural and Marine Sciences, Sultan Qaboos University, Muscat, Oman

Ahmed Al Alawi Department of Food Science and Nutrition, College of Agricultural and Marine Sciences, Sultan Qaboos University, Muscat, Oman

Zaher Al-Attabi Department of Food Science and Nutrition, College of Agricultural and Marine Sciences, Sultan Qaboos University, Muscat, Oman

Amanat Ali Department of Food Science and Nutrition, College of Agricultural and Marine Sciences, Sultan Qaboos University, Muscat, Oman

Hassan Talib Al-Lawati Department for Honey Bee Research, Ministry of Agriculture and Fisheries, Muscat, Oman

Neeru Bhatt Global Science Heritage, Toronto, ON, Canada

Ikram Ali Burney Department of Medicine, Sultan Qaboos University Hospital, Sultan Qaboos University, Muscat, Oman

Richard C. Deth Department of Pharmaceutical Sciences, Nova Southeastern University, Fort Lauderdale, FL, USA

Nejib Guizani Department of Food Science and Nutrition, College of Agricultural and Marine Sciences, Sultan Qaboos University, Muscat, Oman

Matthew Hill Department of Pharmaceutical and Biomedical Sciences, The Raabe College of Pharmacy, Ohio Northern University, Ada, OH, USA

Smitha Padmanabhan Department of Food Science and Nutrition, College of Agricultural and Marine Sciences, Sultan Qaboos University, Muscat, Oman

Preeja Prabhakar Department of Food Science and Nutrition, College of Agricultural and Marine Sciences, Sultan Qaboos University, Muscat, Oman

Pushpendra Pratap Department of Biotechnology, ERA'S Lucknow Medical College & Hospital, ERA University, Lucknow, India

Sanju Pratap Department of Biotechnology, ERA'S Lucknow Medical College & Hospital, ERA University, Lucknow, India

Sivaprasad Punnaveetil Department of Gastroenterology, Starcare Hospital LLC, Muscat, Oman

Mohammad Shafiur Rahman Department of Food Science and Nutrition, College of Agricultural and Marine Sciences, Sultan Qaboos University, Muscat, Oman

Syed Tasleem Raza Department of Biotechnology, ERA'S Lucknow Medical College & Hospital, ERA University, Lucknow, India

Haleama Al Sabbah Health Sciences Department, Zayed University, Dubai, UAE

Amy L. Stockert Department of Pharmaceutical and Biomedical Sciences, The Raabe College of Pharmacy, Ohio Northern University, Ada, OH, USA

Sithara Suresh Department of Food Science and Nutrition, College of Agricultural and Marine Sciences, Sultan Qaboos University, Muscat, Oman

Varna Taranikanti Department of Human and Clinical Anatomy, College of Medicine and Health Sciences, Sultan Qaboos University, Muscat, Oman

Reema F. Tayyem Faculty of Agriculture, Department of Nutrition and Food Technology, University of Jordan, Amman, Jordan

Mostafa I. Waly Department of Food Science and Nutrition, College of Agricultural and Marine Sciences, Sultan Qaboos University, Muscat, Oman

Risk Factors for Cancer: Genetic and Environment

Mohammad Shafiur Rahman, Sithara Suresh, and Mostafa I. Waly

1 Introduction

Today, millions of people are living with cancer or have had cancer. The risk of developing most types of cancer can be reduced by eliminating risk factors of this disease. Often, the sooner a cancer is found and treatment begins, the better are the chances for living for many years. Risk is considered as the chance or probability that a given hazard will occur. Judgement of risk should be made so that level of concern could be made. Severity is the degree of damage one hazard could cause. Based on the calculations of the cumulative risks, it is reported that three in every four men and one in every four women would have cancer before the age of 75 years [1]. Cumulative risk factor can be defined as the combination of threats from exposure to multiple agents or stressors including biochemical, chemical, physical, and psychosocial entities [2]. The risk assessment is a possible tool to analyse, quantify, and ameliorate the combined adverse effects on human health from exposure to many hazards [2, 3]. Currently, there are scarce procedures to analyse the real-world health problems and to conduct risk assessments. This is due to the unavailability of appropriate data, lack of mechanistic understanding, and deficiency of verified analytical frameworks. Exposure to wide range of chemicals and other agents from multiple sources in everyday lives have become a major concern on the cause of several diseases including cancer. Information on the causes of cancer has emerged and it is identified from the investigations of cancer patterns in human populations and induction of tumours in experimental animals with cancer-causing agents [4, 5]. The estimation of human health risk on determining the carcinogenic potency of individual manufactured chemicals from exposure to multiple agents were first

M. S. Rahman (✉) · S. Suresh · M. I. Waly
Department of Food Science and Nutrition, College of Agricultural and Marine Sciences,
Sultan Qaboos University, Muscat, Oman
e-mail: shafiur@squ.edu.om

© Springer International Publishing AG, part of Springer Nature 2018
M. I. Waly, M. S. Rahman (eds.), *Bioactive Components, Diet and Medical Treatment in Cancer Prevention*, https://doi.org/10.1007/978-3-319-75693-6_1

1

employed by the U.S. Environmental Protection Agency (EPA) and the U.S. Food and Drug Administration (FDA) in the 1970s [3]. The majority of assessments conducted by EPA have concentrated on individual chemical agents, distinct sources or source categories, single exposure pathways, environmental media, and routes of exposure. This chapter will provide overview on the risk factors for cancer. This chapter summarizes recent trends in cancer risk factors, in particular the role of genetic and environment.

2 Environmental Risk Factors

Cancer is a multifactorial disease due to a combined effect of both genetic and environmental factors. Therefore, it is important to understand both genetic and environmental risk factors properly since improper understating could lead to take wrong actions towards the reduction of the overall risk. The environmental risk factors include all non-genetic factors such as diet, alcohol consumption, lifestyle, and infectious agents [6].

2.1 Tobacco

The main tobacco plant in the world is *Nicotiana tabacum* and cigarettes represent the main tobacco product worldwide. The industrial production of cigarettes started in the second half of the nineteenth century. Other smoking tobacco products include cigars, cigarillos, pipe, hookah, bidis and many other local products. The use of tobacco is one of the main identified environmental causes of human-cancer-related death worldwide, which invades the lung and other organs like larynx, oral cavity, pharynx, oesophagus, pancreas, kidney and bladder [7]. Higher rates of lung cancer are observed in North America, whereas its incidences in the developing countries are the lowest [8]. In USA, Europe and Japan, 83–92% of lung cancer is observed in men and 57–80% of lung cancers in women and these are related with tobacco consumption [9]. Cigar and pipe smoking habit show a greater risk for oral cavity cancer than cigarette smoking. The risk of oral cavity cancer is double in case of those who smoke and do not drink as compared to those who neither smoke nor drink. The risk of bladder and kidney cancer varies depending on the duration and intensity of smoking, but it is lower than that for lung cancer. Smoking could also lead to other types of cancer such as stomach, liver, nose cancer and myeloid leukaemia. Exposure to environmental tobacco smoke could also lead to lung cancer and laryngeal cancer. However, the incidence of disease is much less as compared to active smokers. Smokeless tobacco products could also lead to increased risk of head and neck cancers. Statistical reports are saying that approximately 25% of cancers in men and 4% in women occur due to tobacco smoking. The prevalence of cancer among women is expected to increase in the future in developing countries and represents a major carcinogenic hazard in the Southern Asian region in both genders [10].

The habit of cigarette smoking or tobacco chewing is common in many communities [11]. The prevalence of smoking varies throughout the world and the proportion of smokers is decreasing among the men in industrialized countries. During the first decades of the twentieth century, more than 70% of men in Europe and North America were addicted to smoking. However, the proportion has decreased in recent times. In contrast, women smoking rates became prevalent in the second half of the twentieth century and is seen as an increasing trend in industrialized countries. In China, the increase is particularly dramatic, it is observed that more than 60% of adult men are estimated to smoke, whereas smokeless tobacco and bidi smoking are common in India and its neighbouring countries [12]. Habit of smoking is also seen increasing in young women. The risk of lung cancer is related to the parameters of tobacco smoking which is determined by the dose of carcinogen, the duration of administration and the intensity of exposure. Hence, the annual lung cancer death rate among 55–64 years old who started smoking at the age of 15 and smoked a daily of 21–39 cigarettes is about three times higher than for those who started at the age 25.

Increase in cancer risks can also be caused by the interaction of other environmental carcinogens, like alcohol consumption, exposure to asbestos, and ionizing radiation, with smoking. The risk of lung cancer is more in individuals exposed to both tobacco smoke and asbestos. The most abundant compound present in cigarette is nicotine (0.1–2.0 mg/cigarette) and includes polycyclic aromatic hydrocarbons [13, 14]. Other carcinogens present are N-nitroso compounds, particularly nitroso derivatives of nicotine and nornicotine. Cancer caused by tobacco smoke is not attributable to any specific chemical compound, but to an overall effect of the complex chemical mixtures. A greater tobacco-related cancer risk is seen from black tobacco cigarette smoking than smoking of blond cigarettes [15]. Similarly, unfiltered and high-tar cigarettes pose a higher risk for tobacco-related cancers compared to filtered and low-tar cigarettes. However, there is no "safe" mode exit for tobacco products.

2.2 Alcohol

Alcohol consumption is another targeted risk factor for developing cancer [16]. Beverages containing alcohol are produced in most countries since ancient times. Most alcoholic beverages can be grouped as beers (5% alcohol), wines (12% alcohol), and spirits (40% alcohol). Official consumption of alcoholic beverages by an adult is equivalent to 4 L of alcohol/year (or 9 g/day) whereas unofficial consumption is estimated to be 20–100% of the official figures depending on the country [17].

Epidemiological studies of case-control type conducted in populations with different level of consumption showed the risk of developing oral cavity, oesophageal, liver, breast, colon and rectal cancers. The carcinogenic effect of alcohol is more potent to oral cavity, pharynx, and oesophagus [18, 19]. Daily consumption of alcohol is proportional to risk of developing a cancer [20]. The risk of developing head and neck cancer is reported to be 5–10 times higher in heavy drinkers, while the breast cancer in women, the risk is approximately twofold. There is a synergistic interaction between alcohol drinking and tobacco smoking in the aetiology of oral cavity, pharynx, larynx and oesophagus cancers. The risk of developing cancers is more in individuals who consume both tobacco and alcohol than in those consuming separately [21, 22]. The pattern of drinking (i.e. intake of moderate quantity or intermittent intake of large quantity) is irrespective in the risk of developing cancer.

The mechanism of cancer causation by alcohol is not well understood. The hypothesis proposed for the increased cancer development due to alcohol is either the presence of chemicals (such as N-nitrosamines) in alcoholic beverages other than ethanol or a solvent action which facilitates the absorption of other carcinogens (from tobacco smoke) or a carcinogenic role of acetaldehyde, a major metabolite of ethanol and a proven carcinogen in experimental animals [23, 24]. Overconsumption of alcohol also leads to several other diseases like alcohol psychosis, chronic pancreatitis, liver cirrhosis, hypertension, haemorrhagic stroke, and low birth weight in babies born to alcoholic mothers. Therefore, a control over alcohol consumption reduces several types of cancer and helps to lead a healthy and quality life.

2.3   Occupational Carcinogens

The link between the cancer risks and working environment were first reported in 1950. The first occupational cancer was mesothelioma due to asbestos and was reported in 1993. Occupational-related cancer is considered as the most significant and preventable causes of cancer. The global burden of occupational cancer was first estimated in 1981 at 2–4% of total cancer cases [25]. Evidences of occupational-related cancer have been obtained mainly in developed countries due to the rise of hazardous industries and the establishment of local industries as a part of rapid global industrialization, especially where health and safety standards and requirements may not be so stringent. The evaluation of cancer risks to humans emerged as a consequence of exposure to chemicals, physical and biological agents such as asbestos, crystalline silica, heavy metals, mustard gas, 2-naphthylamine, dichloromethane, inorganic lead compounds, formaldehyde and 1,3-butadiene [26, 27]. Most of these chemicals have been shown to be carcinogenic in experimental animals and have been associated with an increased cancer risk with a group of agents rather than a single compound. Several individual polycyclic aromatic hydrocarbons are proved to be experimental carcinogens however; human exposure always involves complex mixtures of these chemicals in variable proportions.

An increased risk of cancer has been evaluated from a number of industries and occupations. In some cases, the agents responsible for increased cancer risks are well established, such as wood dust from wood industry whereas the scenario is different for those working in rubber industry or employed as a painter. Here, the risk of cancer would be high but a precise carcinogen is difficult to identify. Exposure of workers mainly to wood dust in furniture and cabinet making industries are shown to cause nasal adenocarcinomas. Leclerc et al. [28] reported an elevated sino-nasal cancer risk by the exposure of wood dust. Bonneterre et al. [29] also reported sino-nasal cancer with exposure to leather dust. Occupational exposure to some of the known or suspected to be carcinogenic pharmaceutical drugs and administration of these drugs to patients by nursing staffs can also occur in pharmacies. Friedman et al. [30] observed the carcinogenic effects of some of the pharmaceutical drugs and reported that 61 out of 105 drugs have shown increased cancer risk.

Other sources of exposure could be by hepatitis B virus in the hospitals, food processors contaminated with aflatoxins from contaminated food, ultraviolet radiation and combustion fumes. By the mid of 1950s, studies were reported that benzidine and 2-napthylamine caused occupational bladder cancer [31]. It was also reported that rubber workers were subjected to malignancy which were attributed to aromatic amines and 4-aminobiphenyl. Dalrymple [32] reported bladder tumours in rubber workers. Later studies on working environmental exposure to aromatic amines have shown that mixtures of compounds were responsible for the malignancy rather than a single agent. Gastric cancer is one of the main causes of significant morbidity and mortality and several occupations in coal and tin mining, metal processing, particularly steel and iron, and rubber manufacturing industries could lead to an increased risk of gastric cancer [33]. Tumours of the urinary bladder in workmen associated in the manufacture and use of certain dye stuff intermediates have been reported frequently. Several million people are believed to work as painters and approximately 0.2 million workers worldwide are employed in paint manufacture. A 40% excess risk of lung cancer has been consistently recorded in painters exposed to hydrocarbon and chlorinated solvents, dyes, polyesters, phenol-formaldehyde and polyurethane resins. Auramine colourants are used for dyeing leather, jute, tanned cotton, and paints, and as dye components in ballpoint pastes, oils and waxes, and carbon paper. The manufacture of auramine has been reported to cause bladder cancer but the causative agent is unknown [34].

Another causative agent responsible for leukaemia is benzene which is used as a solvent and as an intermediate in chemical and petroleum industries [35]. Many studies have reported that exposure to benzene causes non-lymphocytic and myelogenous leukaemia [36, 37]. Khalade et al. [38] showed that exposure to benzene at work increased the risk of leukaemia in a dose-response pattern. Rushton et al. [39] reported that the occurrence of myelodysplastic syndrome was more related with low exposure to benzene and higher lymphoid leukaemia in refinery workers may be due to the diverse exposure to carcinogenic agents than benzene alone. Recognition of asbestos dust as a cancer causative agent has been reported since 1950s. Different forms of asbestos such as chrysotile and the amphibole, crocidolite, are shown to cause lung cancer and mesothelioma, a rare tumour derived from the lining of the peritoneum, pericardium or pleura. A crucial factor responsible for determining the carcinogenicity of asbestos is the fibre size. Pasetto et al. [40]

reported that the number of estimated deaths in 5 years for mesothelioma and for lung, larynx, and ovary cancers attributable to occupational asbestos exposures were, respectively, 735, 233, 29, and 14 for Argentina; 340, 611, 68, and 43 for Brazil; 255, 97, 14, and 9 for Colombia, and 1075, 219, 18, and 22 for Mexico. The risk of incidence of lung cancer is high for those working in chromate producing industries. Studies have shown that the risk is associated with hexavalent chromium compounds. Luippold et al. [41] studied the lung cancer mortality among chromate production workers. The risk is significantly increased at an exposure levels over 1.05 mg/m^3-years. Other metals responsible for increased cancer risks are nickel sulphides, oxides and soluble nickel salts. A variety of occupations involving coal tar, coal gas production and iron founding have been reported to cause skin-related cancers and could also affect the urinary and respiratory systems.

2.4 Environmental Pollution

Environmental pollutants are mainly to a specific subset of cancer-causing environmental factors, namely, air contaminants, water and soil. One characteristic of environmental pollutants is that individuals lack control over their level of exposure. Some of the main carcinogenic pollutants include asbestos (non-occupational exposure), indoor and urban air pollutants, and chlorination by-products and other drinking water contaminants [42, 43]. Estimation of total burden of cancer due to environmental pollutants in developed countries represents 8–9% [44].

Non-occupational exposure to asbestos may occur domestically and as a consequence of localized pollution. Another mode of domestic exposure could be through the installation, degradation, removal and repair of asbestos-containing products in the context of household maintenance. On the other hand, people may be subjected to outdoor pollution as a result of local asbestos mining or manufacture. In both occupational and non-occupational exposure to asbestos resulted in an increased risk of mesothelioma and lung cancer, particularly among smokers in the latter. An example of asbestos exposure carcinogenic risk to inhabitants of villages in Turkey showed a very high incidence of mesothelioma where houses are built from erionite (a zeolite mineral) [45]. Many studies have suggested about the positive dose-response relationship between mesothelioma and exposure to asbestos [46]. Camus [47] reported an excess number of deaths due to pleural cancer and asbestosis and suggested an excess risk of mesothelioma. Another cause of lung cancer could be through ambient air pollution. Air may be polluted through a mixture of complex gases and components with varied concentrations. Some of the atmospheric pollutants leading to cancer include benzo[a]pyrene, benzene, some metals, and possibly ozone. Engine combustion products are another main concern for an increased risk of cancer and other health problems. They include volatile organic compounds (benzene, toluene, xylenes and acetylene), oxides of nitrogen and fine particulates (i.e. carbon, adsorbed organic material and traces of metallic compounds) [48]. Outdoor air pollution is a major concern especially in developing countries than the developed ones due to the usage of poorly regulated use of coal, wood and biomass (e.g. animal dung, crop residues) for electricity production and heating [49].

Many studies reports have also confirmed about the polluted air in the residence in urban areas as compared to the rural areas and the risk driven to lung cancer. Lung cancer is responsible for approximately 31% of all cancer deaths among men and 15% among women. In general, the reports are focusing towards the increased risk of lung cancer in urban areas and its correlation towards specific pollutants such as benzo[a]pyrene, metals and particulate matter, or with mutagenicity of particulate extracts in bacterial assay systems. Widziewics et al. [50] mentioned a strong correlation between the prevalence of lung cancer risk and the ambient concentration of benzo(A)pyrene in polish agglomerations, cities and other areas. Another hazard in terms of localized air pollution is the residences near petroleum refineries, metal manufacturing plants, iron foundries, incinerator plants and smelters. Lin et al. [51] studied lung cancer mortality of residents living near petrochemical industrial complexes. They observed that lung cancer mortality of residents living near petrochemical industrial complexes was 1.03-fold higher than people living far. Another possible targeted air pollutant is chlorofluorocarbons (CFCs) which is indirectly responsible for increased risk of skin cancers. These chemicals include halons, carbon tetrachloride, and methyl chloroform, which are emitted from home air conditioners, foam cushions, and many other products. Chlorofluorocarbons are also carried by winds into the stratosphere, where the action of strong solar radiation releases chlorine and bromine atoms that reacts and thereby eliminate the molecules of ozone which is believed to be responsible for global increases in UVB radiation. The skin cancer mortality rates associated with ozone depletion are expected to increase in the years 2040–2050 [52].

Some reports have revealed about the elevated occurrence of lung cancer in some regions of China and other Asian countries among non-smoking women who spend much of their time at home [53]. Indoor air pollution could be mainly through the combustion sources used for heating and cooking, and may also occur as a consequence of cooking oil vapours. Studies have shown that the carcinogenic hazard is strong for cooking oil vapours from Chinese-style cooking. Kim et al. [54] reported a strong association between cooking conditions, fuel use, oil use and the prevalence of lung cancer in Shanghai region with poor kitchen ventilation. They demonstrated that indoor air pollution from poor ventilation of coal combustion increased the risk of lung cancer. Tobacco smoke is another important source of indoor air pollution. Studies have shown that chronic exposure of adult non-smokers to environmental tobacco smoke increased mortality from lung cancer between 20 and 30%. Exposure of adults to environmental tobacco smoke is linked with increased risk of lung cancer and heart disease whereas in children are affected with respiratory disease, middle ear disease, asthma attacks and sudden infant death syndrome. Vineis et al. [55] investigated the association between environmental tobacco smoke and respiratory cancer and concluded that frequent exposure to environmental tobacco smoke during childhood was associated with lung cancer in adulthood.

Another greatest concern related to infectious disease is the quality of water, which is the basic requirement of human health. Water quality could be influenced by several factors, which include seasons, geology of the soil, and industrial and agricultural discharges [56]. The quality of water is also controlled by disinfection methods that contain chlorine, hypochlorite, chloramine, and ozone. As a consequence, it could result in the contamination of drinking water by several potential carcinogenic agents including the by-products of chlorination and arsenic [43]. The International Agency for Research on Cancer (IARC) has classified inorganic arsenic compounds as carcinogenic to humans and evaluated the carcinogenicity of arsenic in drinking water. Many studies have also suggested about the relationship between chlorinated drinking water and bladder cancer. Bladder cancer is the seventh most frequent type of cancer among men, which is occurring especially in the industrialized regions. Approximately, 261,000 cases are diagnosed annually and about 115,000 deaths are reported globally [57]. Villanueva et al. [58] reported that long-term consumption of chlorinated drinking water is associated with bladder cancer, particularly among men. Smith et al. [59] also reported on the contamination of drinking water with arsenic in Bangladesh. They mentioned that long-term exposure to arsenic (500 µg/L) in groundwater may die from lung, bladder and skin cancers. Several other pollutants of drinking water could also lead to cancer, which includes organic compounds derived from industrial, commercial and agricultural activities and in particular from waste sites, as well as nitrites, nitrates, radionuclides and asbestos. Increased risks of stomach cancer and leukaemia have been frequently reported in areas with high nitrate levels and in areas with elevated levels of radium in drinking water [60]. Sandor et al. [61] studied the association between gastric cancer mortality and nitrate content of drinking water and concluded that high level of nitrate in drinking water is involved in the development of gastric cancer. Another study has also reported a positive association for bladder and ovarian cancer in older women (55–69 years) and the nitrate level in municipal drinking water [62].

3 Diet Risk Factor

3.1 Food Contaminants

Food safety is a critical factor in maintaining the health of the population. A safer food contributes to less illness, and therefore improved livelihood. Diet is thought to play a substantial role in cancer aetiology. Epidemiological and laboratory studies have shown about the undesirable effects of food contaminants and a link between diet and cancer. The primary route of exposure to contaminants could be from multiple sources such as metals, persistent organic pollutants and pesticides [63].

There are primarily four types of potentially carcinogenic compounds that have been examined. The first are natural products that are unavoidable. For example, salted fish contains carcinogens, which cannot be easily avoided. Secondly, natural products that might be contaminated such as contamination of grains with carcinogenic fungal metabolite aflatoxin, which could be eliminated using best practices for grain storage. Thirdly, anthropogenic chemicals may be present in food. For example, 2,3,7,8-tetracholordibenzo-p-dioxin produced during the manufacture of chlorinated hydrocarbons could contaminate the environment, and accumulates in certain foodstuffs. A fourth category is anthropogenic chemicals intentionally added to foods such as saccharin or food colouring.

Fish are rich sources of secondary and tertiary amines, nitrate and nitrite. IARC [64] examined N-nitrosamines levels in uncooked salted fish. Poirier et al. [65] reported the range of N-nitrosodimethylamine in uncooked salted fish from not detected to 388 μg/kg. Other volatile nitrosamines reported were N-nitrosodiethylamine, N-nitrosopyrrolidine and N-nitrosopiperidine, which ranged from not detected to 30 μg/kg. Ho [66] reported that boat people who consumed Chinese-style salted fish in their daily diet is shown to have twice the incidence of nasopharyngeal carcinoma (NPC). NPC is a rare cancer seen among whites in Europe and North America and is one of the most common cancers among Chinese residing in the south-eastern provinces of China. Mimi et al. [67] estimated that over 90% of young NPC cases in Hong Kong Chinese could be attributed to the consumption of Cantonese-style salted fish during childhood. Other studies have shown about the increased risk of gastric cancer and salted foods. Gastric cancer is an important health issue and the second most frequent cause of cancer death. Several risk factors for stomach cancer have been explored, which includes *Helicobacter pylori* infection, salt-preserved foods, dietary nitrite, smoking, alcohol, obesity, radiation, and family history [68]. Strumylaite et al. [69] also reported a strong association between increased risk of gastric cancer and frequent intake of salted or smoked meat and fish. Lin et al. [70] investigated a hospital-based case-control study in China to observe the association between salt processed food and gastric cancer. They concluded that the consumption of salted meat, pickled and preserved vegetables were positively associated with gastric cancer which may be due to N-nitroso compounds. Meat is also an integral part of diet for many people, particularly in the developed world. The average daily intake of total meat by men and women in UK and Ireland are 108 g and 72 g and 168 g and 107 g, respectively [71]. A number of epidemiological studies have associated with red meat and processed meat with cardiovascular disease and colon cancer. The carcinogenicity of the consumption of red meat and processed meat has been evaluated by the International Agency for Research on Cancer (IARC) and the cancer agency of the World Health Organization. The role of westernized dietary pattern in increased incidence of colorectal cancer is a major concern in the developed countries. The possible association between colorectal cancers and consumption of red meat (i.e. beef, pork, lamb, veal and mutton) was first reported in 1975 by determining the per capita meat intake in women from 23 countries [72]. The possible constituents responsible for the development of cancer that have been reported includes fat content, fatty acid composition and the possible formation of carcinogenic compounds, such as heterocyclic amines (HCAs), when cooked at high temperatures [71].

3.2   Aflatoxins

Aflatoxins are the most potent toxic metabolites of *Aspergillus* fungi that can contaminate various foods and feed products. These are acutely toxic, immunosuppres-
sive, mutagenic and carcinogenic compounds targeting mainly the liver [73, 74].
The clinical manifestations of aflatoxicosis include vomiting, abdominal pain, pulmonary oedema, fatty infiltration, and necrosis of the liver [64]. Hepatocellular carcinoma (HCC) accounts for approximately 9.2% of all new cancers worldwide, with
the number increasing year by year. It is the fifth most common cancer in males, and
the seventh in females. Studies have observed that approximately 84% of all new
cases of HCC occur in resource-constrained regions, especially in sub-Saharan
Africa and the Asia-Pacific region than in resource-rich regions. The major causes
of HCC in the high-risk region are due to the chronic hepatitis B virus (HBV) infection and dietary exposure to the toxin. Murugavel et al. [75] studied the prevalence
of aflatoxin B_1 as co-carcinogen using an in-house immunoperoxidase test in 31
liver biopsies and 7 liver-resection specimens from histopathologically proven HCC
and in 15 liver biopsies from cirrhosis patients (control group). Lye et al. [76]
reported that the consumption of aflatoxin-contaminated noodles resulted in acute
hepatic encephalopathy in children in Malaysia. Up to 3 mg of aflatoxin was suspected to be present in a single serving of contaminated noodles. Another outbreak
of acute aflatoxicosis was reported in Kenya in 1981, which was associated with
consumption of maize highly contaminated with aflatoxin [77]. Another outbreak of
aflatoxicosis was also reported in the eastern Kenya in early 2004. The Kenyan
outbreak was followed by a poor harvest of maize due to drought which has been
made susceptible to mould growth. Around, 317 people have approached hospital
treatment for the symptoms of liver failure and 125 people have died due to viral
liver diseases due to acute aflatoxin poisoning. The health officials have examined
the maize samples and ruled out aflatoxin B_1 concentrations as high as 4400 ppb,
which was 220 times the normal Kenyan food limit. Exposure to chronic low level
aflatoxins, especially aflatoxin B_1, is associated with an increased risk of developing
liver cancer, impaired immune function, and malnutrition whereas acute high level
exposure causes early symptoms of diminished appetite, malaise, and low fever.
Later symptoms include vomiting, abdominal pain, hepatitis and potentially fatal
liver failure [78]. The mycotoxins are produced at optimum temperatures of between
25 and 32 °C, moisture contents of greater than 12% but less than 16%, and a relative humidity of 85% [73].

3.3   Chemicals and Pesticides

More than 2500 chemical substances are intentionally added to foods to modify
flavour, colour, stability, texture, or cost, whereas others may unintentionally enter
the food supply through food-packaging materials, processing aids, pesticide

residues, and drugs given to animals. Pesticide residues and industrial pollutants in food are a serious health concern which could lead to cancer risks. Persistent organic pollutants (POPs) are heterogeneous group of chemicals which includes organo-chlorine pesticides, industrial pollutants such as polychlorinated biphenyls (PCBs), and unintentional by-products of chemical manufacturing and combustion processes, such as dioxins and furans. Their long-term persistence and diffusion in the environment open ups the main route of exposure through the diet [79]. Studies have shown that exposure to several naturally occurring and anthropogenic chemicals could influence the initiation and/or progression of tumours in animals and humans. POPs have shown to cause breast cancer, pancreatic cancer, soft tissue sarcoma, non-Hodgkin's lymphoma, and adult onset leukaemia. Breast cancer is the most common cancer seen in women and the highest incidence rates are observed in North America, and lowest risk in Asia and Africa. It is also the most common cancer in females in Europe with the highest incidence rates in Netherlands and Denmark and lowest in the eastern part of Europe. Lee et al. [80] observed the contamination of breast milk by PCBs and organochlorine pesticides in Korea. Bonefeld-Jorgensen et al. [81] also reported the association between POPs and per-fluorinated compounds and breast cancer. Another study was also reported by Zhang et al. [82] about the environmental PCB exposure and breast cancer risk.

3.4   Food Additives

Food additives are the substances that are intentionally added to foods. The use of food additives is controlled based on the international benchmarks, such as the Codex Alimentarius, the European Union and, complementarily, the US Food and Drug Administration. The major concern on the part of public has been focused on artificially added chemicals which are intentionally added to foods to enhance the flavours, nutrient value, shelf life and increased availability. These include food colours, non-nutritive and low-nutrient sweeteners (saccharin, cyclamate, aspartame), antioxidants, and nitrides. Contaminants, sometimes incorrectly included in lists of food additives, present the greatest potential threat to public health. Such contaminants include mycotoxins, nitrosamines, polychlorinated biphenyls (PCBs), and pesticides, which provide a continuing challenge to our regulatory agencies and to public health authorities [83]. Sweeteners are food additives that are added to give the sweet taste without adding calories at any stage of food processing. Among the sweeteners, the use of the artificial sweetener saccharin was originally listed as generally recognized as safe (GRAS), but FDA proposed a ban on saccharin because of an association with bladder cancer in laboratory animals in 1958. Later, in 1996, the ban was withdrawn and in 2000, it was widely used in combination with other sweeteners. The role of sweeteners on cancer risk has been widely debated over the last few decades. But there are major concerns with regard to the safety of saccharin, since it is consumed by millions of people, including children and even foetuses. As per the studies, the genotoxicity and carcinogenity of saccharin is still confusing and should be careful to the consumption [84]. Reuber [85] reported that saccharin is carcinogenic for the urinary bladder in rats and mice. Schernhammer et al. [86] confirmed the detrimental effect of artificial sweetener and sugar containing soda on lymphoma and leukaemia in men and women. There are many studies which indicate a lack of association between artificial sweeteners and cancer risks [87, 88].

4   Genetic Predisposition

Genetic counselling is vital in helping people at high risk for hereditary diseases. Cancer is the most common cause of death after heart disease. Mostly, cancer is caused by both internal factors and environmental factors. The incidence of prostate cancer is 25 times lower and the incidence of breast cancer is ten times lower in Asians as compared to Western countries [89]. Cancer is a genetic disease due to the alterations in the DNA sequences of cells. These alterations may be by mutations, duplications, deletions, or genomic rearrangements or may be inherited in the germ cell line; or may be due to environmental factors. These risk factors could increase the chance of developing certain cancers, but it does not imply that you could get the disease by having a risk factor or even several.

The development of cancer is influenced by genetic mutations. Cell division is a controlled process and cancer develops when mutations lead to uncontrolled cell division. When the cellular processes such as cell fate, cell survival and genomic maintenance are interrupted, the cancerous cells proliferate beyond the capability of a healthy cell. Gene mutation could be inherited from a parent or obtained during a person's lifetime. Mutations that are passed from a parent to child are called hereditary mutations or germ line mutations. If a genetic alteration is inherited in the germ line of a family, a large number of breast cancer cases in women are likely to appear among those family members. The aetiology behind development of breast cancer is multifactorial which includes diet, life style, environmental factors, reproductive factors and hormonal status. However, a greater risk factor is due to genetic predisposition and a positive family history [90]. The overall development of breast cancer risk is 1.9–3.9 times higher in women with an affected mother or sister [91]. Estimation of new cases of breast cancer in 2014 was reported as approximately 235,030 from which 10% are likely to be hereditary. An autosomal dominant pattern of transmission is followed by hereditary cancers and is ascribed to defects in *BRCA1* and *BRCA2* genes. There are additional genetic syndromes other than *BRCA1* and *BRCA2* breast hereditary cancers, such as Li Fraumeni which is associated with abnormalities in the *p53* gene. It is characterized by a wide range of malignancies that is mainly occurring at a remarkably young age. Approximately 1% will be found to carry a *p53* mutation among women diagnosed with a breast cancer before an age of 40 years. Patients could have a 21–49% risk in developing cancer by the age of 30 years once they have been diagnosed with Li Fraumeni syndrome and have 68–93% risk in their lifetime. Another syndrome is Cowden syndrome which is caused by a mutation in phosphatase and tensin homologue deleted from chromosome 10. Women with this syndrome would have a 25–50% chance of risk in developing breast cancer at young age.

A few other hereditary syndromes to consider are Peutz-Jeghers, which is characterized by multiple hamartomatous polyps in the gastrointestinal tract which could lead to cervical and ovarian malignancies. There is a 15-fold increased risk of developing breast cancer in women with Peutz-Jeghers due to *STK11* mutation [92, 93]. Hereditary breast and ovarian cancer (HBOC) is characterized by a young age of onset, multiple primaries, bilateral breast cancer and family history of first- or second-degree kin. The incidence of ovarian and breast carcinoma in United States is estimated to be 21,980 and 232,670, respectively. Of these cases, about 20–25% of ovarian cases and 5–7% of breast carcinoma are thought to be as a result of hereditary predisposition. The scientific studies are supporting about the major role of *BRCA1/2* mutations as the known genetic causes of HBOC. Other than that, *MLH1*, *MSH2*, *MSH6*, and *PMS2* have also been contributing in developing hereditary ovarian carcinoma [94]. Women with *CDH1* mutation (hereditary diffuse gastric cancer) have a high risk of developing lobular breast cancers. Economopoulou et al. [95] studied about breast cancer susceptibility genes that include rare germ line mutations in high penetrant genes such as *TP53* and *PTEN*, and more frequent mutations in moderate penetrant genes such as *CHEK2*, *ATM* and *PALB2* which were responsible for hereditary breast cancer syndromes. There is also an increased risk of developing breast and pancreatic cancers in women with *PALB2* mutation. A study of breast cancer patients with invasive operable breast cancer concluded that patients with a family history were significantly associated with tumour size, age and oestrogen receptor [91]. Several cohort studies have shown the association between long-term post-menopausal hormone use and increased epithelial ovarian cancer [96]. Some studies have suggested a decreased association between a positive family history and breast cancer risk with increasing age, whereas some reports have shown no variation in risk across age groups. A study on a Swedish-based registry study found a non-significant prognosis in women with a family history of breast cancer [97]. Chang et al. [98] also reported a non-significant difference between a positive family history of breast cancer and mortality risk. Another study of breast cancer patients with invasive breast cancer reported a non-significant difference between a positive family history of breast cancer and breast cancer specific mortality risk [90].

There are many evidences that support endometriosis as a risk factor for ovarian cancer. The endometrium is the lining of the uterus and endometriosis is a complex disorder caused by multiple genetic factors and environmental factors. A majority of the cancers that occur in the uterus are endometrial cancers. It is the sixth most common cancer in women worldwide and affects approximately 10% of all women of reproductive age [99]. There is a threefold increased risk of ovarian cancer in women with a first-degree relative with ovarian cancer compared to those with no family history. Simpson et al. [100] studied 123 patients with histologically proved endometriosis which opens the view that the disease may have a genetic background. Endometriosis is considered in risk prediction model for ovarian cancer.

Burghaus et al. [101] studied the genetic risk factors for ovarian cancer and its role for endometriosis risk. They observed that *HNF1B* gene was associated in the aetiology of both endometriosis and ovarian cancer. A case control study of 110 women with ovarian epithelial carcinoma was conducted in Hokkaido, Japan, to identify risk factors for ovarian cancer. They observed a positive and an increased ovarian cancer risk in women with a family history of breast, uterine, or ovarian cancer in a mother or sister [102]. Oesophageal cancer is one of the most aggressive cancers and is the sixth leading cause of cancer death worldwide. Song et al. [103] studied the genomic alterations in the oesophageal squamous cancer cell and identified eight significantly mutated genes. They observed six known tumour associated genes which were *TP53, RB1, CDKN2A, PIK3CA, NOTCH1, NFE2L2* and novel cancer-implicated genes (*ADAM29* and *FAM135B*). They have also noticed alterations in several important histone regulator genes such as *MLL2, ASH1L, MLL3, SETD1B, CREBBP,* and *EP300*.

5 Interrelationship of Genetic Risk and Environmental Risk Factors

The influence of environmental factors, such as lifestyle factors, occupational exposures, and dietary habits, on development of cancer have been discussed. There are multiple external factors combined with internal genetic changes which could lead to human cancers. Individuals with genetic predispositions would be more susceptible to the effects of environmental factors. Studies were supporting the penetrance of *BRCA1/2* associated breast cancer with hormone-related exposures [104]. John et al. [105] reported that breast cancer risks were higher for women with medical radiation exposure at a young age. Both ionizing and non-ionizing radiations could cause leukaemia, lymphoma, thyroid cancers, skin cancers, sarcomas, lung and breast carcinomas [89].

Huang et al. [106] showed that several hormones-related risk factors were associated with an increased risk of breast cancer positive for oestrogen and progesterone. Ali et al. [107] reported that a high correlation was observed between the incidence of oral cancer and life style factors (alcohol and tobacco use). These behaviours could lead to genetic variations in tumour suppressor genes (*APC, p53*), proto-oncogenes (*Myc*), oncogene (*Ras*) and genes controlling normal cellular processes (*EIF3E, GSTM1*) and produces defects in normal cellular processes such as segregation of chromosomes, genomic copy number, regulations of cell-cycle checkpoints, DNA damage repairs and defects in notch signalling pathways.

Studies have discovered that endogenous factors including genetic factors may interact with specific foods or food components that could lead to increased cancer risk. The interactions could be either by genes that could affect the action of compounds of dietary origin by increasing or decreasing the amount needed for good nutritional status and these compounds could affect the action of genes [108]. The role of diet is complex to relate with cancer risk. There are many epidemiological studies supporting the role of foods and food components in scavenging free radicals and reducing the cancer risk [109, 110]. But there are also studies supporting the role of nutrients and how it interacts with genes and the probability in developing cancer. Epidemiological studies have shown a negative correlation between the intakes of carotenoids and the risk of developing cancer. Beta-carotene was found to increase the risk of lung cancer among smokers [111]. Smoking-related malignancies have a high burden of mutations, including in the gene encoding for *p53*. Cancers derived from tissues directly exposed to tobacco smoke is attributed to misreplication of DNA damage caused by tobacco carcinogens together with indirect activation of DNA editing by APOBEC cytidine deaminases and of an endogenous clock-like mutational process [112, 113].

6 Awareness of Risk Factors

Cancer is a disease believed to be preventable by improving the lifestyle and through awareness programmes. Around 90–95% of all cancers can be attributed to the environment and lifestyle factors and the remaining 5–10% due to genetic defects [114]. It is also important to be aware of the risk factors. Ignorance may lead to a low quality of treatment. Public awareness about cancer, its risk factors, symptoms, and promote early health-seeking approach would able to control the disease [115]. Martsevich et al. [116] studied the awareness of cardiovascular disease, its risk factors, and its association with attendance at clinics in acute coronary syndrome patients. They observed that the majority of patients were aware of diabetes. The awareness of arterial hypertension slightly increased with increasing attendance, whereas awareness of dyslipidemia increased dramatically. This was explained by the fact that most patients have an opportunity to check their blood pressure at home, except for those who do not have symptoms of arterial hypertension and do not visit their doctors' clinics, which can draw their attention to this problem. Therefore, attending the clinic could have significant role in increasing the awareness of the risk factors.

Several studies analysed factors associated with patients' unawareness of CVD risk factors. He et al. [117] showed that patients with body mass index ≥24 kg/m^2, family history of dyslipidemia, elderly patients, and retirees were more aware of dyslipidemia. Alcohol drinking, cigarette smoking, and physical activity were associated with a lower level of awareness of dyslipidemia. Wang et al. [118] demonstrated that patients with family history of diabetes mellitus and those who frequently exercise were more likely to be aware of diabetes mellitus. At the same time, alcohol drinkers and cigarette smokers were less likely to be aware of their blood glucose levels. Mendez-Chacon et al. [119] demonstrated that men and smokers were less aware of arterial hypertension. History of ischemic heart disease, stroke, diabetes mellitus, and obesity were associated with patients' awareness of arterial hypertension. Patients who had been home visited by community health workers were less likely to be unaware of their hypertension [116].

Many countries have programmes for citizens with chronic diseases and their risk factors to receive a free consultation and examinations. Al-Azri et al. [120] conducted a survey in three areas of Oman to measure public awareness of cancer risk factors using the Cancer Awareness Measure. They observed a significant association between participant responses and their educational level. The higher educational level made the respondents in this study and identified possible risk factors such as smoking, passive smoking, alcohol drinking, less consumption of fruits and vegetables, and infection with human papilloma virus. They observed that most of the participated respondents were not aware of the cancer risk factors. Therefore, it's very important to educate the public to know about possible cancer risk factors to make their life healthy and safe. Lagerlund et al. [121] carried out a study to compare the awareness of cancer risk factors among Danish and Swedish population. Most of the respondents were aware of smoking and radiation as cancer risk factors. However, a limited awareness about human papilloma virus infection, low consumption of fruits and vegetables, alcohol drinking have been observed in both countries and with increasing age, a decline in awareness have been observed.

Mwaka et al. [115] conducted a survey in northern Uganda about cervical cancer risk factors. They observed that the selected respondents in this study were aware about cervical cancer, risk factors and its symptoms. Preventive measures like human papilloma virus vaccination, cervical screening, routine check-ups for early diagnosis and treatment of cervical cancer symptoms would be suggested to make the awareness into action. Rhazi et al. [122] carried out a population-based cross-sectional study about public awareness of cancer risk factors in Moroccan population. They observed a strong association between participant responses and their educational level. The higher the level of education, the more likely people are aware of cancer risk factors. The result can be used to build-up relevant cancer prevention strategies to enhance people's knowledge about the risk factors. Another awareness study about cancer risk factors was conducted in Karachi, Pakistan [123]. They observed that the population was not aware of the intrinsic risk factors like age and obesity. Therefore, it is very important and relevant to take actions through educational programmes, availability of screening tests, vaccinations, and to avail benefits of early diagnosis.

7   Conclusion

Age specific mortality rates for chronic diseases are controlled by knowledge about risk factors and availability of screening systems and treatment. Cancer is a leading global cause of death. Several factors including exposure to environmental factors and genetic factors contribute to the development of cancers. Several environmental factors include lifestyle behaviours like cigarette smoking, excessive alcohol consumption, poor diet, lack of exercise, excessive sunlight exposure, and others include exposure to medical drugs, hormones, radiation, viruses, bacteria, and environmental chemicals. Genetic alterations in the body cells, abnormal hormone level in the blood stream, or a weakened immune system also could make an individual more susceptible to cancer. However, the majority of the cancers could be controlled by maintaining a quality life. Therefore, government authorities and hospitals should promote certain public awareness programmes, free screening tests for maintain a healthy and long life.

References

1. Schouten LJ, Straatman H, Kiemeney LALM, Verbeek ALM. J Epidemiol Community Health. 1994;48:596–600.
2. Callahan MA, Sexton K. If cumulative risk assessment is the answer, what is the question? Environ Health Perspect. 2007;115(5):799–806.
3. Sexton K. Cumulative risk assessment: an overview of methodological approaches for evaluating combined health effects from exposure to multiple environmental stressors. Int J Environ Res Public Health. 2012;9(2):370–90.
4. Maronpot RR, Flake G, Huff J. Relevance of animal carcinogenesis findings to human cancer predictions and preventions. Toxicol Pathol. 2004;32(1):40–8.
5. Tokar EJ, Benbrahim-Tallaa L, Ward JM, Lunn R, Sams RL, Waalkes MP. Cancer in experimental animals exposed to arsenic and arsenic compounds. Crit Rev Toxicol. 2010;40(10):912–27.
6. Ames BN, Gold LS. The causes and prevention of cancer: the role of environment. Biotherapy. 1998;11:205–20.
7. WHO. Tobacco. 2009. www.who.int/nmh/publications/fact_sheet_tobacco_en.pdf. Accessed 8 Oct 2017
8. Rafiemanesh H, Mehtarpour M, Khani F, Hesami SM, Shamlou R, Towhidi F, Salehiniya H, Makhsosi BR, Moini A. Epidemiology, incidence and mortality of lung cancer and their relationship with the development index in the world. J Thorac Dis. 2016;8(6):1094–102.
9. Cruz CSDC, Tanoue LT, Matthay RA. Lung cancer: epidemiology, etiology, and prevention. Clin Chest Med. 2011;32(4):1–61.
10. WHO. Global status report on noncommunicable diseases. 2010. www.who.int/nmh/publications/fact_sheet_tobacco_en.pdf. Accessed 8 Oct 2017
11. Singh CR, Kathiresan K. Effect of cigarette smoking on human health and promising remedy by mangroves. Asian Pac J Trop Biomed. 2015;5(2):162–7.
12. Mishra S, Joseph RA, Gupta PC, Pezzack B, Ram F, Sinha DN, Dikshit R, Patra J, Jha P. Trends in bidi and cigarette smoking in India from 1998 to 2015, by age, gender and education. BMJ Global Health. 2016;1:1–8.
13. Helen GS, Goniewicz ML, Dempsey D, Wlison M, Jacob P, Bonowitz NL. Exposure and kinetics of polycyclic aromatic hydrocarbons (PAHs) in cigarette smokers. Chem Res Toxicol. 2012;25(4):952–64.
14. Rehman AU, Khan MN, Sarwar A, Bhutto S. Physicochemical analysis of different cigarettes brands available in Pakistan. Pak J Anal Environ Chem. 2014;15(2):26–38.
15. Momas I, Daures JP, Festy B, Bontoux J, Gremy F. Bladder cancer and black tobacco cigarette smoking. Eur J Epidemiol. 1994;10:599–604.
16. Ratna A, Mandrekar P. Alcohol and cancer: mechanisms and therapies. Biomol Ther. 2017;7(61):1–20.
17. WHO. World Cancer Report. 2003.

18. Goldstein BY, Chang SC, Hashibe M, Vecchia CL, Zhang ZF. Alcohol consumption and cancer of the oral cavity and pharynx from 1988 to 2009: an update. Eur J Cancer Prev. 2010;19(6):431–65.
19. Testino G. The burden of cancer attributable to alcohol consumption. Maedica (Buchar). 2011;6(4):313–20.
20. Chang ET, Canchola AJ, Lee VS, Clarke CA, Purdie DM, Reynolds P, Bernstein L, Stram DO, Anton-Culver H, Deapen D, Mohrenweiser H, Peel D, Pinder R, Ross RK, West DW, Wright W, Ziogas A, Horn-Ross PL. Wine and other alcohol consumption and risk of ovarian cancer in the California teachers study cohort. Cancer Causes Control. 2007;18:91–103.
21. Morse DE. Smoking and drinking in relation to oral cancer and oral epithelial dysplasia. Cancer Causes Control. 2007;18(9):919–29.
22. Pelucchi C, Gallus S, Garavello W, Bosetti C, La Vecchia C. Cancer risk associated with alcohol and tobacco use: focus on upper aero-digestive tract and liver. Alcohol Res Health. 2006;29(3):193–8.
23. Scoccianti C, Lauby-Secretan B, Bello PY, Chajes V, Romieu I. Female breast cancer and alcohol consumption: a review of the literature. Am J Prev Med. 2014;46(3):S16–25.
24. Stickel F, Schuppan D, Hahn EG, Seitz HK. Cocarcinogenic effects of alcohol in hepatocarcinogenesis. Gut. 2002;51:132–9.
25. Kim EA, Lee HE, Kang SK. Occupational burden of cancer in Korea. Saf Health Work. 2010;1(1):61–8.
26. Pinar T. Occupation and cancer. Int J Hematol Oncol. 2012;22:202–10.
27. WHO. Occupational Carcinogens. 2004.
28. Leclerc A, Cortes MM, Gerin M, Luce D, Brugere J. Sinonasal cancer and wood dust exposure: results from a case-control study. Am J Epidemiol. 1994;140(4):340–9.
29. Bonneterre V, Deschamps E, Persoons R, Bernardet C, Liaudy S, Maitre A, Gaudemaris R. Sino-nasal cancer and exposure to leather dust. Occup Med. 2007;57:438–43.
30. Friedman GD, Udaltsova N, Chan J, Quesenberry CP, Habel LA. Screening pharmaceuticals for possible carcinogenic effects: initial positive results for drugs not previously screened. Cancer Causes Control. 2009;20(10):1821–35.
31. Clayson DB. Occupational bladder cancer. Prev Med. 1976;5(2):228–44.
32. Dalrymple JO. Bladder tumours in rubber workers. Proc R Soc Med. 1967;60:14–6.
33. Raj A, Mayberry JF, Podas T. Occupation and gastric cancer. Postgrad Med J. 2003;79:252–8.
34. Case RAM, Pearson JT. Tumours of the urinary bladder in workmen engaged in the manufacture and use of certain dyestuff intermediates in the British chemical industry. Br J Ind Med. 1954;11:213–6.
35. Snyder R. Leukemia and Benzene. Int J Environ Res Public Health. 2012;9(8):2875–93.
36. Natelson EA. Benzene-induced acute myeloid leukemia: a clinician's perspective. Am J Hematol. 2007;82:826–30.
37. Sorahan T, Kinlen LJ, Doll R. Cancer risks in a historical UK cohort of benzene exposed workers. Occup Environ Med. 2005;62:231–6.
38. Khalade A, Jaakkola MS, Pukkala E, Jaakkola JJK. Exposure to benzene at work and the risk of leukemia: a systematic review and meta-analysis. Environ Health. 2010;9:31–7.
39. Rushton L, Schnatter AR, Tang G, Glass DC. Acute myeloid and chronic lymphoid leukaemias and exposure to low-level benzene among petroleum workers. Br J Cancer. 2014;110:783–7.
40. Pasetto R, Terracini B, Marsili D, Comba P. Occupational burden of asbestos-related cancer in Argentina, Brazil, Colombia, and Mexico. Ann Glob Health. 2014;80:263–8.
41. Luippold RS, Mundt KA, Austin RP, Liebig E, Panko J, Crump C, Crump K, Proctor D. Lung cancer mortality among chromate production workers. Occup Environ Med. 2003;60:451–7.
42. Boffetta P. Human cancer from environmental pollutants: the epidemiological evidence. Mutat Res Genet Toxicol Environ Mutagen. 2006;608(2):157–62.
43. Boffetta P, Nyberg F. Contribution of environmental factors to cancer risk. Br Med Bull. 2003;68(1):71–94.

44. Briggs D. Environmental pollution and the global burden of disease. Br Med Bull. 2003;68(1):1–24.
45. Carbone M, Baris YI, Bertino P, Brass B, Comertpay S, Dogan AU, Gaudino G, Jube S, Kanodia S, Partridge CR, Pass HI, Rivera ZS, Steele I, Tuncer M, Way S, Yang H, Miller A. Erionite exposure in North Dakota and Turkish villages with mesothelioma. Proc Natl Acad Sci. 2011;108(33):13618–23.
46. Hillerdal G. Mesothelioma: cases associated with non-occupational and low dose exposures. Occup Environ Med. 1999;56:505–13.
47. Camus M. Nonoccupational exposure to chrysotile asbestos and the risk of lung cancer. N Engl J Med. 1998;338:1565–71.
48. Nikic D, Stankovic A. Air pollution as a risk factor for lung cancer. Arch Oncol. 2005;13(2):79–82.
49. Mannucci PM, Franchini M. Health effects of ambient air pollution in developing countries. Int J Environ Res Public Health. 2017;14:2–8.
50. Widziewics K, Rogula-Kozlowska W, Majewski G. Lung cancer risk associated with exposure to benzo(a)pyrene in polish agglomerations, cities, and other areas. Int J Environ Res. 2017;11:685–93.
51. Lin CK, Hung HY, Christiani DC, Forastiere F, Lin RT. Lung cancer mortality of residents living near petrochemical industrial complexes: a meta-analysis. Environ Health. 2017;16:101–10.
52. Slaper H, Elzen MGJD, Woerd HJVD. Ozone depletion and skin cancer incidence: an integrated modeling approach and scenario study. In: Biggs RH, Joyner MEB, editors. Stratospheric ozone depletion/UV-B radiation in the biosphere, NATO ASI series (series I: global environmental change), vol. 18. Berlin: Springer; 1994. p. 1–52.
53. Seow WJ, Hu W, Vermeulen R, Hosgood HD, Downward GS, Chapman RS, He X, Bassig BA, Kim C, Wen C, Rothman N, Lan Q. Household air pollution and lung cancer in China: a review of studies in Xuanwei. Chin J Cancer. 2014;33(10):471–5.
54. Kim C, Gao YT, Xiang YB, Barone-Adesi F, Zhang Y, Hosgood HD, Ma S, Shu X, Ji BT, Chow WH, Seow WJ, Bassig B, Cai Q, Zheng W, Rothman N, Lan Q. Home kitchen ventilation, cooking fuels, and lung cancer risk in a prospective cohort of never smoking women in Shanghai, China. Int J Cancer. 2015;136:632–8.
55. Vineis P, Airoldi L, Veglia F, Olgiati L, Pastorelli R, Autrup H, Dunning A, Garte S, Gormally E, Hainaut P, Malaveille C, Matullo G, Peluso M, Overvad K, Tjonneland A, Clavel-Chapelon F, Boeing H, Krogh V, Palli D, Panico S, Tumino R, Bueno-De-Mesquita B, Peeters P, Berglund G, Hallmans G, Saracci R, Riboli E. Environmental tobacco smoke and risk of respiratory cancer and chronic obstructive pulmonary disease in former smokers and never smokers in the EPIC prospective study. Br Med J. 2005;330:277–82.
56. Khatri N, Tyagi S. Influences of natural and anthropogenic factors on surface and groundwater quality in rural and urban areas. Front Life Sci. 2014;8(1):23–39.
57. Meliker JR, Nriagu JO. Arsenic in drinking water and bladder cancer: review of epidemiological evidence. Trace Met Other Contam Environ. 2007;9:551–84.
58. Villanueva C, Fernandez F, Malats N, Grimalt J, Kogevinas M. Meta-analysis of studies on individual consumption of chlorinated drinking water and bladder cancer. J Epidemiol Community Health. 2003;57(3):166–73.
59. Smith AH, Lingas EO, Rahman M. Contamination of drinking-water by arsenic in Bangladesh: a public health emergency. Bull World Health Organ. 2000;78(9):1093–103.
60. Hoffmann W, Kranefeld A, Schmitz-Feuerhake I. Radium-226-contaminated drinking water: hypothesis on an exposure pathway in a population with elevated childhood leukemia. Environ Health Perspect. 1993;101(3):113–5.
61. Sandor J, Kiss I, Farkas O, Ember I. Association between gastric cancer mortality and nitrate content of drinking water: ecological study on small area inequalities. Eur J Epidemiol. 2001;17(5):443–7.

62. Weyer PJ, Cerhan JR, Kross BC, Hallberg GR, Kantamneni J, Breuer G, Jones MP, Zheng W, Lynch CF. Municipal drinking water nitrate level and cancer risk in older women: the Iowa women's health study. Epidemiology. 2001;11(3):327–38.
63. Vogt R, Bennett D, Cassady D, Frost J, Ritz B, Picciotto IH. Cancer and non-cancer health effects from food contaminant exposures for children and adults in California: a risk assessment. Environ Health. 2012;11:83–96.
64. IARC. In: Wild CP, Miller JD, Groopman JD, editors. Effects of aflatoxins on aflatoxicosis and liver cancer. Lyon; 2015.
65. Poirier S, Bouvier G, Malaveille C, Ohshima H, Shao YM, Hubert A, Zeng Y, de The G, Bartsch H. Volatile nitrosamine levels and genotoxicity of food samples from high-risk areas for nasopharyngeal carcinoma before and after nitrosation. Int J Cancer. 1989;44:1088–94.
66. Ho JH. Nasopharyngeal carcinoma in Hong Kong. In: Muir CS, Shanmugaratnam K, editors. Cancer of the nasopharynx. Copenhagen: Munksgaard; 1967. p. 58–63.
67. Mimi CY, John HCH, Lai SH, Henderson BE. Cantonese-style salted fish as a cause of nasopharyngeal carcinoma: report of a case-control study in Hong Kong. Cancer Res. 1986;46:956–61.
68. Wang XQ, Terry PD, Yan H. Review of salt consumption and stomach cancer risk: epidemiological and biological evidence. World J Gastroenterol. 2009;15(18):2204–13.
69. Strumylaite L, Zickute J, Dudzevicius J, Dregval L. Salt-preserved foods and risk of gastric cancer. Medicina (Kaunas). 2006;42(2):164–70.
70. Lin SH, Li YH, Leung K, Huang CY, Wang XR. Salt processed food and gastric cancer in a Chinese population. Asian Pac J Cancer Prev. 2014;15(13):5293–8.
71. McAfee AJ, McSorley EM, Cuskelly GJ, Moss BW, Wallace JMW, Bonham MP, Fearon AM. Red meat consumption: an overview of the risks and benefits. Meat Sci. 2010;84:1–13.
72. Aykan NF. Red meat and colorectal cancer. Oncol Rev. 2015;9(1):288–94.
73. Kew MC. Aflatoxins as a cause of hepatocellular carcinoma. J Gastrointestin Liver Dis. 2013;22(3):305–10.
74. Wolde M. Effects of aflatoxin contamination of grains in Ethiopia. Int J Agric Sci. 2017;7(4):1298–308.
75. Murugavel KG, Naranatt PP, Shankar EM, Mathews S, Raghuram K, Rajasambandam P, Jayanthi V, Surendran R, Murali A, Srinivas U, Palaniswami KR, Srikumari D, Thyagarajan SP. Prevalence of aflatoxin B1 in liver biopsies of proven hepatocellular carcinoma in India determined by an in-house immunoperoxidase test. J Med Microbiol. 2007;56:1455–9.
76. Lye MS, Ghazali AA, Mohan J, Alwin N, Nair RC. An outbreak of acute hepatic encephalopathy due to severe aflatoxicosis in Malaysia. Am J Trop Med Hyg. 1995;53(1):68–72.
77. Ngindu A, Kenya PR, Ocheng DM, Omondi TN, Ngare W, Gatei D, Johnson BK, Ngira JA, Nandwa H, Jansen AJ, Kaviti JN, Siongok TA. Lancet. 1982;319:1346–8.
78. Barrett JR. Liver cancer and aflatoxin: new information from the Kenyan outbreak. Environ Health Perspect. 2005;113(12):A837–8.
79. Fattore E, Fanelli R, Vecchia CL. Persistent organic pollutants in food: public health implications. J Epidemiol Community Health. 2002;56:831–2.
80. Lee S, Kim S, Lee HK, Lee IS, Park J, Kim HJ, Lee JJ, Choi S, Kim S, Kim SY, Choi K, Kim S, Moon HB. Contamination of polychlorinated biphenyls and organochlorine pesticides in breast milk in Korea: time-course variation, influencing factors, and exposure assessment. Chemosphere. 2013;93(8):1578–85.
81. Bonefeld-Jorgensen EC, Long M, Bossi R, Ayotte P, Asmund G, Kruger T, Ghisari M, Mulvad G, Kern P, Nzulumiki P, Dewailly E. Perfluorinated compounds are related to breast cancer risk in greenlandic inuit: a case control study. Environ Health. 2011;10:88–102.
82. Zhang J, Huang Y, Wang X, Lin K, Wu K. Environmental polychlorinated biphenyl exposure and breast cancer risk: a meta-analysis of observational studies. PLoS One. 2015;10(11):1–18.
83. Newberne PM, Conner MW. Food additives and contaminants. An update. Cancer. 1986;58(8):1851–62.

84. Ucar A, Yilmaz S. Saccharin genotoxicity and carcinogenicity: a review. Advances in food. Sciences. 2015;37(3):138–42.
85. Reuber MD. Carcinogenicity of saccharin. Environ Health Perspect. 1978;25:173–200.
86. Schernhammer ES, Bertrand KA, Birmann BM, Sampson L, Willett WC, Feskanich D. Consumption of artificial sweetener- and sugar-containing soda and risk of lymphoma and leukemia in men and women. Am J Clin Nutr. 2012;96(6):1419–28.
87. Gallus S, Scotti L, Negri E, Talamini R, Franceschi S, Montella M, Giacosa A, Dal Maso L, La Vecchia C. Artificial sweeteners and cancer risk in a network of case-control studies. Ann Oncol. 2007;18(1):40–4.
88. Lim U, Subar AF, Mouw T, Hartge P, Morton LM, Stolzenberg-Solomon R, Campbell D, Hollenbeck AR, Schatzkin A. Consumption of aspartame-containing beverages and incidence of hematopoietic and brain malignancies. Cancer Epidemiol Biomark Prev. 2006;15(9):1654–9.
89. Parihar A. Genetic and environmental factors in cancer pathogenesis. Int J Res Granthaalayah. 2015;3(9):1–3.
90. Melvin JC, Wulaningsih W, Hana Z, Purushotham AD, Pinder SE, Fentiman I, Gillett C, Mera A, Holmberg L, Hemelrijck MV. Family history of breast cancer and its association with disease severity and mortality. Cancer Med. 2016;5(5):942–9.
91. Molino A, Giovannini M, Pedersini R, Frisinghelli M, Micciolo R, Mandara M, Pavarana M, Cetto GL. Correlations between family history and cancer characteristics in 2256 breast cancer patients. Br J Cancer. 2004;91(1):96–8.
92. Boland CR, Jung B, Carethers JM. Cancer of the colon and gastrointestinal tract. In: Rimoin DL, Pyeritz RE, Korf B, editors. Emery and Rimoin's principles and practice of medical genetics. Boston: Elsevier; 2013. p. 1–35.
93. Chae HD, Jeon CH. Peutz-Jeghers syndrome with germline mutation of STK11. Ann Surg Treat Res. 2014;86(6):325–30.
94. Minion LE, Dolinsky JS, Chase DM, Dunlop CL, Chao EC, Monk BJ. Hereditary predisposition to ovarian cancer, looking beyond *BRCA1/BRCA2*. Gynecol Oncol. 2015;137:86–92.
95. Economopoulou P, Dimitriadis G, Psyrri A. Beyond BRCA: new hereditary breast cancer susceptibility genes. Cancer Treat Rev. 2015;41(1):1–8.
96. Danforth KN, Tworoger SS, Hecht JL, Rosner BA, Coldit GA, Hankinson SE. A prospective study of postmenopausal hormone use and ovarian cancer risk. Br J Cancer. 2007;96:151–6.
97. Thalib L, Wedrén S, Granath F, Adami HO, Rydh B, Magnusson C, Hall P. Breast cancer prognosis in relation to family history of breast and ovarian cancer. Br J Cancer. 2004;90(7):1378–81.
98. Chang ET, Milne RL, Phillips KA, Figueiredo JC, Sangaramoorthy M, Keegan THM, Andrulis IL, Hopper JL, Goodwin PJ, Malley FPO, Weerasooriya N, Apicella C, Southey MC, Friedlander ML, Giles GG, Whittemore AS, West DW, John EM. Family history of breast cancer and all-cause mortality after breast cancer diagnosis in the Breast Cancer Family Registry. Breast Cancer Res Treat. 2009;117(1):167–76.
99. Vigano P, Parazzini F, Somigliana E, Vercellini P. Endometriosis: epidemiology and aetiological factors. Best Pract Res Clin Obstet Gynaecol. 2004;18(2):177–200.
100. Simpson JL, Elias S, Malinak LR, Buttram VC. Heritable aspects of endometriosis: I. Genetic studies. Am J Obstetr Gynaecol. 1980;137(3):327–31.
101. Burghaus S, Fasching PA, Haberle L, Rubner M, Buchner K, Blum S, Engel A, Ekici AB, Hartmann A, Hein A, Beckmann MW, Renner SP. Genetic risk factors for ovarian cancer and their role for endometriosis risk. Gynecol Oncol. 2017;145(1):142–7.
102. Mori M, Harabuchi I, Miyake H, Casagrande JT, Henderson BE, Ross RK. Reproductive, genetic, and dietary risk factors for ovarian cancer. Am J Epidemiol. 1988;128(4):771–7.
103. Song Y, Li L, Ou Y, Gao Z, Li E, Li X, Zhang W, Wang J, Xu L, Zhou Y, Ma X, Liu L, Zhao Z, Huang X, Fan J, Dong L, Chen G, Ma L, Yang J, Chen L, He M, Li M, Zhuang X, Huang k, Qiu K, Yin G, Guo G, Feng Q, Chen P, Wu Z, Wu J, Ma L, Zhao J, Luo L, Fu M, Xu B, Chen

B, Li Y, Tong T, Wang M, Liu Z, Lin D, Zhang X, Yang H, Wang J, Zhan Q. Identification of genomic alterations in oesophageal squamous cell cancer. Nature. 2014;509:91–5.

104. Rebbeck TR, Wang Y, Kantoff PW, Krithivas K, Neuhausen SL, Godwin AK, Daly MB, Narod SA, Brunet JS, Vesprini D, Garber JE, Lynch HT, Weber BL, Brown M. Modification of BRCA1- and BRCA2-associated breast cancer risk by AIB1 genotype and reproductive history. Cancer Res. 2001;61:5420–4.

105. John EM, Phipps AI, Knight JA, Milne RL, Dite GS, Hopper JL, Andrulis IL, Southey M, Giles GG, West DW, Whittemore AS. Medical radiation exposure and breast cancer risk: findings from the Breast Cancer Family Registry. Int J Cancer. 2007;121:386–94.

106. Huang WY, Newman B, Millikan RC, Schell MJ, Hulka BS, Moorman PG. Hormone-related factors and risk of breast cancer in relation to estrogen receptor and progesterone receptor status. Am J Epidemiol. 2000;151:703–14.

107. Ali J, Sabiha B, Jan HU, Haider SA, Khan AA, Ali SS. Genetic etiology of oral cancer. Oral Oncol. 2017;70:23–8.

108. Freudenheim JL, Gower E. Interaction of genetic factors with nutrition in cancer. In: Coulston AM, Boushey CJ, Ferruzzi M, Delahanty L, editors. Nutrition in the prevention and treatment of disease. New York: Academic Press; 2017. p. 733–47.

109. Syed DN, Chamcheu JC, Adhami VM, Mukhtar H. Pomegranate extracts and cancer prevention: molecular and cellular activities. Anti Cancer Agents Med Chem. 2013;13(8):1149–61.

110. Waly MI, Ali A, Guizani N, Al-Rawahi AS, Farooq SA, Rahman MS. Pomegranate (*Punica granatum*) peel extract efficacy as a dietary antioxidant against azoxymethane-induced colon cancer in rat. Asian Pac J Cancer Prev. 2012;13(8):4051–5.

111. Alpha-Tocopherol, Beta Carotene Cancer Prevention Study Group. The effect of vitamin E and beta carotene on the incidence of lung cancer and other cancers in male smokers. N Engl J Med. 1994;330(15):1029–35.

112. Alexandrov LB, Ju YS, Haase K, Loo PV, Martincorena I, Nik-Zainal S, Totoki Y, Fujimoto A, Nakagawa H, Shibata T, Campbell PJ, Vineis P, Phillips DH, Stratton MR. Mutational signatures associated with tobacco smoking in human cancer. Science. 2016;354:618–22.

113. Gibbons DL, Byers LA, Kurie JM. Smoking, *p53* mutation, and lung cancer. Mol Cancer Res. 2014;12(1):3–13.

114. Anand P, Kunnumakara AB, Sundaram C, Harikumar KB, Tharakan ST, Lai OS, Sung B, Aggarwal BB. Cancer is a preventable disease that require major lifestyle changes. Pharm Res. 2008;25(9):2097–116.

115. Mwaka AD, Orach CG, Were EM, Lyratzopoulos G, Wabinga H, Roland M. Awareness of cervical cancer risk factors and symptoms: cross-sectional community survey in post-conflict northern Uganda. Health Expect. 2015;19(4):854–67.

116. Martsevich SY, Semenova YV, Kutishenko NP, Zagrebelnyy AV, Ginzburg ML. Awareness of cardiovascular disease, its risk factors, and its association with attendance at outpatient clinics in acute coronary syndrome patients. Integr Med Res. 2017;6(3):240–4.

117. He H, Yu Y, Li Y, Kou CG, Li B, Tao YC, et al. Dyslipidemia awareness, treatment, control and influence factors among adults in the Jilin province in China: a cross-sectional study. Lipids Health Dis. 2014;13:122.

118. Wang C, Yu Y, Zhang X, Li Y, Kou C, Li B, et al. Awareness, treatment, control of diabetes mellitus and the risk factors: survey results from Northeast China. PLoS One. 2014;9:e103594.

119. Mendez-Chacon E, Santamaria-Ulloa C, Rosero-Bixby L. Factors associated with hypertension prevalence, unawareness and treatment among Costa Rican elderly. BMC Public Health. 2008;8:275.

120. Al-Azri M, Al-Rasbi K, Al-Hinai M, Davidson R, Al-Maniri A. Awareness of risk factors for cancer among Omani adults—a community based study. Asian Pac J Cancer Prev. 2014;15(3):5401–6.

121. Lagerlund M, Hvidberg L, Hajdarevic S, Pedersen AF, Runesdotter S, Vedsted P, Tishelman C. Awareness of risk factors for cancer: a comparative study of Sweden and Denmark. BMC Public Health. 2015;15:1156–63.

122. Rhazi KE, Bennani B, Fakir SE, Boly A, Bekkali R, Zidouh A, Nejjari C. Public awareness of cancer risk factors in the Moroccan population: a population-based cross-sectional study. BMC Cancer. 2014;14:695–700.
123. Bhurgri H. Awareness of cancer risk factors among patients and attendants presenting to a tertiary care hospital in Karachi, Pakistan. J Pak Med Assoc. 2008;58(10):584–8.

Anticancer Potential of Dietary Polyphenols

Amy L. Stockert and Matthew Hill

1 Introduction

Numerous compounds found in dietary sources have been correlated to decreased cancer incidence, a statement endorsed by the National Cancer Institute and the American Institute for Cancer Research. These include but are in no way limited to: red wine, ginger, cauliflower, brussel sprouts, turmeric, onion, cabbage, soy bean, green tea, tomato, and potato [1–8]. Of these some of the most well-studied and promising dietary compounds are the polyphenols. Natural polyphenols are as diverse in number as the plant sources which create them. These plant-derived phenolic compounds have been used for centuries both spiritually and medicinally in their whole or extracted form [9]. Medicinal herb use has been limited in modern western medicine in the last century despite anecdotal and historical evidence of efficacy [10–13]. The reluctance to use herbal medicine in modern western medicine stems from concerns over purity to lack of evidence in mechanisms of action. Lack of correlation between in vitro and in vivo studies also cause skepticism [10, 14]. However as modern trends sometimes favor "natural" medicine and the cost of healthcare and pharmaceutics increases, the popularity of herbal medicine has blossomed. Our decade-long knowledge of the human genome compounded by an increased appreciation for epigenetics has sparked interest in the research world. Numerous studies have shown the benefits of healthy lifestyle and nutritious foods in cancer prevention and stimulated a whole new level of research targets. Studies have linked the impact on human health to the individual's ability to absorb and metabolize polyphenols; thus an understanding of the structure, classification, and

A. L. Stockert (✉) · M. Hill
Department of Pharmaceutical and Biomedical Sciences, The Raabe College of Pharmacy,
Ohio Northern University, Ada, OH, USA
e-mail: a-stockert@onu.edu

© Springer International Publishing AG, part of Springer Nature 2018
M. I. Waly, M. S. Rahman (eds.), *Bioactive Components, Diet and Medical Treatment in Cancer Prevention*, https://doi.org/10.1007/978-3-319-75693-6_2

bioavailability of polyphenols is essential to understanding the potential of polyphenols to exhibit anticancer activity [15].

2 Properties of Polyphenols

2.1 Structural Classifications of Polyphenols

The chemical structure of the bioactive plant-based polyphenols varies in both size and linkages, but as the name suggests, all contain multiple hydroxyl (–OH) groups. In most cases these hydroxyl groups are linked to a(n) aromatic phenyl(s) or benzene based rings [16]. Polyphenols are generally classified as flavonoids and non-flavonoids [17]. Flavonoid polyphenols are further segregated into six subclasses based on the methyl group substitution and hydroxyl group position. These six classes include catechins, anthocyanidins, flavanones, flavones, flavonoid, and isoflavones. The second group of polyphenols, the non-flavonoids has fewer subclasses with each group differing primarily in carbon skeleton structure. The three subclasses include hydroxycinnamates (C6-C3), stilbenes (C6-C2-C6), and the hydroxybenzoates (C6-C3) [17]. It is important to note that although several dietary sources have many of these flavonoids, they are not all available in their bioactive form nor can we be certain that our metabolism can convert them into the most absorbable and bioactive form [18–20].

The bioactivity of polyphenols compounds relies heavily on the position of hydroxyl groups and relative ease of substituent modification. In general antioxidant capacity of the compound increases with the number of hydroxyl groups available. As expected polyphenols with a large number of methylations will exhibit less antioxidant potential [21, 22]. Although there have been in vivo studies in mammals for several polyphenols, a large amount of the available research was completed in vitro, leading to potential concerns over translational use of the data. Irrespective of the study design, polyphenols have been clearly linked to anticancer activities both as preventative measures and as therapeutic. Therapeutic uses have been explored as conjunctive therapy with currently used chemotherapies as well as studied for their effectiveness as an independent therapy [23, 24].

2.2 Variability of Bioactivity and Bioavailability

The bioactivity of these polyphenols is extremely variable. Research has demonstrated beneficial antioxidant behavior under some conditions and prooxidant conditions under other conditions, possibly even toxic or carcinogenic activity [22, 25, 26]. Activity can be affected by harvest time, soil cultivation, plant location, surrounding plant environment, weather fluctuations, storage, and preparation [27–31]. Environment, other drug exposures, general health, and genetic variants of some metabolic genes can alter the activity from one individual to another. Bioactivity is highly sensitive to methylation, a modification that depends highly on the epigenome of the individual.

The dietary polyphenols are naturally derived by plants. Nearly all the polyphenolic compounds in plants exist in a glycosylates form rather than the agylcone form [32]. Flavonoids always exist as an alpha or beta glycoside in plants, the O- and C- glycosides of true flavanols being the highest proportion in foods [33, 34]. Plant flavonoid glycoside biosynthesis results in increased solubility and stability making the enzymatic synthesis of these polyphenol glycosides of interest in the development of supplements for human consumption. Glycosylation can be accomplished by chemical synthesis but much attention has been shifted towards the use of microbial enzymes to accomplish glycosylation efficiently, affordably, and environmentally friendly [32]. Research has explored the use of different microbes to selectively and specifically make these modifications with great success. Synthesis enzymes from different microbes exhibit different specificities for the variety of polyphenol tested.

2.3   Relationship of the Gut Microbiome to Polyphenol Activity

Finally another layer of variance is added when one considers the differences from individuals' microbiome and the epigenetic modifications to the microbial genome [35]. An individual's lifestyle, genotypes, standard diet, and physiological homeostasis can greatly affect the microbiome composition [36]. The importance of the gut microbiome cannot be overstated as the success of any potential benefit to dietary polyphenols is reliant on the enzymes hosted by the microorganisms that allow bioconversion of the dietary compounds by modifications including dihydroxylation, demethylation, and metabolite formation [37]. It is well known that bioactivation of many dietary polyphenols is most prevalent in the colon, and as indicated previously the success of this activation is highly dependent on the diversity and population size of the human gut microbiota [35]. One such example is the bioconversion of flavonoids. Individuals can be classified as high or low flavonoid converters based primarily on the relative composition of gut microbiota [36, 38–41]. Although much effort has been made to study the effects of the human gut biome on cancer prevalence and metabolite changes, the sheer diversity in composition makes this very challenging [42]. Human studies that have demonstrated success at this challenge have focused primarily on absorption, distribution, metabolism, and excretion (ADME) and metabolomics. These studies were able to clearly analyze data collected and categorize variation of absorption between individuals [43, 44]. A well-designed study examined the effects of standardizing the diet for a prolonged period of time in an attempt to normalize the human metabolome. This study was one of few that have been able to successfully moderate control of the major variable in human diet-microbiota relationship during human trials. A key component of this study was admittance to a clinical research center for a 2-week period. Daily serum and urine samples were drawn and analyzed. A 2-week follow-up draw was also included. Data analysis showed that standardization did occur based on the similar profiles observed between subjects even within 24 h period. The importance of this study was the successful demonstration of variable control that is possible and necessary for studies on bioavailability and bioactivity of dietary components [45].

2.4 Polyphenol Effects on Endogenous Metabolites

Another important consideration of both bioactivity and metabolism of the polyphenols is the effect of polyphenols on metabolite modifications. Numerous studies have examined the effects of catechins on modifications of endogenous metabolites [46–50]. Although metabolite involvement in cancer has been explored for some time, the more recent explosion of the omics fields have enabled metabolomics to identify correlation between metabolite concentrations and cancer prevalence [35, 51, 52]. One such study identified increase in multiple metabolites including valine, tyrosine, 2-methylguanosine, 2-aminobutyric acid, and ornithine following consumption of the equivalent of 5 cups of tea catechins. Production of urea was decreased in these subjects [53]. Another human study examined changes in metabolite concentrations upon supplementation of 6 g per day of green tea, black tea, or caffeine for 2 days. Succinate, oxaloacetate, and 2-oxoglutarate all increased potentially due to a stimulation in oxidative metabolism [54]. The basis of studying the metabolome stems from two directions. First, addressing the question of whether changes in metabolite levels can be used as markers of cancer, and second, whether metabolite changes can be inductive of cancer. Considering the use of metabolite levels as a marker of cancer is useful simply because the metabolic needs of cancer cells are much different than standard cells. Cancer cells rely on higher levels of glucose metabolism to meet the energy demand of cell division [55, 56]. Several potential drugs have been designed with a therapeutic target of limiting glucose to the cancer cell or limiting energy metabolism. These include metformin, oligomycin, and resveratrol, to name a few [56–60].

3 Polyphenols and Its Effects on Cancer

3.1 Polyphenols and Cancer Prevention and Treatment

Upon consideration of the variable conditions in which plants produce and microorganisms modify polyphenols, it is easy to surmise that the mechanisms of anticancer activity of polyphenols is at least as diverse as the polyphenols themselves. Polyphenols are a very rich and varied aspect of the human diet. This coupled with growing research indicating their potential effectiveness in cancer treatment has led to a substantial increase in research studies looking to their preventative effects in cancer treatment [61]. Literature citing the effects of polyphenols in cancer prevention is vast. As discussed many of the effects are highly individual. Despite the diversity of individual response to the many polyphenols, evidence both for cancer prevention and for lack of correlation stand out in epidemiological studies [62]. Some studies showed benefits to intake of certain polyphenols, most commonly the flavanol and flavones, for some cancers but not others [63, 64]. One large randomized controlled trial referred to as the Polyp Prevention Trial failed to demonstrate a correlation between flavonoid intake and colorectal cancer risk [65]. However, much of the epidemiological comparisons recognize obvious limitations to the studies, including poor biomarker availability, lack of controlled exposure to the polyphenols, influence of other dietary components, lifestyle factors such as smoking, and little information regarding subject gut health [65]. Few studies, both in vivo and in vitro, have addressed the synergistic effects from multiple dietary phytochemicals, potentially leading to data misinterpretation [64, 66]. The lack of definitive answers regarding cancer prevention with polyphenols is to be expected with the unprecedented number of variables involved in even a well-designed animal or human study. Advancement can only be made with open consideration of all studies, both preclinical and clinical. The ability of a preclinical study to control certain variables may highlight the projects weakness in physiological relevance, but it also stands out as an advantage for improving design of the clinical studies by indicating target biomarkers or potential for drug development. The potential for future research is therefore driven by inconclusive results. Although not yet solidified, the potential mechanisms of action of polyphenol prevention highlight both current knowledge and future research.

Many studies have been completed looking at the in vitro effects of polyphenols on cancer prevention. Of these studies numerous polyphenols emerge with potential cancer prevention activity, however some polyphenols seem to have demonstrated the most promise in part due to the number of studies completed testing effects of these promising polyphenols. One such frequently studied polyphenol is (−)-epigallocatechin-3-gallate or EGCG. Green tea has some of the largest quantities of EGCG, although it can also be found in smaller quantities in other teas, pecans, hazelnuts, cranberries, and pistachios.

3.2   Potential Mechanisms of Polyphenol Anticancer Activities

Although many mechanisms of cancer prevention from polyphenols likely exist, there are a few that stand out in multiple studies. Cancer prevention mechanisms include inhibition of cell proliferation and metastasis, antioxidant protection from cell damage, mediation of signaling pathways, immune response modulation, mitochondrial dysfunction, and inhibition of enzyme activities important in carcinogenesis [67–78]. Due to the large number of potential mechanisms and the overlapping nature of effects of signaling pathways, it is highly likely that the cancer prevention potential of polyphenols is due to multiple molecular mechanisms rather than one isolated action. The multi-targeted molecular action may explain, in part, why results from multiple studies appear to contradict each other occasionally. It may also shed light on the criticism of correlation between the in vitro and in vivo experiments. Expression levels of some oncogenes seem dependent on the expression of other oncogenes, making conclusions based on isolated molecular actions on gene targets observable only under certain conditions [79]. Although much research shows overlap into multiple areas, attempts to separate the current knowledge into some categorical understanding is important. The majority of the work currently available can be separated into either polyphenol based cancer prevention or treatment, although the diversity of polyphenol action sometimes still allows both to be evaluated simultaneously. For that reason, it is more convenient to present current research in terms of action of the polyphenol. Current research will be divided into the following categories based on polyphenol actions: antioxidant activity, prooxidant activity, mediation of cellular signaling, epigenetic modifications, glycolytic inhibition, and adjunctive therapy.

3.2.1   Antioxidant Activity

Polyphenol compounds are well suited to function effectively as an antioxidant due to the large number of hydroxyl groups attached to the compounds. Generally speaking, the more hydroxyl groups attached, the greater the antioxidant potential. The preventative effect of antioxidants is highly dependent on the type of cancer and is commonly considered most effective for cancers in the digestive tract, although recent research has also shown benefits of polyphenol antioxidant activity in other cancers as well. The antioxidant based cancer prevention mechanism primarily involves scavenging of free radicals, thus protecting cellular components from reactive oxygen species [80–84]. Scavenging of free radicals can be accomplished directly by the polyphenols, thus reducing the free radicals available to generate reactive oxygen species. Protection from reactive oxygen species results from either reduced production, due to free radical scavenging, or from increased inactivation of already existing reactive oxygen species. In either case, the net result is protection of oxidation sensitive cellular components including free lipids, membrane lipids, proteins, and DNA.

The effects of polyphenols on lipid peroxidation have been a popular target of study in the past two decades. Lipid peroxidation is of importance because not only does it affect free lipids but also membrane lipids. More recently the oxidation status of membrane lipids, particularly those in the mitochondria, have been linked to the relative metabolic health of the cell [85–90]. Mitochondrial dysfunction is related to numerous disease states including cancer, heart disease, type 2 diabetes, and neurodegenerative diseases [91–95]. Decreases in lipid peroxidation due to polyphenol supplementation were identified in adults with type 2 diabetes, but the same effects were not observed in healthly individuals [96]. Studies in healthy human subjects consuming 500 mg per day of tea catechins over a month long period demonstrated a nearly 20% reduction in oxidized low density lipoprotein (LDL) found in the plasma [97]. Decreases in C-reactive protein and inflammation markers have been identified in patients with a similar catechin intake level [98]. Polyphenols have been demonstrated in numerous studies to decrease lipid peroxidation in patients taking medications with typical oxidizing potential, such as antipsychotics and doxirubicin, or with metabolic diseases including metabolic syndrome and diabetes [99–101].

As metabolic health and disease development result from mitochondrial dysfunction, it is clear that the health of the mitochondria can play a role in initiation of apoptosis [102–104]. The initiation of apoptosis can be cancer preventative by stimulating cell death when damage has occurred, but can also provide avenues for potential cancer therapies. Protection from lipid peroxidation provides some anticancer effects, but another obvious cell component sensitive to damage is the DNA. Studies have evaluated the oxidative damage in both nuclear and mitochondrial DNA and both seem equally important in terms of cancer prevention. Polyphenol protection from DNA damage was characterized by evaluating levels of urinary 8-hydroxyldeoxy-2′-deoxyguanosine (8-OHdg) in smokers followed by 4 months supplementation with approximately 300 mg of catechins per day divided in 4 doses of green tea. This study demonstrated a 31% decrease in 8-OHdg [105]. Similarly, green tea polyphenol has decreased the formation of pyrimidine dimers formed as a result of ultraviolet light exposure [106] as well as reducing the levels of UVB-induced inflammation [107].

Although many studies have explored the scavenging ability of polyphenol supplements, antioxidant activity is also prevalent from regulation of expression of genes encoding antioxidant enzymes. Table 1 summarizes the dietary polyphenols that have shown antioxidant activity by modifying either expression or activity of enzymes related to oxidative stress.

In a study completed in rats treated with EGCG, antioxidant and antioxidant enzyme levels were increased in the liver, skeletal muscle, and brain; however, this increase was only observed in older rats exposed to oxidant stress and not the younger relatively stress free rats [108, 109]. The major antioxidant enzymes protect the body from oxidative damage and include glutathione peroxidase, catalase, and superoxide dismutase. Gene expression studies of cells treated with reactive oxygen species have identified the glutathione peroxidase/reductase antioxidant enzyme system as one of the most inducible via oxidative stress in muscle [110]. The expression level of glutathione peroxidase (GPx) is so variable in cancer cells that it has been successfully used as a predictor of prognosis and response to chemotherapeutics [111]. Expression, translocation, and function of the glutathione peroxidase enzyme vary based on isoform. At least seven isoforms have been identified for the GPx enzymes differing in tissue location and presumably enzyme function [112]. In addition to modulating expression in response to exposure to reactive oxygen species, the gene exhibits translational control via inclusion of secretory factors that appear to stabilize the messenger RNA in response to available selenium, a required element for GPx function [113, 114]. Downregulation of matrix metalloproteinases via polyphenol action has been

Table 1 Dietary polyphenols altering expression or activity of antioxidant enzyme systems

Polyphenol	Enzyme(s) affected	Level of evidence
EGCG, ECG, EGC	12- and 15-lipoxygenase (recombinant) [108], lipoxygenase [109], cyclooxygenase [109]	Conditions: in vitro [108, 109]
		Specificity: nonhuman mammal [108]; human [109]
		Tissue/Cell: smooth muscle/ J774A.1 cells [108]; colon mucosa and colon tumor [109]
Resveratrol	SOD [110], MPO [110], GR [110]	Conditions: ex vivo [110]
		Specificity: nonhuman mammal [110]
		Tissue/Cell: skin [110]
Quercetin	SOD [111, 112], CAT [112], GSH [112], Gpx [111], GR [112]	Conditions: in vivo [112]; in vitro [111]
		Specificity: nonhuman mammal [112]; human [111]
		Tissue/Cell: liver [111, 112]
Curcumin	GSTP2 [113], CAT [114], SOD [114], MPO [114]	Conditions: in vivo [113, 114]
		Specificity: human [113]; rat [114]
		Tissue/Cell: liver [113, 114]
Catechin Proanthocyanidin B4	CAT [115], GST [115], SOD [115]	Conditions: in vitro [115]
		Specificity: rat [115]
		Tissue/Cell: cardiac H9C2 [115]

EGCG (−)-epigallocatechin-3-gallate, *ECG* epigallocatechin, *EGC* Epigallocatechin, *SOD* superoxide dismutase, *MPO* myeloperoxidase, *GR* glutathione reductase, *CAT* catalase, *GSH* glutathione, *GPx* Glutathione peroxidase, *GSTP2* glutathione S-transferase P2

attributed to a decrease in lipid peroxidation as well, suggesting that decreasing expression of genes associated with damaging effects can also be accomplished by polyphenol treatment [115].

3.2.2 Prooxidant Activity

It is clear that polyphenols offer antioxidant potential on multiple levels that relate to cancer prevention; however, polyphenols are sensitive to oxidation themselves, which under certain conditions can generate reactive oxygen species [116–120]. There is evidence that reactive oxygen species generated by the polyphenols may activate nuclear factor erythroid 2 related factor 2 (Nrf2) which is part of a pathway that is triggered in response to oxidative stress to activate antioxidant enzymes [121–124].

Human subjects treated for 4 weeks following a washout period with 800 mg EGCG per day exhibited significant increase in glutathione S-transferase activity in blood lymphocytes drawn under fasting conditions. Glutathione 2-transferase activity was increased from 30.7 ± 12.2 to 35.1 ± 14.3 nmol/min/mg protein corresponding to a p-value of 0.058 or 0.004 when analyzed against baseline activity. The baseline comparison represents an 80% increase in subjects with baseline activity in the lowest tertile [125]. These studies indicated that even under prooxidant conditions polyphenols, specifically EGCG and resveratrol, can function to protect the cell from oxidative stress. However, few large-scale clinical studies have been conducted that address potential hazards of over supplementation. Reported case studies have demonstrated potential for liver toxicity when extracted tea polyphenols have been supplemented in large quantities, beyond what would ordinarily be consumed from drinking tea. The patient exhibited aspartate aminotransferase (AST) level of 1783 U/L (reference 17–39 U/L), alanine aminotransferase (ALT) level of 1788 U/L (reference 8–30 U/L), and alkaline phosphatase level of 238 U/L (reference 39–113 U/L) following consumption of a tea extract based weight loss supplement for 4 months [126]. In vitro experiments in lung cancer cells have suggested that incubation with 1 mmol/L EGCG resulted in hydrogen peroxide production in the amount of 334 µmol/L. Importantly, cell death was inhibited in these cells upon addition of catalase [127, 128].

Cell viability was decreased in lung, esophageal, and liver cells treated with high doses (20–200 µmol/L) of EGCG; however, in these cases addition of superoxide dismutase and catalase reversed the effects of EGCG, at least in part [116, 129]. Animal studies of toxicity following polyphenol intake have shown varied results ranging from multi-organ toxicity to an absence of clinical adverse effects. One of the most alarming animal studies examined short-term effects of high doses of EGCG on organ toxicity [130]. This study examined effects of a variety of administration methods including topical, divided- and single- oral dosing.

A single oral dose of 200 mg EGCG/kg resulted in no toxicity, while a single dose of 2000 mg EGCG/kg was lethal to rats. No toxicity was observed with daily dosing of up to 500 mg/kg for 13 weeks in rats or dogs. However dosing the dogs in a fasting state at this level caused morbidity [130]. Conversely, rats fed quercetin ranging from 20–40 g/kg diet showed no signs of clinical adverse effects from supplementation, although pathological evidence suggests some nephropathy [131]. A large portion of polyphenols obtained through diet are attributed to phenolic acids, which when consumed at high doses have been shown to induce carcinogenesis through DNA damage [132]. Stability of the genome is altered by direct DNA damage as well as chromosome translocation [118, 132–134]. These studies together illustrate the importance of establishing upper limits for polyphenol consumption as well as emphasizing careful dose response studies to determine levels at which the benefits out weigh the detriments. Although in vitro studies are well suited to study dose response, direct translation to humans is impossible. Careful attention should be made to calculate appropriate human dosing based on in vitro results as well as emphasizing the importance of continuing to clinical studies.

3.2.3   Mediation of Cellular Signaling

Polyphenols have the unique ability to interact with cellular components in a variety of ways. These include binding to receptors, traversing the membrane to bind to components of a signaling pathway, interacting with various cytokines, and moderating activity of enzymes involved in signaling cascades [135–142].

3.2.4   Mediation of Cellular Signaling: Immunomodulation

Interestingly, evidence exists for high affinity binding (Kd ~ 10 nmol/L) of EGCG to the T-cell receptor CD4 demonstrating not only evidence for potential cancer prevention but also as a prevention of HIV-1 infection [135]. Furthermore, studies that involved the polyphenols found in bee propolis have linked polyphenols to immunomodulation, suggesting that the propolis compounds exhibit anticancer activity by activation of macrophages in addition to other tumor inhibition mechanisms [143]. Resveratrol has been implicated in the reversible reduction of antigen-specific cytotoxic T lymphocytes developed in response to mitogen, IL-2, and alloantigen. Likewise, resveratrol irreversibly inhibited production of cytokines IFN-γ and IL-2 from splenic lymphocytes and tumor necrosis factor α (TNF-α) and IL-12 from peritoneal macrophages [144]. These studies collectively suggested that polyphenols have the potential to modulate immune response specifically to damaged cells, thus providing a preventative measure against cancer.

3.2.5   Mediation of Cellular Signaling: Nuclear Factor-$\kappa\beta$ (NF-κB) Inhibition

Nuclear factor-$\kappa\beta$ (NF-κB) functions as a transcription factor sensitive to stress. It is present in functional amount endogenously and therefore provides rapid control of transcription upon cellular stimulus from a variety of factors including reactive oxygen species, TNF-α, inflammatory interleukins, and bacterial infection. NF-κB therefore plays a significant role in chronic disease state, especially those that are inflammatory in nature, including cancer. It is believed that NF-κB is primarily responsible for induction of a variety of cancer-promoting molecules including adhesion molecules, growth factors, angiogeneic proteins, cell proliferative proteins, and inflammatory cytokines [139]. It is relevant, therefore, to consider the effects of polyphenols on the NF-κB pathway. During non-stimulatory conditions cytosolic inhibitory proteins, known as IκBs, bind NF-κB excluding it from the nucleus. Upon stimulation these inhibitory proteins are targeted for degradation and NF-κB is translocated into the nucleus [145]. Regulatory points in this activation of NF-κB include inhibition of IκB kinase (IKK) activation and inhibition of IκB phosphorylation and degradation, all of which can be influenced by polyphenols [139]. Figure 1 shows the interactions of inhibitory proteins with NF-κB and potential levels of polyphenol control. Inhibition of IKK activation and IκB degradation by

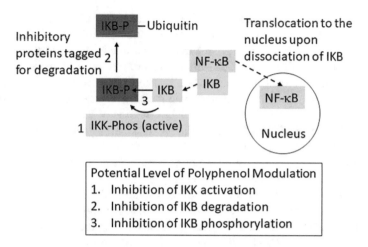

Fig. 1 The potential points of polyphenol mediated inhibition of the NF-κB pathway

EGCG have been demonstrated in vitro [146]. Inhibition of the NF-κB pathway has been demonstrated with other polyphenols as well. Flavonoids appear to limit NF-κB activation by regulating the levels of oxidants in the cell as well as interfering with IKK activation. Evidence also suggests that flavonoids may interfere with the binding of NF-κB to DNA [147]. Inflammation was also inhibited on multiple levels with quercetin treatment, one of which included the inhibition of IκB phosphorylation, which differs from the EGCG results [148].

3.2.6 Mediation of Cellular Signaling: Mitogen-Activated Protein Kinase (MAPK) Pathway Modulation

Another major pathway sensitive to polyphenol interaction is the mitogen-activated protein kinase (MAPK) pathway. The MAPK pathway is responsible for control of processes such as cell growth, differentiation, proliferation, and death. In brief, the MAPK pathway signal is initiated by mitogen binding membrane bound receptors such as the epithelial growth factor receptor (EGFR) which triggers G-protein Ras to activate Raf (MAP3K), which activates MEK ½ (MAP2K/ERK) and finally MEK1/2 activates MAPK (Erk). MAPK when active can phosphorylate transcription factors including c-Myc, cAMP response element B (CREB), and c-Fos. Each of these transcription factors have been linked to cellular processes that have potential for development of cancer. A mutant version of the gene encoding phosphoprotein c-Myc generates a constitutive faulty transcription factor enhancing cell proliferation [149–151]. CREB is a transcription factor that interacts with an enhancer region known as cAMP response element (CRE), which has been associated with formation of long-term memories, drug addiction, major depressive disorder, and cell survival. Research has suggested that the involvement of CREB in cancer is somewhat tissue specific, but due to the central signaling location of CREB it is well suited as an overlapping target for inhibition of proliferation and differentiation [152]. C-Fos is a transcription factor responsible for both positive and negative regulation of cell proliferation, differentiation, and survival genes with direct links to the development of cancer when induced [153]. Numerous studies have shown polyphenol potential to interact with the MAPK pathways. In HaCaT cells treated with TNF-α, curcumin inhibited the expression of IL-6, IL-1β, TNF-α, and cyclin E. Activation of NF-κB and multiple MAP kinases including JNK, p38, and ERK was also inhibited [154].

In addition to the MAPK pathway, polyphenols have been heavily researched for effects on the PI3K/Akt pathway both directly and indirectly. Polyphenols extracted from cocoa have been shown in vitro to directly inhibit PI3K activity by binding and inactivating its activity [155]. Effectiveness of the cocoa polyphenols are enhanced by additional interference in the signaling cascade by inhibiting TNF-α dependent phosphorylation of Akt and TNF-α dependent activity of MEK1, although no evidence was found for suppression of the TNF-α dependent phosphorylation of MEK1 [155]. It suffices to say that suppression of Akt activation, either by inhibiting inflammatory factors dependent phosphorylation or by PI3K mediated activation of Akt, shows promise for the use of polyphenols in cancer prevention and therapy. EGCG and TF from green and black tea, respectively, decrease PI3K and phospho-Akt while increasing Erk1/2 [156]. Typically activation of Erk1/2 stimulates cell survival but under specific conditions can also induce proapoptotic signals [157, 158]. Despite extensive research it is still relatively unclear how Erk1/2 activation results in two drastically different effects, but it has been suggested with some evidence that the levels of Erk1/2 and even the activity of this MAPK subgroup may direct cellular outcome as well as the cellular localization of the Erk1/2 protein [157]. The modulation of signal amplitude and the variability of cellular localization could potentially explain the activated Erk1/2 anticancer effects exhibited by polyphenols.

Although mediation of numerous signaling pathways overlaps with all mechanisms of both prevention and management of cancer, some studies with specific targets of metastasis are important to consider individually. Japanese researchers studied the effects of certain polyphenols, Epigallocatechin (EGC) and EGCG, on prevention of cancer metastasis. Of particular interest is the migration and invasion pathways induced by heregulin-β1 (HRG-B1), and how these catechins could potentially inhibit this activating peptide [159]. HRG-B1 is a peptide growth factor that can work by binding to ErbB3, allowing it to form a heterodimer with ErbB2. ErbB proteins are a family of tyrosine receptor kinases, also referred to as human epidermal growth factor receptors (HER). This leads to downstream phosphorylation and activation of the PI3K/AKT/mTOR pathway that can lead to cancer metastasis. To perform this experiment, MCF-7 breast cancer cells were treated with 30 μM of EGC, EGCG, or a vehicle control and incubated for times 0, 2, 4, 8, and 12 h in a media containing 50 ng/mL HRG-B1 protein. Western blots were then run to measure for protein and phosphorylation (activation) levels of ErbB2 and ErbB3, tyrosine receptor kinases activated by HRG-B1, for each study set [159]. HRG-B1

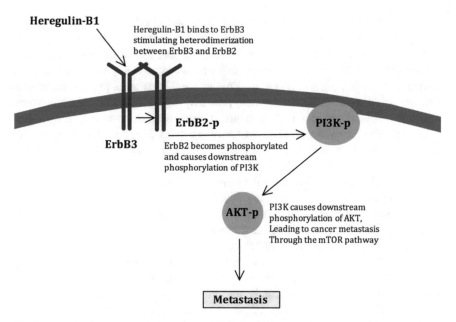

Fig. 2 The activation of Akt by HRG-B1 [161]

has been shown to increase heterodimerization of ErbB3 and ErbB2 as well as phosphorylation (activation) of both kinases [160, 161]. Both of these processes lead to recruitment of phosphoinositol-3-kinase (PI3K) and downstream activation of Akt, and ultimately cell migration and cancer metastasis [162]. Figure 2 summarizes the effects of HRG-B1 on Akt activation.

Researchers found that EGCG treatment was able to effectively reduce phosphorylation and heterodimerization levels of both ErbB2 and ErbB3; however, similar results were not seen in EGC treatment [159]. No hypothesis was given as to why these results were differing between the two treatments, but the potential effectiveness of using polyphenolic compounds for inhibition of HRG-induced migration was evident [159].

3.2.7 Mediation of Cellular Signaling: Cell Cycle Arrest

A crucial aspect of tumorigenesis is cell cycle dysregulation. This predominantly occurs when the checkpoints along the cell cycle lose their natural function due to unmediated activation of cyclin-dependent kinases (CDKs), which is associated with different cyclins and/or cyclin-dependent kinase inhibitors (CDKIs) to cause downstream effects that lead to cell cycle progression or arrest [163]. Because dysregulation of these vital checkpoints in the cell cycle is such a crucial step in tumorigenesis, it has become a popular target for cancer prevention focused research [164].

Many polyphenols have been shown to have strong effects in aiding in proper cell cycle regulation and even promoting cell cycle arrest when it becomes dysregulated. One heavily studied polyphenol source is grape seed extract. Grape seed extract contains flavonoids, flavanols, and various catechins, procyanidin dimers, trimers, and higher polyprocyanidins. Proanthocyanidins are a class of flavonoids that are polymers of various catechins, primarily catechin and epicatechin. These proanthocyanidins are major components of grape seed extract [165, 166]. When tested in different colorectal and pancreatic cell lines in vitro, grape seed extract resulted in inhibition of cell cycle growth at the G_1 phase and led to increased levels of cellular apoptosis [165]. The mechanism of grape seed extract polyphenols has yet to be confirmed, but data from the same studies have shown that CDK4/CDK6 interactions with cyclin D were decreased in both time- and concentration-dependent manners with grape seed extract treatment [165]. Since CDK4/CDK6 association with cyclin D is the primary trigger for cell cycle progression, this has been proposed as a possible mechanism for cell cycle regulation by grape seed extract [167].

Another promising result identified by researchers working with colorectal cell lines was that grape seed extract increased Cip1/p21 protein expression [165]. Cip1/p21, a CDKI, is a complex protein that has proapoptotic and anti-proliferative effects by binding to proliferating cell nuclear antigen (PCNA) to inhibit DNA replication and entry into mitosis [168]. Cip1/p21 expression is normally triggered and upregulated by p53 tumor suppressor protein [167]. In this case, however, the line of colorectal cells that were being studied, HT29, had a loss of function point mutation in the gene that coded for p53. Researchers hypothesize that grape seed extract polyphenols may have properties that allow it to perform p53 independent functions, leading to cellular apoptosis [165]. Interestingly, research has also shown the EGCG has the ability to reactivate epigenetically silenced Cip1/p21 and p16^{INK3a}, another tumor suppressor gene, by demethylation and acetylating histones associated with the gene loci, thus allowing expression of the tumor suppressor genes in human skin cancer cells [169]. Together these results indicate a multi-faceted ability of polyphenols to enhance gene expression of tumor suppressors.

3.2.8 Mediation of Cellular Signaling: Apoptotic Pathway Induction

Cell cycle regulation is a common focal point in cancer prevention research. Many natural polyphenols have been shown to perform certain actions in vitro that can aid in regulation as well as help promote apoptosis [170]. Both extrinsic and intrinsic apoptosis initiation have been studied, but both will ultimately lead to caspase-3 activation downstream, resulting in DNA fragmentation and cell death [171].

Quercetin is one polyphenol that has been shown to exhibit many of these activating effects. Many studies have shown that it will not only activate caspase-3, -8, and -9, but it can also upregulate expression of Bax, a proapoptotic protein, and downregulate expression of Bcl-2, an anti-apoptotic protein [170, 172]. Therefore, quercetin demonstrates both mitochondrial and death protein signaling pathways indicating that it participates in both intrinsic and extrinsic apoptotic pathways

[172]. Moreover, the number of apoptotic NCI-H209 cells increased by 60% between concentrations of 0 and 10 μM when treated with quercetin for 48 h in vitro [170].

Other notable polyphenols that contribute to cell apoptosis mediation are theaflavins (TF) and thearubigins (TR), prominent black tea polyphenols. These compounds are known to cause several different effects to interfere with carcinogenesis, however, one of the most notable is their effect on p-Akt levels [173]. Treatment with TF and TR have been shown to decrease the presence of p-Akt, which can lead to many downstream effects such as downregulation of CDK4 through p27 activation and upregulation of cyclin D1, both of which contribute to prolonged cell survival, cell cycle dysregulation, and, ultimately, tumorigenesis [173, 174].

3.2.9 Epigenetic Modifications

Although initially much emphasis was placed on utilizing polyphenols for cancer prevention, the emerging knowledge of the cancer epigenome has influenced experiments in polyphenols as anticancer therapeutics both singly and as adjunctive therapies. Polyphenols have an inert ability to regulate reactive oxygen species. The protective effect leads to disease prevention via scavenging and decreases in inflammatory factors [9, 11, 71, 80, 139, 175, 176]. Mediation of reactive oxygen species can also modulate epigenetic changes in the genome that result from cancerous cell growth. Epigenetic changes in the genome are so predictive of cancer outcome that analysis of methylation states of specific cancer genes are now used as both markers of cancer and cancer survival predictors [177–182]. One such example is the human ovarian cancer study where the methylation state of the BRCA1 promoter was analyzed. Patient cohorts exhibited similar clinical factors but differences in methylation status of the BRCA1 promoter. This study demonstrated a shorter median disease free interval for patients with the methylated promoter (9.8 months) than patients' carrying the BRCA1 mutation (39.5 months). This disease free interval difference was significant with a p-value of 0.04. A significant difference ($P = 0.02$) was also found between the methylated promoter group and mutation group for the median overall survival. Patients carrying the mutation as well as having a methylated promoter had significantly shorter survival than wild-type patients [181]. The promise of this study is that facilitating demethylation of the BRCA1 promoter, in either the wild-type or mutant genotype patient, could increase survival time and decrease re-occurrence significantly in patients. Furthermore, this phenomenon translates into breast cancer as well where BRCA1 promoter methylation was identified in triple negative tumors with large significance ($P < 0.0001$). Methylation status was also related to increased lymph vessel invasion and higher nuclear grade [182].

Various polyphenols have been reported to carry the ability to reverse CpG methylation in promoters of numerous genes, making polyphenols possible adjunct therapy treatments that could increase survival in many cancers [183–185]. Research has shown that inflammatory conditions lead to epigenetic modifications including inactivation of tumor suppressor genes, silencing of antioxidant genes, and activation of cancer-promoting genes [186, 187]. Evidence has suggested that even after cancerous conditions develop, control of the relatively high level of reactive oxygen species allows for reversal of these epigenetic modifications. Expression of glutathione-2 transferase P1 can be re-stimulated in human prostate cancer cells by demethylation of the promoter via the polyphenols found in green tea [188]. Furthermore EGCG inhibited DNA methyltransferases (DNMT) in vitro [189]. Curcumin, for example, has been shown to reverse promoter methylation of glutathione-s-transferase, allowing decreased oxidative stress [183]. This decrease in oxidative stress is both due to direct scavenging and increased expression of antioxidant system genes. These conditions have allowed natural cellular death gene expression. Similarly, reduced oxidative stress have also positively influenced the effectiveness of known chemotherapeutics.

Inhibition of methyltransferase enzymes DNMT by multiple polyphenols has been demonstrated. Evidence suggests that histone acetylation is also affected as some histone acetylases (HAT) are inactivated and histone deaceytlases (HDAC) are activated. Epigenetic modulation relies on these enzymes and the ability to control them makes polyphenols of interest not only for anticancer activity but also for antiaging and general disease prevention. Possibilities of polyphenols to affect health, both negatively and positively, via these mechanisms are essentially limitless.

3.2.10   Glycolytic Inhibition

Cancer cells, like all cells, rely heavily on their metabolic capabilities for energy production. However, unlike most cells, cancer cells often rely more on aerobic glycolysis rather than oxidative phosphorylation to produce the majority of its ATP [190]. Even though, oxidative phosphorylation is largely more efficient than glycolysis, glycolysis produces ATP much more rapidly which can be helpful for rapidly proliferating cells [190]. Inhibition of glycolysis has thus been considered as a means for cancer treatment and management.

Resveratrol, a polyphenol largely found in different types of grapes and berries, has been increasingly studied for its effects on cell metabolism. It has the ability to cause inhibition of 6-phosphofructo-1-kinase (PFK), an important regulatory enzyme in cell metabolism which converts fructose-6-phosphate (F6P) to fructose-1,6-bisphosphate (F-1,6-BP) [191]. Researchers have found that, when treated with varying concentrations of resveratrol from 1 to 100 μM, MCF-7 breast cancer cell line showed as low as a 16% reduction in ATP production at 1 μM, and as high as a 50% reduction at concentrations of 100 μM [191]. To confirm the mechanism, they took their tests further to analyze changes in PFK activity in relation to the varying resveratrol concentrations. Ratios of intracellular F6P to F1,6BP showed that PFK was affected in a similar concentration-dependent manner to ATP production with approximately a 65% reduction at 100 μM [191]. While these are significant findings and potentially an effective agent against cancerous activity, we must be careful

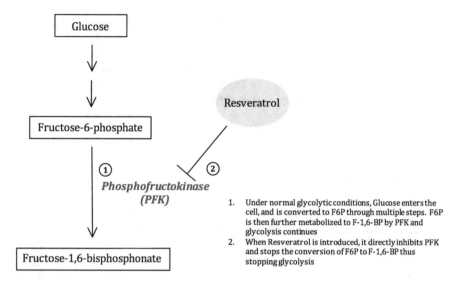

Fig. 3 Effects of resveratrol on glycolysis

in this approach as to not damage or impair the metabolism of healthy cells. Figure 3 demonstrates the effects of resveratrol on the glycolytic pathway.

4 Adjunctive Therapy

The concept of adjunctive therapy has expanded in recent years. Research has shown that treating with polyphenols in conjunction with chemotherapeutics can not only ease the damage of the treatment to healthy cells but also selectively target and sensitize cancer cells to the treatment. The ability to selectively sensitize cancer cells that have developed resistance to common chemotherapeutics has the potential to expand the efficacy and the crossover usage of therapeutics. One such example is the use of selenium supplementation with cisplatin for colon cancer. Although not a polyphenol, selenium is required for the glutathione peroxidase and reductase anti-oxidant enzyme system. Addition of selenium decreased the level of reactive oxygen species in the HT-29 colon cancer cell line and facilitated cisplatin efficacy in a cancer cell line typically refractive to cisplatin [192]. Likewise, RGCG has been shown to reverse cisplatin resistance in the A549/DDP cell line via demethylation [193]. Treatment with curcumin facilitated epigenetic decrease in expression of microRNA-186, a short RNA sequence associated with resistance and poor survival, in A549/DDP cells that allowed for induction of apoptosis [194]. Curcumin has also been shown to inhibit the multidrug resistant p-glycoprotein transporter [195]. Direct inhibition of this ABC type transporter limits efflux of the drug thereby increasing the cellular concentration and improving efficacy of the drug against otherwise resistant cells. Although it is possible for the cells to evolve a drug efflux transporter that is also resistant to inhibition by polyphenols, the success would be limited by the predicted relative nonspecific binding of the polyphenols to the transporter. Computational models have identified multiple polyphenol molecules binding in one active site with numerous binding poses of nearly equal affinity [196]. Evolution to counteract such flexible and variant binding of multi-molecular interactions is unlikely.

5   Conclusion

Although the research surrounding the anticancer potential of polyphenol compounds is extensive and numerous mechanisms have been identified, no such study exists that can explore the multitude of effects that polyphenols can have in the overlapping mechanisms by which they act. The sheer diversity of the available polyphenols and the variation in bioavailability complicate this need for an all-inclusive study evaluating the safety and efficacy of polyphenol use for anticancer prevention and treatment. Available research methods limit the ability to monitor multiple variables simultaneously while controlling appropriately for any modifications in cell process, thus research is limited to evaluation of single (or few) changes per experiment. Polyphenols have been shown to interact in cellular processes at so many levels, in so many different cells or tissues, in so many different pathways, that it may never be possible to predict human interaction with polyphenols with certainty.

Clinical trials and in vivo studies have begun to show trends in effectiveness of polyphenol use, but results are still and always will be dependent on influence of the individual's environment and health status in a way that few main-stream drugs have faced. Currently, the closest comparison for a therapy with such individuality would be the incorporation of pharmacogenomics testing and clinically actionable therapeutic modifications based on the individual genotype. However, even pharmacogenomics has not achieved full implementation.

The difficulty in correlating between human studies with an unprecedented number of variables and preclinical studies will continue. The potential benefits of polyphenols must continue to be explored preclinically as well as clinically in order to further test and generate research hypotheses. Although much has been learned from the numerous experiments conducted on polyphenol anticancer activities, there is still not a "one size fits all" conclusion in regard to the translational benefits in human therapy. There is clear evidence for benefits to polyphenol incorporation in human preventative therapy, but the number of precautions to consider have placed the onus of the decision on the individual rather incorporating the therapy decision as common physician protocol. Evidence also exists for polyphenol use as a cancer treatment or adjunctive therapy, however concerns over the effectiveness will always exist. The risk versus benefit analysis favors polyphenol use as an adjunctive therapy, while with prevention the analysis is not as clear.

References

1. Levine M, et al. Criteria and recommendations for vitamin C intake. JAMA. 1999;281(15):1415–23.
2. Levi F. Cancer prevention: epidemiology and perspectives. Eur J Cancer. 1999;35(7):1046–58.
3. Lee KW, Lee HJ. The roles of polyphenols in cancer chemoprevention. Biofactors. 2006;26(2):105–21.
4. Knekt P, et al. Flavonoid intake and risk of chronic diseases. Am J Clin Nutr. 2002;76(3):560–8.
5. Knekt P, et al. Dietary flavonoids and the risk of lung cancer and other malignant neoplasms. Am J Epidemiol. 1997;146(3):223–30.
6. Garcia-Closas R, et al. Intake of specific carotenoids and flavonoids and the risk of gastric cancer in Spain. Cancer Causes Control. 1999;10(1):71–5.
7. Cao G, et al. Serum antioxidant capacity is increased by consumption of strawberries, spinach, red wine or vitamin C in elderly women. J Nutr. 1998;128(12):2383–90.
8. Surh Y-J. Cancer chemoprevention with dietary phytochemicals. Nat Rev Cancer. 2003;3(10):768–80.
9. Quideau S, et al. Plant polyphenols: chemical properties, biological activities, and synthesis. Angew Chem Int Ed. 2011;50(3):586–621.
10. Asensi M, et al. Natural polyphenols in cancer therapy. Crit Rev Clin Lab Sci. 2011;48(5–6):197–216.
11. Dai J, Mumper RJ. Plant phenolics: extraction, analysis and their antioxidant and anticancer properties. Molecules. 2010;15(10):7313.
12. Sies H. Polyphenols and health: update and perspectives. Arch Biochem Biophys. 2010;501(1):2–5.
13. Bravo L. Polyphenols: chemistry, dietary sources, metabolism, and nutritional significance. Nutr Rev. 1998;56(11):317–33.
14. Scalbert A, et al. Dietary polyphenols and the prevention of diseases. Crit Rev Food Sci Nutr. 2005;45(4):287–306.
15. Scalbert A, et al. Absorption and metabolism of polyphenols in the gut and impact on health. Biomed Pharmacother. 2002;56(6):276–82.
16. Manach C, et al. Polyphenols: food sources and bioavailability. Am J Clin Nutr. 2004;79(5):727–47.
17. Tsao R. Chemistry and biochemistry of dietary polyphenols. Forum Nutr. 2010;2(12):1231.
18. Kroon PA, et al. How should we assess the effects of exposure to dietary polyphenols in vitro? Am J Clin Nutr. 2004;80(1):15–21.
19. Landis-Piwowar KR, et al. Methylation suppresses the proteasome-inhibitory function of green tea polyphenols. J Cell Physiol. 2007;213(1):252–60.
20. Tapiero H, et al. Polyphenols: do they play a role in the prevention of human pathologies? Biomed Pharmacother. 2002;56(4):200–7.
21. Dugas AJ, et al. Evaluation of the total peroxyl radical-scavenging capacity of flavonoids: structure–activity relationships. J Nat Prod. 2000;63(3):327–31.
22. Heim KE, Tagliaferro AR, Bobilya DJ. Flavonoid antioxidants: chemistry, metabolism and structure-activity relationships. J Nutr Biochem. 2002;13(10):572–84.
23. Shin SY, et al. Polyphenols bearing cinnamaldehyde scaffold showing cell growth inhibitory effects on the cisplatin-resistant A2780/Cis ovarian cancer cells. Bioorg Med Chem. 2014;22(6):1809–20.
24. Dominique D, Jianbo X. EDITORIAL (hot topic: natural polyphenols properties: chemopreventive and chemosensitizing activities). Anti Cancer Agents Med Chem. 2012;12(8):835.
25. Lee SH, Oe T, Blair IA. Vitamin C-induced decomposition of lipid hydroperoxides to endogenous genotoxins. Science. 2001;292(5524):2083–6.
26. Lee KW, et al. Vitamin C and cancer chemoprevention: reappraisal. Am J Clin Nutr. 2003;78(6):1074–8.

27. Kevers C, et al. Influence of cultivar, harvest time, storage conditions, and peeling on the antioxidant capacity and phenolic and ascorbic acid contents of apples and pears. J Agric Food Chem. 2011;59(11):6165–71.
28. Wang SY, Zheng W. Effect of plant growth temperature on antioxidant capacity in strawberry. J Agric Food Chem. 2001;49(10):4977–82.
29. Chandra S, et al. Assessment of total phenolic and flavonoid content, antioxidant properties, and yield of aeroponically and conventionally grown leafy vegetables and fruit crops: a comparative study. Evid Based Complement Alternat Med. 2014;2014:9.
30. Winardiantika V, et al. Effects of cultivar and harvest time on the contents of antioxidant phytochemicals in strawberry fruits. Hortic Environ Biotechnol. 2015;56(6):732–9.
31. Cogo SLP, et al. Low soil water content during growth contributes to preservation of green colour and bioactive compounds of cold-stored broccoli (Brassica oleraceae L.) florets. Postharvest Biol Technol. 2011;60(2):158–63.
32. Xiao J, Muzashvili TS, Georgiev MI. Advances in the biotechnological glycosylation of valuable flavonoids. Biotechnol Adv. 2014;32(6):1145–56.
33. Kozlowska A, Szostak-Wegierek D. Flavonoids—food sources and health benefits. Rocz Panstw Zakl Hig. 2014;65(2):79–85.
34. de Pascual-Teresa S, Moreno DA, García-Viguera C. Flavanols and anthocyanins in cardiovascular health: a review of current evidence. Int J Mol Sci. 2010;11(4):1679–703.
35. van Duynhoven J, et al. Metabolic fate of polyphenols in the human superorganism. Proc Natl Acad Sci. 2011;108(Suppl 1):4531–8.
36. Turnbaugh PJ, et al. A core gut microbiome in obese and lean twins. Nature. 2009;457(7228):480.
37. Cermak R, et al. In vitro degradation of the flavonol quercetin and of quercetin glycosides in the porcine hindgut. Arch Anim Nutr. 2006;60(2):180–9.
38. Zoetendal EG, Vaughan EE, De Vos WM. A microbial world within us. Mol Microbiol. 2006;59(6):1639–50.
39. Blaut M, Clavel T. Metabolic diversity of the intestinal microbiota: implications for health and disease. J Nutr. 2007;137(3):751S–5S.
40. Simons AL, et al. Human gut microbial degradation of flavonoids: structure–function relationships. J Agric Food Chem. 2005;53(10):4258–63.
41. Erlund I. Review of the flavonoids quercetin, hesperetin, and naringenin. Dietary sources, bioactivities, bioavailability, and epidemiology. Nutr Res. 2004;24(10):851–74.
42. Roowi S, et al. Yoghurt impacts on the excretion of phenolic acids derived from colonic breakdown of orange juice flavanones in humans. Mol Nutr Food Res. 2009;53(S1):S68–75.
43. van Velzen EJ, et al. Phenotyping tea consumers by nutrikinetic analysis of polyphenolic endmetabolites. J Proteome Res. 2009;8(7):3317–30.
44. van Dorsten FA, et al. The metabolic fate of red wine and grape juice polyphenols in humans assessed by metabolomics. Mol Nutr Food Res. 2010;54(7):897–908.
45. Winnike JH, et al. Effects of a prolonged standardized diet on normalizing the human metabolome. Am J Clin Nutr. 2009;90(6):1496–501.
46. Seyfried T. Cancer as a mitochondrial metabolic disease. Front Cell Dev Biol. 2015;3:43.
47. Seyfried TN, Shelton LM. Cancer as a metabolic disease. Nutr Metab. 2010;7(1):7.
48. Denkert C, et al. Metabolite profiling of human colon carcinoma—deregulation of TCA cycle and amino acid turnover. Mol Cancer. 2008;7(1):72.
49. Denkert C, et al. Mass spectrometry–based metabolic profiling reveals different metabolite patterns in invasive ovarian carcinomas and ovarian borderline tumors. Cancer Res. 2006;66(22):10795–804.
50. Struck-Lewicka W, et al. Urine metabolic fingerprinting using LC–MS and GC–MS reveals metabolite changes in prostate cancer: a pilot study. J Pharm Biomed Anal. 2015;111:351–61.
51. Slupsky CM, et al. Urine metabolite analysis offers potential early diagnosis of ovarian and breast cancers. Clin Cancer Res. 2010;16:5835.

52. Dang L, et al. Cancer-associated IDH1 mutations produce 2-hydroxyglutarate. Nature. 2009;462(7274):739.
53. Xie G, et al. Metabolic fate of tea polyphenols in humans. J Proteome Res. 2012;11(6):3449–57.
54. Van Dorsten FA, et al. Metabonomics approach to determine metabolic differences between green tea and black tea consumption. J Agric Food Chem. 2006;54(18):6929–38.
55. Locasale JW, Cantley LC. Altered metabolism in cancer. BMC Biol. 2010;8(1):88.
56. Zhang Y, Yang J-M. Altered energy metabolism in cancer: a unique opportunity for therapeutic intervention. Cancer Biol Ther. 2013;14(2):81–9.
57. Cao X, et al. Glucose uptake inhibitor sensitizes cancer cells to daunorubicin and overcomes drug resistance in hypoxia. Cancer Chemother Pharmacol. 2007;59(4):495–505.
58. Riccio A, et al. Glucose and lipid metabolism in non-insulin-dependent diabetes. Effect of metformin. Diabetes Metab. 1991;17(1 Pt 2):180–4.
59. Wolvetang EJ, et al. Mitochondrial respiratory chain inhibitors induce apoptosis. FEBS Lett. 1994;339(1–2):40–4.
60. Baur JA, Sinclair DA. Therapeutic potential of resveratrol: the in vivo evidence. Nat Rev Drug Discov. 2006;5(6):493–506.
61. Zhou Q, Bennett LL, Zhou S. Multifaceted ability of naturally occurring polyphenols against metastatic cancer. Clin Exp Pharmacol Physiol. 2016;43(4):394–409.
62. Arts IC, Hollman PC. Polyphenols and disease risk in epidemiologic studies. Am J Clin Nutr. 2005;81(1):317S–25S.
63. Yang CS, Wang Z-Y. Tea and cancer. J Natl Cancer Inst. 1993;85(13):1038–49.
64. Liu RH. Potential synergy of phytochemicals in cancer prevention: mechanism of action. J Nutr. 2004;134(12):3479S–85S.
65. Nimptsch K, et al. Habitual intake of flavonoid subclasses and risk of colorectal cancer in 2 large prospective cohorts. Am J Clin Nutr. 2016;103(1):184–91.
66. Liu RH. Health benefits of fruit and vegetables are from additive and synergistic combinations of phytochemicals. Am J Clin Nutr. 2003;78(3):517S–20S.
67. Yang CS, et al. Cancer prevention by tea: animal studies, molecular mechanisms and human relevance. Nat Rev Cancer. 2009;9(6):429–39.
68. Adhami VM, et al. Dietary flavonoid fisetin: a novel dual inhibitor of PI3K/Akt and mTOR for prostate cancer management. Biochem Pharmacol. 2012;84(10):1277–81.
69. de Kok TM, van Breda SG, Manson MM. Mechanisms of combined action of different chemopreventive dietary compounds: a review. Eur J Nutr. 2008;47(Suppl 2):51–9.
70. de Oliveira MR, et al. Resveratrol and the mitochondria: from triggering the intrinsic apoptotic pathway to inducing mitochondrial biogenesis, a mechanistic view. Biochim Biophys Acta. 2016;1860(4):727–45.
71. Ferguson LR, Philpott M. Cancer prevention by dietary bioactive components that target the immune response. Curr Cancer Drug Targets. 2007;7(5):459–64.
72. He Z, et al. Selecting bioactive phenolic compounds as potential agents to inhibit proliferation and VEGF expression in human ovarian cancer cells. Oncol Lett. 2015;9(3):1444–50.
73. Keijer J, et al. Bioactive food components, cancer cell growth limitation and reversal of glycolytic metabolism. Biochim Biophys Acta. 2011;1807(6):697–706.
74. Malavolta M, et al. Modulators of cellular senescence: mechanisms, promises, and challenges from in vitro studies with dietary bioactive compounds. Nutr Res. 2014;34(12):1017–35.
75. Mileo AM, Miccadei S. Polyphenols as modulator of oxidative stress in cancer disease: new therapeutic strategies. Oxidative Med Cell Longev. 2016;2016:6475624.
76. Nichenametla SN, et al. A review of the effects and mechanisms of polyphenolics in cancer. Crit Rev Food Sci Nutr. 2006;46(2):161–83.
77. Roy P, et al. Tea polyphenols inhibit cyclooxygenase-2 expression and block activation of nuclear factor-kappa B and Akt in diethylnitrosoamine induced lung tumors in Swiss mice. Investig New Drugs. 2010;28(4):466–71.
78. Thomas E, et al. A novel resveratrol based tubulin inhibitor induces mitotic arrest and activates apoptosis in cancer cells. Sci Rep. 2016;6:34653.

79. Weinstein IB, Joe A. Oncogene addiction. Cancer Res. 2008;68(9):3077–80.
80. Terao J. Dietary flavonoids as antioxidants. Forum Nutr. 2009;61:87–94.
81. Afrin S, et al. Chemopreventive and therapeutic effects of edible berries: a focus on colon cancer prevention and treatment. Molecules. 2016;21(2):1–40.
82. Brückner M, et al. Green tea polyphenol epigallocatechin-3-gallate shows therapeutic antioxidative effects in a murine model of colitis. J Crohn's Colitis. 2012;6(2):226–35.
83. Gresele P, et al. Resveratrol, at concentrations attainable with moderate wine consumption, stimulates human platelet nitric oxide production. J Nutr. 2008;138(9):1602–8.
84. Karlsen A, et al. Bilberry juice modulates plasma concentration of NF-κB related inflammatory markers in subjects at increased risk of CVD. Eur J Nutr. 2010;49(6):345–55.
85. Kappus H, Sies H. Toxic drug effects associated with oxygen metabolism: redox cycling and lipid peroxidation. Experientia. 1981;37(12):1233–41.
86. Wilhelm J. Metabolic aspects of membrane lipid peroxidation. Acta Univ Carol Med Monogr. 1990;137:1–53.
87. Jiang Y, Huang B. Drought and heat stress injury to two cool-season turfgrasses in relation to antioxidant metabolism and lipid peroxidation. Crop Sci. 2001;41(2):436–42.
88. Paradies G, et al. Lipid peroxidation and alterations to oxidative metabolism in mitochondria isolated from rat heart subjected to ischemia and reperfusion. Free Radic Biol Med. 1999;27(1):42–50.
89. Vladimirov YA, et al. Lipid peroxidation in mitochondrial membrane. Adv Lipid Res. 1980;17:173–249.
90. Wallace DC. A mitochondrial paradigm of metabolic and degenerative diseases, aging, and cancer: a dawn for evolutionary medicine. Annu Rev Genet. 2005;39:359–407.
91. Lin MT, Beal MF. Mitochondrial dysfunction and oxidative stress in neurodegenerative diseases. Nature. 2006;443(7113):787.
92. Chicco AJ, Sparagna GC. Role of cardiolipin alterations in mitochondrial dysfunction and disease. Am J Phys Cell Phys. 2007;292(1):C33–44.
93. Lesnefsky EJ, et al. Mitochondrial dysfunction in cardiac disease: ischemia–reperfusion, aging, and heart failure. J Mol Cell Cardiol. 2001;33(6):1065–89.
94. Wallace DC. Mitochondrial diseases in man and mouse. Science. 1999;283(5407):1482–8.
95. Boland ML, Chourasia AH, Macleod KF. Mitochondrial dysfunction in cancer. Front Oncol. 2013;3:292.
96. Basu A, et al. Pomegranate polyphenols lower lipid peroxidation in adults with type 2 diabetes but have no effects in healthy volunteers: a pilot study. J Nutr Metab. 2013;2013:1–7.
97. Inami S, et al. Tea catechin consumption reduces circulating oxidized low-density lipoprotein. Int Heart J. 2007;48(6):725–32.
98. Hsu SP, et al. Chronic green tea extract supplementation reduces hemodialysis-enhanced production of hydrogen peroxide and hypochlorous acid, atherosclerotic factors, and proinflammatory cytokines. Am J Clin Nutr. 2007;86(5):1539–47.
99. Dietrich-muszalska A, Olas B. Inhibitory effects of polyphenol compounds on lipid peroxidation caused by antipsychotics (haloperidol and amisulpride) in human plasma in vitro. World J Biol Psychiatry. 2010;11(2_2):276–81.
100. Shabalala S, et al. Polyphenols, autophagy and doxorubicin-induced cardiotoxicity. Life Sci. 2017;180:160–70.
101. Kojadinovic MI, et al. Consumption of pomegranate juice decreases blood lipid peroxidation and levels of arachidonic acid in women with metabolic syndrome. J Sci Food Agric. 2017;97(6):1798–804.
102. Letai A, et al. Distinct BH3 domains either sensitize or activate mitochondrial apoptosis, serving as prototype cancer therapeutics. Cancer Cell. 2002;2(3):183–92.
103. Tabit CE, et al. Endothelial dysfunction in diabetes mellitus: molecular mechanisms and clinical implications. Rev Endocr Metab Disord. 2010;11(1):61–74.

104. Keller JN, et al. Mitochondrial manganese superoxide dismutase prevents neural apoptosis and reduces ischemic brain injury: suppression of peroxynitrite production, lipid peroxidation, and mitochondrial dysfunction. J Neurosci. 1998;18(2):687–97.
105. Hakim IA, et al. Effect of increased tea consumption on oxidative DNA damage among smokers: a randomized controlled study. J Nutr. 2003;133(10):3303s–9s.
106. Katiyar SK, Perez A, Mukhtar H. Green tea polyphenol treatment to human skin prevents formation of ultraviolet light B-induced pyrimidine dimers in DNA. Clin Cancer Res. 2000;6(10):3864–9.
107. Nichols JA, Katiyar SK. Skin photoprotection by natural polyphenols: anti-inflammatory, antioxidant and DNA repair mechanisms. Arch Dermatol Res. 2010;302(2):71–83.
108. Srividhya R, et al. Attenuation of senescence-induced oxidative exacerbations in aged rat brain by (−)-epigallocatechin-3-gallate. Int J Dev Neurosci. 2008;26(2):217–23.
109. Senthil Kumaran V, et al. Repletion of antioxidant status by EGCG and retardation of oxidative damage induced macromolecular anomalies in aged rats. Exp Gerontol. 2008;43(3):176–83.
110. Franco AA, Odom RS, Rando TA. Regulation of antioxidant enzyme gene expression in response to oxidative stress and during differentiation of mouse skeletal muscle. Free Radic Biol Med. 1999;27(9):1122–32.
111. Jardim BV, et al. Glutathione and glutathione peroxidase expression in breast cancer: an immunohistochemical and molecular study. Oncol Rep. 2013;30(3):1119–28.
112. Jurkovič S, Osredkar J, Marc J. Molecular impact of glutathione peroxidases in antioxidant processes. Biochem Med. 2008;18(2):162–74.
113. Chada S, Whitney C, Newburger PE. Post-transcriptional regulation of glutathione peroxidase gene expression by selenium in the HL-60 human myeloid cell line. Blood. 1989;74(7):2535–41.
114. Tan M, et al. Transcriptional activation of the human glutathione peroxidase promoter by p53. J Biol Chem. 1999;274(17):12061–6.
115. Liu C-W, et al. Polyphenol-rich longan (Dimocarpus longan Lour.)-flower-water-extract attenuates nonalcoholic fatty liver via decreasing lipid peroxidation and downregulating matrix metalloproteinases-2 and -9. Food Res Int. 2012;45(1):444–9.
116. Hou Z, et al. Mechanism of action of (−)-epigallocatechin-3-gallate: auto-oxidation-dependent inactivation of epidermal growth factor receptor and direct effects on growth inhibition in human esophageal cancer KYSE 150 cells. Cancer Res. 2005;65(17):8049–56.
117. Yang GY, et al. Inhibition of growth and induction of apoptosis in human cancer cell lines by tea polyphenols. Carcinogenesis. 1998;19(4):611–6.
118. Lambert JD, Elias RJ. The antioxidant and pro-oxidant activities of green tea polyphenols: a role in cancer prevention. Arch Biochem Biophys. 2010;501(1):65–72.
119. Yen G-C, Chen H-Y, Peng H-H. Antioxidant and pro-oxidant effects of various tea extracts. J Agric Food Chem. 1997;45(1):30–4.
120. Martin KR, Appel CL. Polyphenols as dietary supplements: a double-edged sword. Nutr Diet Suppl. 2010;2:1–12.
121. Na HK, Surh YJ. Modulation of Nrf2-mediated antioxidant and detoxifying enzyme induction by the green tea polyphenol EGCG. Food Chem Toxicol. 2008;46(4):1271–8.
122. DeNicola GM, et al. Oncogene-induced Nrf2 transcription promotes ROS detoxification and tumorigenesis. Nature. 2011;475(7354):106–9.
123. Jaiswal AK. Nrf2 signaling in coordinated activation of antioxidant gene expression. Free Radic Biol Med. 2004;36(10):1199–207.
124. Kode A, et al. Resveratrol induces glutathione synthesis by activation of Nrf2 and protects against cigarette smoke-mediated oxidative stress in human lung epithelial cells. Am J Phys Lung Cell Mol Phys. 2008;294(3):L478–88.
125. Chow HH, et al. Modulation of human glutathione s-transferases by polyphenon e intervention. Cancer Epidemiol Biomark Prev. 2007;16(8):1662–6.
126. Bonkovsky HL. Hepatotoxicity associated with supplements containing Chinese green tea (Camellia sinensis). Ann Intern Med. 2006;144(1):68–71.

127. Halliwell B. Are polyphenols antioxidants or pro-oxidants? What do we learn from cell culture and in vivo studies? Arch Biochem Biophys. 2008;476(2):107–12.
128. Weisburg JH, et al. In vitro cytotoxicity of epigallocatechin gallate and tea extracts to cancerous and normal cells from the human oral cavity. Basic Clin Pharmacol Toxicol. 2004;95(4):191–200.
129. Galati G, et al. Cellular and in vivo hepatotoxicity caused by green tea phenolic acids and catechins. Free Radic Biol Med. 2006;40(4):570–80.
130. Isbrucker R, et al. Safety studies on epigallocatechin gallate (EGCG) preparations. Part 2: dermal, acute and short-term toxicity studies. Food Chem Toxicol. 2006;44(5):636–50.
131. Dunnick JK, Hailey JR. Toxicity and carcinogenicity studies of quercetin, a natural component of foods. Fundam Appl Toxicol. 1992;19(3):423–31.
132. Ferguson LR. Role of plant polyphenols in genomic stability. Mutat Res. 2001;475(1):89–111.
133. Strick R, et al. Dietary bioflavonoids induce cleavage in the MLL gene and may contribute to infant leukemia. Proc Natl Acad Sci. 2000;97(9):4790–5.
134. Lambert JD, Sang S, Yang CS. Possible controversy over dietary polyphenols: benefits vs risks. Chem Res Toxicol. 2007;20(4):583–5.
135. Williamson MP, et al. Epigallocatechin gallate, the main polyphenol in green tea, binds to the T-cell receptor, CD4: potential for HIV-1 therapy. J Allergy Clin Immunol. 2006;118(6):1369–74.
136. Gehm BD, et al. Resveratrol, a polyphenolic compound found in grapes and wine, is an agonist for the estrogen receptor. Proc Natl Acad Sci. 1997;94(25):14138–43.
137. Williams RJ, Spencer JP, Rice-Evans C. Flavonoids: antioxidants or signalling molecules? Free Radic Biol Med. 2004;36(7):838–49.
138. Kang NJ, et al. Polyphenols as small molecular inhibitors of signaling cascades in carcinogenesis. Pharmacol Ther. 2011;130(3):310–24.
139. Santangelo C, et al. Polyphenols, intracellular signalling and inflammation. Ann Ist Super Sanita. 2007;43(4):394.
140. Crespo I, et al. A comparison of the effects of kaempferol and quercetin on cytokine-induced pro-inflammatory status of cultured human endothelial cells. Br J Nutr. 2008;100(5):968–76.
141. Yu R, et al. Activation of mitogen-activated protein kinases by green tea polyphenols: potential signaling pathways in the regulation of antioxidant-responsive element-mediated phase II enzyme gene expression. Carcinogenesis. 1997;18(2):451–6.
142. Chen C, et al. Activation of antioxidant-response element (ARE), mitogen-activated protein kinases (MAPKs) and caspases by major green tea polyphenol components during cell survival and death. Arch Pharm Res. 2000;23(6):605.
143. Oršolić N, et al. Immunomodulatory and antimetastatic action of propolis and related polyphenolic compounds. J Ethnopharmacol. 2004;94(2):307–15.
144. Gao X, et al. Immunomodulatory activity of resveratrol: suppression of lymphocyte proliferation, development of cell-mediated cytotoxicity, and cytokine production. Biochem Pharmacol. 2001;62(9):1299–308.
145. Haddad JJ. Redox regulation of pro-inflammatory cytokines and IκB-α/NF-κB nuclear translocation and activation. Biochem Biophys Res Commun. 2002;296(4):847–56.
146. Wheeler DS, et al. Epigallocatechin-3-gallate, a green tea-derived polyphenol, inhibits IL-1β-dependent proinflammatory signal transduction in cultured respiratory epithelial cells. J Nutr. 2004;134(5):1039–44.
147. Mackenzie GG, et al. Epicatechin, catechin, and dimeric procyanidins inhibit PMA-induced NF-κB activation at multiple steps in Jurkat T cells. FASEB J. 2004;18(1):167–9.
148. De Stefano D, et al. Lycopene, quercetin and tyrosol prevent macrophage activation induced by gliadin and IFN-γ. Eur J Pharmacol. 2007;566(1):192–9.
149. Ciribilli Y, et al. Decoding c-Myc networks of cell cycle and apoptosis regulated genes in a transgenic mouse model of papillary lung adenocarcinomas. Oncotarget. 2015;6(31):31569–92.
150. Dolezal JM, et al. Sequential adaptive changes in a c-Myc-driven model of hepatocellular carcinoma. J Biol Chem. 2017;292(24):10068–86.

151. Wang H, et al. Coordinated activities of multiple Myc-dependent and Myc-independent biosynthetic pathways in hepatoblastoma. J Biol Chem. 2016;291(51):26241–51.
152. Daniel P, et al. Selective CREB-dependent cyclin expression mediated by the PI3K and MAPK pathways supports glioma cell proliferation. Oncogene. 2014;3:e108.
153. Tulchinsky E. Fos family members: regulation, structure and role in oncogenic transformation. Histol Histopathol. 2000;15(3):921–8.
154. Cho J-W, Lee K-S, Kim C-W. Curcumin attenuates the expression of IL-1β, IL-6, and TNF-α as well as cyclin E in TNF-α-treated HaCaT cells; NF-κB and MAPKs as potential upstream targets. Int J Mol Med. 2007;19(3):469–74.
155. Kim J-E, et al. Cocoa polyphenols suppress TNF-α-induced vascular endothelial growth factor expression by inhibiting phosphoinositide 3-kinase (PI3K) and mitogen-activated protein kinase kinase-1 (MEK1) activities in mouse epidermal cells. Br J Nutr. 2010;104(7):957–64.
156. Siddiqui IA, et al. Modulation of phosphatidylinositol-3-kinase/protein kinase B-and mitogen-activated protein kinase-pathways by tea polyphenols in human prostate cancer cells. J Cell Biochem. 2004;91(2):232–42.
157. Mebratu Y, Tesfaigzi Y. How ERK1/2 activation controls cell proliferation and cell death: is subcellular localization the answer? Cell Cycle. 2009;8(8):1168–75.
158. Lu Z, Xu S. ERK1/2 MAP kinases in cell survival and apoptosis. IUBMB Life. 2006;58(11):621–31.
159. Kushima Y, et al. Inhibitory effect of (−)-epigallocatechin and (−)-epigallocatechin gallate against heregulin β1-induced migration/invasion of the MCF-7 breast carcinoma cell line. Biol Pharm Bull. 2009;32(5):899–904.
160. Wallasch C, et al. Heregulin-dependent regulation of HER2/neu oncogenic signaling by heterodimerization with HER3. EMBO J. 1995;14(17):4267.
161. Stoica GE, et al. Heregulin-b1 regulates the estrogen receptor-a gene expression and activity via the ErbB2/PI 3-K/Akt pathway. Oncogene. 2005;24:1964.
162. Chausovsky A, et al. Molecular requirements for the effect of neuregulin on cell spreading, motility and colony organization. Oncogene. 2000;19(7):878.
163. Golias C, Charalabopoulos A, Charalabopoulos K. Cell proliferation and cell cycle control: a mini review. Int J Clin Pract. 2004;58(12):1134–41.
164. Amararathna M, Johnston MR, Rupasinghe H. Plant polyphenols as chemopreventive agents for lung cancer. Int J Mol Sci. 2016;17(8):1352.
165. Kaur M, et al. Grape seed extract inhibits in vitro and in vivo growth of human colorectal carcinoma cells. Clin Cancer Res. 2006;12(20):6194–202.
166. Shi J, et al. Polyphenolics in grape seeds-biochemistry and functionality. J Med Food. 2003;6(4):291–9.
167. Sherr CJ, Roberts JM. CDK inhibitors: positive and negative regulators of G1-phase progression. Genes Dev. 1999;13(12):1501–12.
168. Chen A, et al. The role of p21 in apoptosis, proliferation, cell cycle arrest, and antioxidant activity in UVB-irradiated human HaCaT keratinocytes. Med Sci Monit Basic Res. 2015;21:86.
169. Nandakumar V, Vaid M, Katiyar SK. (−)-Epigallocatechin-3-gallate reactivates silenced tumor suppressor genes, Cip1/p21 and p 16[INK4a] , by reducing DNA methylation and increasing histones acetylation in human skin cancer cell. Carcinogenesis. 2011;32(4):537–44.
170. Yang J-H, et al. Inhibition of lung cancer cell growth by quercetin glucuronides via G2/M arrest and induction of apoptosis. Drug Metab Dispos. 2006;34(2):296–304.
171. Green DR, Amarante-Mendes GP. The point of no return: mitochondria caspases , and the commitment to cell death. Apoptosis Mech Role Dis. 1998;24:45.
172. Pradhan D, et al. Inhibition of proteasome activity by the dietary flavonoid Quercetin associated with growth inhibition in cultured breast cancer cells and xenografts. J Young Pharm. 2015;7(3):225.
173. Halder B, Das Gupta S, Gomes A. Black tea polyphenols induce human leukemic cell cycle arrest by inhibiting Akt signaling. FEBS J. 2012;279(16):2876–91.

174. Basso AD, et al. Ansamycin antibiotics inhibit Akt activation and cyclin D expression in breast cancer cells that overexpress HER2. Oncogene. 2002;21(8):1159.
175. Colotta F, et al. Cancer-related inflammation, the seventh hallmark of cancer: links to genetic instability. Carcinogenesis. 2009;30:1073.
176. Coussens LM, Werb Z. Inflammation and cancer. Nature. 2002;420:860.
177. Palmisano WA, et al. Predicting lung cancer by detecting aberrant promoter methylation in sputum. Cancer Res. 2000;60(21):5954–8.
178. Gonzalgo ML, et al. Prostate cancer detection by GSTP1 methylation analysis of postbiopsy urine specimens. Clin Cancer Res. 2003;9(7):2673–7.
179. Esteller M, et al. A gene hypermethylation profile of human cancer. Cancer Res. 2001;61(8):3225–9.
180. Tsou JA, et al. DNA methylation analysis: a powerful new tool for lung cancer diagnosis. Oncogene. 2002;21(35):5450.
181. Chiang JW, Karlan BY, Baldwin RL. BRCA1 promoter methylation predicts adverse ovarian cancer prognosis. Gynecol Oncol. 2006;101(3):403–10.
182. Sharma P, et al. The prognostic value of BRCA1 promoter methylation in early stage triple negative breast cancer. J Cancer Ther Res. 2014;3(1):2.
183. Kumar U, Sharma U, Rathi G. Reversal of hypermethylation and reactivation of glutathione S-transferase pi 1 gene by curcumin in breast cancer cell line. Tumor Biol. 2017;39(2):1010428317692258.
184. Thakur VS, et al. Plant phytochemicals as epigenetic modulators: role in cancer chemoprevention. AAPS J. 2014;16(1):151–63.
185. Aggarwal R, et al. Natural compounds: role in reversal of epigenetic changes. Biochem Mosc. 2015;80(8):972–89.
186. Lim SO et al. Epigenetic changes induced by reactive oxygen species in hepatocellular carcinoma: methylation of the E-cadherin promoter. Gastroenterology. 2008;135(6):2128–40, 2140.e1–8.
187. Wu Q, Ni X. ROS-mediated DNA methylation pattern alterations in carcinogenesis. Curr Drug Targets. 2015;16(1):13–9.
188. Pandey M, Shukla S, Gupta S. Promoter demethylation and chromatin remodeling by green tea polyphenols leads to re-expression of GSTP1 in human prostate cancer cells. Int J Cancer. 2010;126(11):2520–33.
189. Fang M, Chen D, Yang CS. Dietary polyphenols may affect DNA methylation. J Nutr. 2007;137(1):223S–8S.
190. Mocanu M-M, Nagy P, Szöllősi J. Chemoprevention of breast cancer by dietary polyphenols. Molecules. 2015;20(12):22578–620.
191. Gomez LS, et al. Resveratrol decreases breast cancer cell viability and glucose metabolism by inhibiting 6-phosphofructo-1-kinase. Biochimie. 2013;95(6):1336–43.
192. Stockert A, et al. Improving the efficacy of cisplatin in colon cancer HT-29 cells via combination therapy with selenium. Austin J Pharmacol Ther. 2014;2(2):6.
193. Zhang Y, et al. Green tea polyphenol EGCG reverse cisplatin resistance of A549/DDP cell line through candidate genes demethylation. Biomed Pharmacother. 2015;69:285–90.
194. Zhang J, et al. Curcumin promotes apoptosis in A549/DDP multidrug-resistant human lung adenocarcinoma cells through an miRNA signaling pathway. Biochem Biophys Res Commun. 2010;399(1):1–6.
195. Shukla S, et al. Curcumin inhibits the activity of ABCG2/BCRP1, a multidrug resistance-linked ABC drug transporter in mice. Pharm Res. 2009;26(2):480–7.
196. Brennemen M, Mahfouz T, Stockert A. Cooperative binding of cinnamon polyphenols as activators of Sirtuin-1 protein in the insulin signaling pathway. FASEB J. 2017;31(1 Supplement):761.25.

Natural Products and Their Benefits in Cancer Prevention

Nejib Guizani, Mostafa I. Waly, Mohammad Shafiur Rahman, and Zaher Al-Attabi

1 Introduction

The search for new sources of natural antioxidants from plant material may have beneficial therapeutic potential for those diseases associated with oxidative stress, including cancer. Natural products are rich in flavonoids, phenolic, alkaloids carotenoids, and organosulfur compounds, these bioactive components are known to combat oxidative stress-mediated diseases pathogenesis, including cancer. A novel approach for preventing cancer is chemoprevention using natural products for suppression, prevention, or reversion premalignancy before the induction of aggressive cancer. Natural products are fruits, vegetables, grains, spices, nuts, herbs, and medicinal plants. During the last few decades, it was found that cancer risk is decreased by having a diet rich in fruits, vegetables, green tea, and legumes and has led research to discover many plant constituents specially phytochemicals that might help in the protection against oxidative stress and blocking specific carcinogenic pathways.

Oxidative stress has been reported to be a major risk factor for cancer, and antioxidants have proved to possess cytotoxic potential effect in various cancer models, in vitro and in vivo. Although there are hundreds of synthetic chemicals that are currently used as a cancer chemotherapeutic agents, yet they have side effects to the normal cells. Therefore, it is essential to search for natural products that have antioxidants and anticancer properties. Natural plants contain phytochemicals that effectively inhibit cancer proliferation by scavenging free radicals, inhibit oxidative stress and thereby extending protective effects against cancer.

N. Guizani (✉) · M. I. Waly · M. S. Rahman · Z. Al-Attabi
Department of Food Science and Nutrition, College of Agricultural and Marine Sciences, Sultan Qaboos University, Muscat, Oman
e-mail: guizani@squ.edu.om

© Springer International Publishing AG, part of Springer Nature 2018
M. I. Waly, M. S. Rahman (eds.), *Bioactive Components, Diet and Medical Treatment in Cancer Prevention*, https://doi.org/10.1007/978-3-319-75693-6_3

In recent years the complementary and alternative medicine have gained greater emphasis; there are at least 1000 indigenous plants that possess medicinal properties for treating chronic human diseases, including cancer. These plants have the ability to prevent the risk of developing various forms of cancer and cancer treatment by modifying tumor behavior. Medicinal plants are important elements of indigenous medical system that have persisted in developing countries. Many of the botanical chemopreventions are currently used as potent anticancer agents; this chapter aims to present the antioxidant properties and chemopreventive effect of a wide variety of natural plants. The chapter summarizes the anticancer effects of phytochemicals as it exhibits in vitro and in vivo anti-proliferation, anti-metastasis, antiangiogenesis, anti-multidrug resistance, and autophagy regulation actions.

2 Antioxidant Properties of Natural Plants

Human used a wide variety of plants as treatment approximately 60,000 years ago [1]. Several scientific evidence have proven that oxidative stress induces the formation of lipid peroxides and other reactive oxygen species that play an important role in cancer pathogenesis [2]. Products of lipid peroxides result in the formation of highly reactive products such as malondialdehyde, which can bind to cellular proteins leading to pleiotropic effects and mutagenicity [3]. Several clinical studies suggested that various natural products are rich in phytochemicals and protect against oxidative stress insults and carcinogenesis [4, 5]. Phytochemicals are bioactive compounds present in plants where they are produced as secondary metabolites to protect themselves from several pathogenic agents. Most bioactive phytochemicals belong to one of five groups: polyphenols, carotenoids, alkaloids, nitrogen-containing compounds, and organosulfur compounds [6].

Oxidative stress insults increased oxidation of thiol (sulfhydryl) groups of different proteins, and subsequent proteins modification and inhibition of cellular antioxidant enzymes [7]. Serum thiol groups, including glutathione, are often diminished in subjects with different types of cancers [8, 9]. A large number of experimental and epidemiological studies have indicated that the reactive oxygen species contribute to organ injury in many systems [10]. As a consequence, different types of molecules, such as proteins, lipids, and nucleic acids, can be damaged, resulting in severe metabolic dysfunction, including lipid peroxidation, protein oxidation, membrane disruption, and DNA damage [11].

Plant products like vegetables, fruits, flowers, and grains are potential source of natural antioxidants and other phytochemicals [12]. The majority of antioxidants are phenolic compounds [13]. These antioxidants differ in structure like the number of phenolic hydroxyl groups and their location, causing difference in their antioxidative ability [14]. Antioxidants are capable to scavenge the free radicals causing reduction in oxidative stress caused by photons and oxygen [15]. Accordingly, they are responsible for the potent of antioxidant action of plants which are essential for optimal well-being [16].

Antioxidants act as the first line of defense against oxidative stress by inhibiting the formation of reactive nitrogen and oxygen species and prevent damage to biologically essential molecules like protein, DNA, and lipid [17]. Phytonutrients such as phenolic acids and flavonoids consider antioxidant and anti-inflammatory properties which can decrease the inflammatory process associated with chronic conditions like cancer [18]. Phenolic compounds are responsible for significant mechanisms of actions including scavenging of free radicals, blocking reactive oxygen species production, detoxifying enzymes, impacting cell cycle, suppression of tumors, apoptosis, modulation of signal transduction and metabolism [19]. There is strong scientific evidence for the protective effect of dietary intake of natural products and medicinal plants against human chronic diseases, including cancer [20]. Natural plants are rich in bioactive ingredients and are considered as the most widespread form of medication for a multitude of health problems in populations throughout the world [21]. These protective effects with potential health benefits are mainly due to the presence of phytochemicals [22]. Molecular mechanism-based cancer chemoprevention by phytochemicals seems to be vital in delaying or preventing the incidence of cancer [23].

3 Anticancer Properties of Selected Natural Products

Acridocarpus orientalis plant showed potential antioxidant activities [24]. Numerous studies have shown that *Allium cepa* or onion has sulfur-containing amino acid, S-methyl cysteine sulphoxide, which is shown to prompt powerful antioxidant activity. Studies indicated that this plant is rich in a constituent called diallyl trisulfide that inhibits growth of cultured human prostate cancer cells in association with apoptosis induction [25]. In cultured human prostate cancer cells, diallyl trisulfide treatment has been shown to cause cell cycle arrest, apoptosis induction, and transcriptional repression of androgen receptor. Furthermore, diallyl trisulfide treatment inhibited angiogenesis in human umbilical vein endothelial cells. Studies have provided novel insights into the molecular circuitry of apoptotic cell death resulting from diallyl trisulfide exposure in human prostate cancer cells [26–28].

Caralluma tuberculata possesses moderate cytotoxic activity on breast cancer and other cancer cells in vitro, which may indicate a source of activity in vivo of interest to future drug design [29]. *Caralluma* species are natural sources of a wide variety of pregnane glycosides, which induce caspase-dependent apoptosis in cancer cells [30, 31].

Carica papaya L. is a potent antioxidant and has an in vitro and in vivo protective effect against oxidizing agent in cancer experimental models [26, 27, 32]. Papaya peel extract is rich in phenolic contents that combat oxidative stress by increasing antioxidant enzymatic activities that are impaired during cancer pathogenesis [33, 34].

Curcuma longa plant has been commonly perceived in decreasing lipid peroxides and free radicals attack in cancer models [35]. In human cancer cell lines, curcumin has been shown to decrease ornithine decarboxylase activity, a rate-limiting enzyme in polyamine biosynthesis that is frequently upregulated in cancer and other rapidly proliferating tissues. Numerous studies have demonstrated that pre-treatment with curcumin can abrogate carcinogen-induced tumorigenesis in different models and organs [36]. The cell proliferation assay indicated that extracts from the *Curcuma longa* exerted anti-proliferative activity in cancer cells, the molecular mechanisms underlying this protective effect is that certain pro-apoptotic molecules, including caspase-3, checkpoint kinase 2, and tumor protein 53, exhibited increased activity in cancer cells, but when treated with the *Curcuma longa* extract, the cells exhibited an opposite effect [26, 27].

Dodonaea viscosa shows high free radical scavenging activity [37]. They are rich in naturally derived triterpenoid saponins (ginsenosides and saikosaponins) and steroid saponins (dioscin, polyphyllin, and timosaponin) that demonstrate various pharmacological effects against mammalian diseases [38].

Haplophyllum tuberculatum contains phenolic compounds as main phytochemicals which exhibit antioxidant potential properties [39]. In cancer cell line, CCRF-CEM, it has cytotoxic effects in a mechanisms involved cell cycle distribution, apoptosis, caspases activities and mitochondrial function [40].

Momordica charantia is rich in polyphenols and carotenoids and exhibits a wide range of biological effects, including anti-inflammatory, antiaging, anti-atherosclerosis, and anticancer [38]. It showed powerful DPPH radical scavenging activity comparing to vitamin E; it also exhibited enhanced iron chelating activity than vitamin E, but they were weaker than vitamin E in free radical scavenging, xanthine oxidase inhibitory, and anti-lipid peroxidation activities [41]. Some studies have reported that oral administration of the *Momordica charantia* juice or seed powder showed a significant reduction in oxidative stress [42].

Moringa oleifera trees grow well in Jamaica and their parts are popularly used locally for various purposes and ailments. Antioxidant activities in *Moringa oleifera* samples from different parts of the world have different ranges [43]. Extracts from the *Moringa oleifera* leaves, root core, and outer parts have protective activity against hepatocarcinoma and breast and colorectal cancer cell lines, as all extracts kill the different cancer cells with different ratios, suggesting its therapeutic use as a natural source of anticancer compounds [44, 45].

Moringa peregrine reduced radicals significantly and showed strong antioxidant activity; it is a tropical tree growing in southeast of Iran. All parts of this plant have nutritional uses and pharmacological activities [46]. All Moringa leaf and seed extracts showed pronounced antioxidant activities in a dose-dependent manner and the effects depend strongly on the solvent used for extraction. Extracts of both leaves and seeds of Moringa exhibit antioxidant potential by combating superoxide anion radicals suggesting that *M. peregrina* is a promising plant with antioxiant therapeutic effect [47, 48].

Oxalis corniculata is an important herbaceous and subtropical plant from the genus *Oxalis*, and has a therapeutic effect and medicinal uses like treatment for cancer [49]; this is based on the antioxidant properties of active compounds such as vitamin C, isoorientin, isovitexin, and swertisin [50]. Phytochemical studies of

Oxalis corniculata have shown the presence of a combination of oleic, linoleic, linolenic, stearic acids, palmitic acid, and tannins [51].

Phyllanthus emblica L. exhibited inhibitory activities against melanogenesis in a mechanism involving selective cytotoxicity to cancer cells with no or low toxicity to the normal wild-type cells [52]. Every part of this plant possesses high medicinal value, where the polyphenols found in *E. officinalis*, especially tannins and flavonoids, are key responsible elements for major bioactivities and pharmacological activities through various mode of actions including antioxidant, anticancer, and cytoprotective properties [53, 54].

Portulaca oleracea provides the basis for the therapeutic importance of studied plants as inhibitors of oxidative stress and antitumor cell proliferation based on its high content of bioactive compounds such as cinnamic acids, caffeic acid, alkaloids, cardiac glycosides, coumarins, flavonoids, glycosides, alanine, saponins, anthraquinone, catechol, and tannins [55, 56]. *P. oleracea* extract inhibits the growth of colon cancer stem cells and it may elicit its effects through regulatory and target genes that mediate the tumor formation in colon cancer stem cells [57].

Prosopis cineraria extract produced an increase in nonenzymatic antioxidants and enzymatic antioxidants [58]. This plant has potency to scavenge the cellular free radicals, mainly hydrogen peroxide, and the results showed that this plant extract had the maximum efficacy to inhibit lipid peroxidation and DNA damage and was found to be potent and possessed significant cytotoxicity towards Ehrlich ascites carcinoma tumor model [59].

Punica granatum peel extract protects against cancer diseases by combating reactive oxygen species generation in experimental cancer model [60]. Pomegranate (*Punica granatum*) is rich in polyphenols, particularly anthocyanins and tannins which have antagonistic interactions against cancer and used in dietary-based cancer chemoprevention and treatment.

Rubus occidentalis has a wide variety of polyphenolics, ellagic acid, sanguiin H-6, and flavonol derivatives with different phytonutrient profiles [61]. Numerous in vitro studies have confirmed the activity of this fruit extract against certain types of human cancers [62]. Bioactive compounds of berry have significant anticancer effects through various complementary mechanisms of action including the induction of metabolizing enzymes, modulation of gene expression, and their effects on cell proliferation, apoptosis, and subcellular signaling pathway [63]. In vitro evidence from different cancer models suggested that berry polyphenols may modulate cellular processes essential for cancer cell survival, such as proliferation and apoptosis [64].

Teucrium stocksianum is a natural herbicide with a strong antioxidant activity and high total phenolic content, and cytotoxicity and phytotoxicity assays indicated that it is rich in saponins, n-hexane, and chloroform fractions that might play a vital role in the treatment of neoplasia [65]. The plant extract also displayed marked phytochemical and antioxidant activity and produce substantial number of antioxidant potential properties [66]. Phytochemical composition of this plant are flavonoids, tannins, saponins, anthraquinone, steroid, phlobatannin, terpenoid, glycoside, and reducing sugars which collectively have free radical scavenging properties against oxidative stress-mediated carcinogenesis [67].

Vaccinium myrtillus exhibited significant antioxidant capacity and is commonly used as an ingredient for the design of new food products or food supplements; it is rich in phenolic compounds such as anthocyanins from blueberry [68]. Several research studies indicate that this fruit is rich in bioactive compounds, including flavonoids, anthocyanin, β-carotenoids, vitamins, and phenolic acids, which protect DNA, and thus it has a therapeutic effectiveness during chemotherapy [69–71].

Zingiber officinale extract administration in animal cancer experimental studies had significantly reduced oxidative stress-induced cancer models [72]. The anticancer properties were ascribed to the free radical scavenging activity of *Z. officinale* and thereby combating oxidative stress-mediated carcinogenesis [73]. In silico investigation demonstrated that the synergetic effects of β-phellandrene with other compounds in *Z. officinale* might be responsible for its anticancerous activity [73].

Zizyphus spina-christi is a rich source of bioactive compounds with medicinal properties in chemoprevention of cancer by ameliorating the intracellular glutathione depletion as well as abrogating pro-apoptotic events associated with cancer [74]. The anticancer effect of *Ziziphus spina-christi* on breast cancer cells was investigated, and providing a scientific basis for its utility in traditional medicine [75]. The cytotoxic activity of *Z. spina-christi* extracts against the early stage of carcinogenesis in tumor cell lines is by preventing oxidative stress, and it can be concluded that *Z. spina-christi* is a good candidate for new cytotoxic chemopreventive agents [76].

4 Conclusion

Phytochemicals containing foods cause a decline in the risk of different types of cancers, and gained considerable recognition as a functional food in the modern era. Experimental studies and human clinical trials illustrated that natural products are rich in polyphenols isoflavones, flavanoid, catechins, carotenoids, and many other constituents that help in protecting against the deleterious impact of reactive oxygen species and its associated carcinogenesis. High intake of natural products counteract the oxidative stress-mediated carcinogenesis, and hence represent a therapeutic effectiveness during chemotherapy of cancer patients as supported by results of case-control studies. Natural products supplements in the diet represent a section of whole health program, along with an increased intake of vegetables and hence to help in the primary prevention of cancer initiation.

References

1. Sheikh BY, Sarker MMR, Kamarudin MNA, Ismail A. Prophetic medicine as potential functional food elements in the intervention of cancer: a review. Biomed Pharmacother. 2017;95:614–48. https://doi.org/10.1016/j.biopha.2017.08.043.
2. Tapsell LC, Hemphill I, Cobiac L, Patch CS, Sullivan DR, Fenech M, Roodenrys S, Keogh JB, Clifton PM, Williams PG, Fazio VA, Inge KE. Health benefits of herbs and spices: the past, the present, the future. Med J Aust. 2006;185(4 Suppl):S4–24.
3. Eoff RL, Stafford JB, Szekely J, Rizzo CJ, Egli M, Guengerich FP, Marnett LJ. Structural and functional analysis of Sulfolobus solfataricus Y-family DNA polymerase Dpo4-catalyzed bypass of the malondialdehyde-deoxyguanosine adduct. Biochemistry. 2009;48(30):7079–88.
4. Russnes KM, Möller E, Wilson KM, Carlsen M, Blomhoff R, Smeland S, Adami HO, Grönberg H, Mucci LA, Bälter K. Total antioxidant intake and prostate cancer in the Cancer of the Prostate in Sweden (CAPS) study. A case control study. BMC Cancer. 2016;16:438. https://doi.org/10.1186/s12885-016-2486-8.
5. Waly MI, Al-Rawahi AS, Al Riyami M, Al-Kindi MA, Al-Issaei HK, Farooq SA, Al-Alawi A, Rahman MS. Amelioration of azoxymethane induced-carcinogenesis by reducing oxidative stress in rat colon by natural extracts. BMC Complement Altern Med. 2014a;14:60. https://doi.org/10.1186/1472-6882-14-60.
6. Rizwanullah M, Amin S, Mir SR, Fakhri KU, MMA R. Phytochemical based nanomedicines against cancer: current status and future prospects. J Drug Target. 2017;December:1–22. https://doi.org/10.1080/1061186X.2017.1408115.
7. Dunning S, Ur Rehman A, Tiebosch MH, Hannivoort RA, Haijer FW, Woudenberg J, van den Heuvel FA, Buist-Homan M, Faber KN, Moshage H. Glutathione and antioxidant enzymes serve complementary roles in protecting activated hepatic stellate cells against hydrogen peroxide-induced cell death. Biochim Biophys Acta. 2013;1832(12):2027–34. https://doi.org/10.1016/j.bbadis.2013.07.008.
8. Blokhina O, Virolainen E, Fagerstedt KV. Antioxidants, oxidative damage and oxygen deprivation stress: a review. Ann Bot. 2003;91 Spec No: 179-94.
9. Valko M, Rhodes CJ, Moncol J, Izakovic M, Mazur M. Free radicals, metals and antioxidants in oxidative stress-induced cancer. Chem Biol Interact. 2006;160(1):1–40.
10. Jomova K, Valko M. Advances in metal-induced oxidative stress and human disease. Toxicology. 2011;283(2–3):65–87. https://doi.org/10.1016/j.tox.2011.03.001.
11. He L, He T, Farrar S, Ji L, Liu T, Ma X. Antioxidants maintain cellular redox homeostasis by elimination of reactive oxygen species. Cell Physiol Biochem. 2017;44(2):532–53. https://doi.org/10.1159/000485089.
12. Chikara S, Nagaprashantha LD, Singhal J, Horne D, Awasthi S, Singhal SS. Oxidative stress and dietary phytochemicals: role in cancer chemoprevention and treatment. Cancer Lett. 2018;413:122–34. https://doi.org/10.1016/j.canlet.2017.11.002.
13. Shu L, Cheung KL, Khor TO, Chen C, Kong AN. Phytochemicals: cancer chemoprevention and suppression of tumor onset and metastasis. Cancer Metastasis Rev. 2010;29(3):483–502. https://doi.org/10.1007/s10555-010-9239-y.
14. Thakur VS, Deb G, Babcook MA, Gupta S. Plant phytochemicals as epigenetic modulators: role in cancer chemoprevention. AAPS J. 2014;16(1):151–63. https://doi.org/10.1208/s12248-013-9548-5.
15. Shankar E, Kanwal R, Candamo M, Gupta S. Dietary phytochemicals as epigenetic modifiers in cancer: promise and challenges. Semin Cancer Biol. 2016 Oct;40–41:82–99. https://doi.org/10.1016/j.semcancer.2016.04.002.
16. Shukla S, Meeran SM, Katiyar SK. Epigenetic regulation by selected dietary phytochemicals in cancer chemoprevention. Cancer Lett. 2014;355(1):9–17. https://doi.org/10.1016/j.canlet.2014.09.017.

17. Tan AC, Konczak I, Sze DM, Ramzan I. Molecular pathways for cancer chemoprevention by dietary phytochemicals. Nutr Cancer. 2011;63(4):495–505. https://doi.org/10.1080/01635581 .2011.538953.
18. Surh YJ, Kundu JK, Na HK, Lee JS. Redox-sensitive transcription factors as prime targets for chemoprevention with anti-inflammatory and antioxidative phytochemicals. J Nutr. 2005;135(12 Suppl):2993S–3001S.
19. Surh YJ. NF-kappa B and Nrf2 as potential chemopreventive targets of some anti-inflammatory and antioxidative phytonutrients with anti-inflammatory and antioxidative activities. Asia Pac J Clin Nutr. 2008;17(Suppl 1):269–72.
20. Xing C, Johnson TE, Limburg PJ. Diets, phytochemicals, and chemoprevention of tumorigenesis. J Diet Suppl. 2008;5(2):95–105. https://doi.org/10.1080/19390210802332877.
21. Saunders FR, Wallace HM. On the natural chemoprevention of cancer. Plant Physiol Biochem. 2010;48(7):621–6. https://doi.org/10.1016/j.plaphy.2010.03.001.
22. Nishino H, Satomi Y, Tokuda H, Masuda M. Cancer control by phytochemicals. Curr Pharm Des. 2007;13(33):3394–9.
23. Priyadarsini RV, Nagini S. Cancer chemoprevention by dietary phytochemicals: promises and pitfalls. Curr Pharm Biotechnol. 2012;13(1):125–36.
24. Ksiksi T, Hamza AA. Antioxidant, lipoxygenase and histone deacetylase inhibitory activities of Acridocarbus orientalis from Al Ain and Oman. Molecules. 2012;17(11):12521–32. https://doi.org/10.3390/molecules171112521.
25. Hussain J, Ali L, Khan AL, Rehman NU, Jabeen F, Kim JS, Al-Harrasi A. Isolation and bio-activities of the flavonoids morin and morin-3-O-β-D-glucopyranoside from Acridocarpus orientalis—a wild Arabian medicinal plant. Molecules. 2014;19(11):17763–72. https://doi.org/10.3390/molecules191117763.
26. Wang HC, Chu YL, Hsieh SC, Sheen LY. Diallyl trisulfide inhibits cell migration and invasion of human melanoma a375 cells via inhibiting integrin/facal adhesion kinase pathway. Environ Toxicol. 2017a;32(11):2352–9. https://doi.org/10.1002/tox.22445.
27. Wang Y, Li J, Guo J, Wang Q, Zhu S, Gao S, Yang C, Wei M, Pan X, Zhu W, Ding D, Gao R, Zhang W, Wang J, Zang L. Cytotoxic and antitumor effects of Curzerene from Curcuma longa. Planta Med. 2017b;83(1–02):23–9. https://doi.org/10.1055/s-0042-107083.
28. Wen SY, Tsai CY, Pai PY, Chen YW, Yang YC, Aneja R, Huang CY, Kuo WW. Diallyl trisulfide suppresses doxorubicin-induced cardiomyocyte apoptosis by inhibiting MAPK/NF-κB signaling through attenuation of ROS generation. Environ Toxicol. 2018;33(1):93–103. https://doi.org/10.1002/tox.22500.
29. Waheed A, Barker J, Barton SJ, Khan GM, Najm-Us-Saqib Q, Hussain M, Ahmed S, Owen C, Carew MA. Novel acylated steroidal glycosides from Caralluma tuberculata induce caspase-dependent apoptosis in cancer cells. J Ethnopharmacol. 2011;137(3):1189–96. https://doi.org/10.1016/j.jep.2011.07.049.
30. Abdallah HM, Osman AM, Almehdar H, Abdel-Sattar E. Acylated pregnane glycosides from Caralluma quadrangula. Phytochemistry. 2013;88:54–60. https://doi.org/10.1016/j.phytochem.2012.12.005.
31. Al-Massarani SM, Bertrand S, Nievergelt A, El-Shafae AM, Al-Howiriny TA, Al-Musayeib NM, Cuendet M, Acylated WJL. pregnane glycosides from Caralluma sinaica. Phytochemistry. 2012;79:129–40. https://doi.org/10.1016/j.phytochem.2012.04.003.
32. Siddique S, Nawaz S, Muhammad F, Akhtar B, Aslam B. Phytochemical screening and in-vitro evaluation of pharmacological activities of peels of Musa sapientum and Carica papaya fruit. Nat Prod Res. 2017:1–4. https://doi.org/10.1080/14786419.2017.1342089.
33. Rivera-Pastrana DM, Gardea AA, Yahia EM, Martínez-Téllez MA, González-Aguilar GA. Effect of UV-C irradiation and low temperature storage on bioactive compounds, antioxidant enzymes and radical scavenging activity of papaya fruit. J Food Sci Technol. 2014a;51(12):3821–9. https://doi.org/10.1007/s13197-013-0942-x.

34. Oboh G, Olabiyi AA, Akinyemi AJ. Inhibitory effect of aqueous extract of different parts of unripe pawpaw (Carica papaya) fruit on Fe^{2+}-induced oxidative stress in rat pancreas in vitro. Pharm Biol. 2013a;51(9):1165–74. https://doi.org/10.3109/13880209.2013.782321.

35. Murray-Stewart T, Casero RA. Regulation of polyamine metabolism by curcumin for cancer prevention and therapy. Med Sci (Basel). 2017;5(4). https://doi.org/10.3390/medsci5040038.

36. Lopes-Rodrigues V, Oliveira A, Correia-da-Silva M, Pinto M, Lima RT, Sousa E, Vasconcelos MH. A novel curcumin derivative which inhibits P-glycoprotein, arrests cell cycle and induces apoptosis in multidrug resistance cells. Bioorg Med Chem. 2017;25(2):581–96. https://doi.org/10.1016/j.bmc.2016.11.023.

37. Cao S, Brodie P, Callmander M, Randrianaivo R, Razafitsalama J, Rakotobe E, Rasamison VE, TenDyke K, Shen Y, Suh EM, Kingston DG. Antiproliferative triterpenoid saponins of Dodonaea viscosa from the Madagascar dry forest. J Nat Prod. 2009;72(9):1705–7. https://doi.org/10.1021/np900293x.

38. Xu DP, Li Y, Meng X, Zhou T, Zhou Y, Zheng J, Zhang JJ, Li HB. Natural antioxidants in foods and medicinal plants: extraction, assessment and resources. Int J Mol Sci. 2017;18(1). https://doi.org/10.3390/ijms18010096.

39. Eissa TF, González-Burgos E, Carretero ME, Gómez-Serranillos MP. Biological activity of HPLC-characterized ethanol extract from the aerial parts of Haplophyllum tuberculatum. Pharm Biol. 2014;52(2):151–6. https://doi.org/10.3109/13880209.2013.819517.

40. Kuete V, Wiench B, Alsaid MS, Alyahya MA, Fankam AG, Shahat AA, Efferth T. Cytotoxicity, mode of action and antibacterial activities of selected Saudi Arabian medicinal plants. BMC Complement Altern Med. 2013;13:354. https://doi.org/10.1186/1472-6882-13-354.

41. Ali MM, Borai IH, Ghanem HM, Abdel-Halim AH, Mousa FM. The prophylactic and therapeutic effects of Momordica charantia methanol extract through controlling different hallmarks of the hepatocarcinogenesis. Biomed Pharmacother. 2017;98:491–8. https://doi.org/10.1016/j.biopha.2017.12.096.

42. Jia S, Shen M, Zhang F, Xie J. Recent advances in Momordica charantia: functional components and biological activities. Int J Mol Sci. 2017;18(12). https://doi.org/10.3390/ijms18122555.

43. Vergara-Jimenez M, Almatrafi MM, Fernandez ML. Bioactive components in Moringa oleifera leaves protect against chronic disease. Antioxidants (Basel). 2017;6(4). https://doi.org/10.3390/antiox6040091.

44. Rehana D, Mahendiran D, Kumar RS, Rahiman AK. Evaluation of antioxidant and anticancer activity of copper oxide nanoparticles synthesized using medicinally important plant extracts. Biomed Pharmacother. 2017;89:1067–77. https://doi.org/10.1016/j.biopha.2017.02.101.

45. Wright RJ, Lee KS, Hyacinth HI, Hibbert JM, Reid ME, Wheatley AO, Asemota HN. An investigation of the antioxidant capacity in extracts from Moringa oleifera plants grown in Jamaica. Plants (Basel). 2017;6(4). https://doi.org/10.3390/plants6040048.

46. Safaeian L, Asghari G, Javanmard SH, Heidarinejad A. The effect of hydroalcoholic extract from the leaves of Moringa peregrina (Forssk.) Fiori. on blood pressure and oxidative status in dexamethasone-induced hypertensive rats. Adv Biomed Res. 2015;4:101. https://doi.org/10.4103/2277-9175.156681.

47. Al-Dabbas MM. Antioxidant activity of different extracts from the aerial part of Moringa peregrina (Forssk.) Fiori, from Jordan. Pak J Pharm Sci. 2017;30(6):2151–7.

48. Dehshahri S, Wink M, Afsharypuor S, Asghari G, Mohagheghzadeh A. Antioxidant activity of methanolic leaf extract of Moringa peregrina (Forssk.) Fiori. Res Pharm Sci. 2012;7(2):111–8.

49. Salahuddin H, Mansoor Q, Batool R, Farooqi AA, Mahmood T, Ismail M. Anticancer activity of cynodon dactylon and oxalis corniculata on Hep2 cell line. Cell Mol Biol (Noisy-le-Grand). 2016;62(5):60–3.

50. Gao Y, Huang R, Gong Y, Park HS, Wen Q, Almosnid NM, Chippada-Venkata UD, Hosain NA, Vick E, Farone A, Altman E. The antidiabetic compound 2-dodecyl-6-methoxycyclohexa-2,5-diene-1,4-dione, isolated from Averrhoa carambola L., demonstrates significant antitumor potential against human breast cancer cells. Oncotarget. 2015;6(27):24304–19.

51. Saghir SA, Sadikun A, Al-Suede FS, Majid AM, Murugaiyah V. Antihyperlipidemic, antioxidant and cytotoxic activities of methanolic and aqueous extracts of different parts of star fruit. Curr Pharm Biotechnol. 2016;17(10):915–25.
52. Zhang J, Miao D, Zhu WF, Xu J, Liu WY, Kitdamrongtham W, Manosroi J, Abe M, Akihisa T, Feng F. Biological activities of phenolics from the fruits of Phyllanthus emblica L. (Euphorbiaceae). Chem Biodivers. 2017;14(12). https://doi.org/10.1002/cbdv.201700404.
53. Guo XH, Ni J, Xue JL, Wang X. Phyllanthus emblica Linn. fruit extract potentiates the anticancer efficacy of mitomycin C and cisplatin and reduces their genotoxicity to normal cells in vitro. J Zhejiang Univ Sci B. 2017;18(12):1031–45. https://doi.org/10.1631/jzus.B1600542.
54. Zhao T, Sun Q, Marques M, Witcher M. Anticancer properties of Phyllanthus emblica (Indian Gooseberry). Oxidative Med Cell Longev. 2015;2015:950890. https://doi.org/10.1155/2015/950890.
55. Nile SH, Nile AS, Keum YS. Total phenolics, antioxidant, antitumor, and enzyme inhibitory activity of Indian medicinal and aromatic plants extracted with different extraction methods. 3 Biotech. 2017;7(1):76. https://doi.org/10.1007/s13205-017-0706-9.
56. Zhao R, Zhang T, Ma B, Li X. Antitumor activity of Portulaca oleracea L. polysaccharide on HeLa cells through inducing TLR4/NF-κB signaling. Nutr Cancer. 2017;69(1):131–9. https://doi.org/10.1080/01635581.2017.1248294.
57. Jin H, Chen L, Wang S, Chao D. Portulaca oleracea extract can inhibit nodule formation of colon cancer stem cells by regulating gene expression of the notch signal transduction pathway. Tumour Biol. 2017;39(7):1010428317708699. https://doi.org/10.1177/1010428317708699.
58. Jinu U, Gomathi M, Saiqa I, Geetha N, Benelli G, Venkatachalam P. Green engineered biomolecule-capped silver and copper nanohybrids using Prosopis cineraria leaf extract: enhanced antibacterial activity against microbial pathogens of public health relevance and cytotoxicity on human breast cancer cells (MCF-7). Microb Pathog. 2017;105:86–95. https://doi.org/10.1016/j.micpath.2017.02.019.
59. Robertson S, Narayanan N, Raj Kapoor B. Antitumour activity of Prosopis cineraria (L.) Druce against Ehrlich ascites carcinoma-induced mice. Nat Prod Res. 2011;25(8):857–62. https://doi.org/10.1080/14786419.2010.536159.
60. Waly MI, Ali A, Guizani N, Al-Rawahi AS, Farooq SA, Rahman MS. Pomegranate (Punica granatum) peel extract efficacy as a dietary antioxidant against azoxymethane-induced colon cancer in rat. Asian Pac J Cancer Prev. 2012;13(8):4051–5.
61. George BP, Abrahamse H, Hemmaragala NM. Anticancer effects elicited by combination of Rubus extract with phthalocyanine photosensitiser on MCF-7 human breast cancer cells. Photodiagn Photodyn Ther. 2017;19:266–73. https://doi.org/10.1016/j.pdpdt.2017.06.014.
62. Grochowski DM, Paduch R, Wiater A, Dudek A, Pleszczyńska M, Tomczykowa M, Granica S, Polak P, Tomczyk M. In vitro antiproliferative and antioxidant effects of extracts from Rubus caesius leaves and their quality evaluation. Evid Based Complement Alternat Med. 2016;2016:5698685. https://doi.org/10.1155/2016/5698685.
63. Kula M, Krauze-Baranowska M. Rubus occidentalis: the black raspberry its potential in the prevention of cancer. Nutr Cancer. 2016;68(1):18–28. https://doi.org/10.1080/01635581.2016.1115095.
64. Kaume L, Howard LR, Devareddy L. The blackberry fruit: a review on its composition and chemistry, metabolism and bioavailability, and health benefits. J Agric Food Chem. 2012;60(23):5716–27. https://doi.org/10.1021/jf203318p.
65. Shah SM, Sadiq A, Shah SM, Khan S. Extraction of saponins and toxicological profile of Teucrium stocksianum boiss extracts collected from District Swat, Pakistan. Biol Res. 2014;47:65. https://doi.org/10.1186/0717-6287-47-65.
66. Shah SM, Shah SM. Phytochemicals, antioxidant, antinociceptive and anti-inflammatory potential of the aqueous extract of Teucrium stocksianum bioss. BMC Complement Altern Med. 2015;15:351. https://doi.org/10.1186/s12906-015-0872-4.
67. Shah SM, Ullah F, Shah SM, Zahoor M, Sadiq A. Analysis of chemical constituents and antinociceptive potential of essential oil of Teucrium Stocksianum bioss collected from

the North West of Pakistan. BMC Complement Altern Med. 2012;12:244. https://doi. org/10.1186/1472-6882-12-244.

68. Dróżdż P, Šěžienė V, Pyrzynska K. Phytochemical properties and antioxidant activities of extracts from wild blueberries and lingonberries. Plant Foods Hum Nutr. 2017;72(4):360–4. https://doi.org/10.1007/s11130-017-0640-3.

69. Alhosin M, León-González AJ, Dandache I, Lelay A, Rashid SK, Kevers C, Pincemail J, Fornecker LM, Mauvieux L, Herbrecht R, Schini-Kerth VB. Bilberry extract (Antho 50) selectively induces redox-sensitive caspase 3-related apoptosis in chronic lymphocytic leuke-mia cells by targeting the Bcl-2/Bad pathway. Sci Rep. 2015;5:8996. https://doi.org/10.1038/srep08996.

70. Esselen M, Fritz J, Hutter M, Teller N, Baechler S, Boettler U, Marczylo TH, Gescher AJ, Marko D. Anthocyanin-rich extracts suppress the DNA-damaging effects of topoisomerase poisons in human colon cancer cells. Mol Nutr Food Res. 2011;55(Suppl 1):S143–53. https://doi.org/10.1002/mnfr.201000315.

71. Hara S, Morita R, Ogawa T, Segawa R, Takimoto N, Suzuki K, Hamadate N, Hayashi SM, Odachi A, Ogiwara I, Shibusawa S, Yoshida T, Shibutani M. Tumor suppression effects of bil-berry extracts and enzymatically modified isoquercitrin in early preneoplastic liver cell lesions induced by piperonyl butoxide promotion in a two-stage rat hepatocarcinogenesis model. Exp Toxicol Pathol. 2014;66(5–6):225–34. https://doi.org/10.1016/j.etp.2014.02.002.

72. Ajith TA, Hema U, Aswathi S. Zingiber officinale Roscoe ameliorates anticancer antibiotic doxorubicin-induced acute cardiotoxicity in rat. J Exp Ther Oncol. 2016;11(3):171–5.

73. Usha T, Pradhan S, Goyal AK, Dhivya S, Kumar HPP, Singh MK, Joshi N, Basistha BC, Murthy KRS, Selvaraj S, Middha SK. Molecular simulation-based combinatorial modeling and antioxidant activities of Zingiberaceae family rhizomes. Pharmacogn Mag. 2017;13(Suppl 3):S715–22. https://doi.org/10.4103/pm.pm_82_17.

74. Guizani N, Waly MI, Singh V, Rahman MS. Nabag (Zizyphus spina-christi) extract prevents aberrant crypt foci development in colons of azoxymethane-treated rats by abrogating oxida-tive stress and inducing apoptosis. Asian Pac J Cancer Prev. 2013;14(9):5031–5.

75. Farmani F, Moein M, Amanzadeh A, Kandelous HM, Ehsanpour Z, Salimi M. Antiproliferative evaluation and apoptosis induction in MCF- 7 cells by Ziziphus spina christi leaf extracts. Asian Pac J Cancer Prev. 2016;17(1):315–21.

76. Jafarian A, Zolfaghari B, Shirani K. Cytotoxicity of different extracts of arial parts of Ziziphus spina-christi on Hela and MDA-MB-468 tumor cells. Adv Biomed Res. 2014;3:38. https://doi. org/10.4103/2277-9175.125727.

Cinnamon as a Cancer Therapeutic Agent

Neeru Bhatt

1 Introduction

Multidisciplinary scientific investigations are continuously making efforts to combat this dreaded disease, but the perfect cure is yet to be brought into world medicine. Many types of cancer treatments are available depending on the type and stage of cancer and preference of the patient. The main types of cancer treatment include surgery, radiation therapy, chemotherapy, immunotherapy, target therapy, hormone therapy, adjuvant therapy, growth signal inhibitors, endogenous angioinhibitors, stem cell therapy, and precision medicine [1]. Each therapy has its own advantages and disadvantages. Some people prefer only one treatment, but most people have a combination of treatments, such as surgery along with chemotherapy and/or radiation therapy. If the disease has become metastasized and the targeted cancer cells are floating around in the bloodstream, multiple strategies should be adopted to get rid of the cancer.

Plant-based drugs were given utmost importance and have been successfully used in cancer treatment from ancient time whether it was Ayurveda, or ancient Chinese medicine, or ancient Egyptian medicine or ancient Greece medicine. In recent years the complementary and alternative medicine has gained greater emphasis to deal with cancer.

There are at least 250,000 species of plants out of which more than 1000 plants have been found to possess a diverse and promising resource for treating chronic human diseases, including cancer, cardiovascular disease, diabetes, and Alzheimer [2–5]. More than 25% of drugs used during the last 20 years are directly derived from plants, while the other 25% are chemically altered natural products [6, 7]. Epidemiological and experimental studies have consistently presented a correlation between regular consumption of fruits and vegetables and prevention of developing lifestyle disorders, such as obesity, diabetes, cardiovascular disorders, and cancer [8, 9]. Phytochemicals,

N. Bhatt (✉)
Global Science Heritage, Toronto, ON, Canada

© Springer International Publishing AG, part of Springer Nature 2018
M. I. Waly, M. S. Rahman (eds.), *Bioactive Components, Diet and Medical Treatment in Cancer Prevention*, https://doi.org/10.1007/978-3-319-75693-6_4

such as polyphenols and flavonoids which are abundant in fruits and vegetables, seem to possess many of the desirable qualities for preventing cancer and could have great potential as chemopreventive and antiproliferative agents [10–14].

A number of studies from all over the world are aiming to culinary herbs and other botanicals as sources of antioxidants and other substances that have anticancer characteristics. These plants may have the ability to prevent the risk of developing various forms of cancer and some can even modify tumor behavior [15]. However, the use of herbal medicine as an anticancer agent requires extensive research and strict criteria for standardization, safety, quality control, toxicity, and clinical trials [16]. A wide variety of plants have proved to possess cytotoxic potential against various cancers in vitro and in vivo. The following are just a few selected examples of the plants with cytotoxic potential: *Curcuma longa, Withania somnifera, Achyranthes aspera, Allium sativum, Annona muricata, Bolbostemma paniculatum, Cannabis sativa, Centaurea ainetensis, Camellia sinensis, Daphne mezereum, Gossypium hirsutum, Hydrocotyle asiatica, Hypericum perforatum, Nervilia fordii, Oroxylum indicum, Picrorrhiza kurroa, Rubia cordifolia, Salvia miltiorrhiza, various Scutellaria species, Silybum marianum, Smilax china, Strychnos nuxvomica, Taraxacum officinale, Zingiber officinale,* etc. Certain plants have shown to possess immunomodulatory effect to kill cancer cells, which include *Tinosporia cordifolia, Apis mellifera, Bidens pilosa, Andrographis paniculata, and Mangifera indica* [17]. Some tetrandrine (from root of *Stephenia tetrandra*), withaferin-A (from *Withania somnifera*), echitamine chloride (from stem bark of *Astonia scholaris*), rohitukine (from *Amoora rohituka*); curcumin (from *Curcuma longa*), and perillyl alcohol and berberine (from *Tinospora cordifolia*) have shown the chemo- and radio-sensitizing activities [18, 19]. To control the harmful side effects of chemo- and radiotherapy, Ayurvedic anticancer medicines can be used as adjuvants to improve the quality of life [20–23].

The Ayurvedic semisolid pharmaceutical preparation *Rasayana avaleha* improves the quality of life, if taken as adjuvant along with chemo- or radiotherapy [23]. Classical Indian Ayurvedic drugs such as *Amritaprasham, Ashwagandha Rasayana, Brahma Rasayana, Chyavanprasha, Narasimha asayana,* and *Triphala Churna* were found to be radio-protective in cancer treatment [24]. Cinnamon is one such natural produce with exceptional culinary, cosmetic, medicinal, and healing properties.

2   Cinnamon as a Cancer Prevention

2.1   Species of Cinnamon

Cinnamon is derived from the Greek word kinnamon that means sweet wood. It belongs to family Lauraceae, many of whose members produce wonderful spices [25, 26]. This genus contains about 250–350 species worldwide, distributed in tropical and subtropical regions of North America, Central America, South America, Southeast Asia, and Australia [27, 28]. Two main varieties of cinnamon are found in nature, one is Ceylon

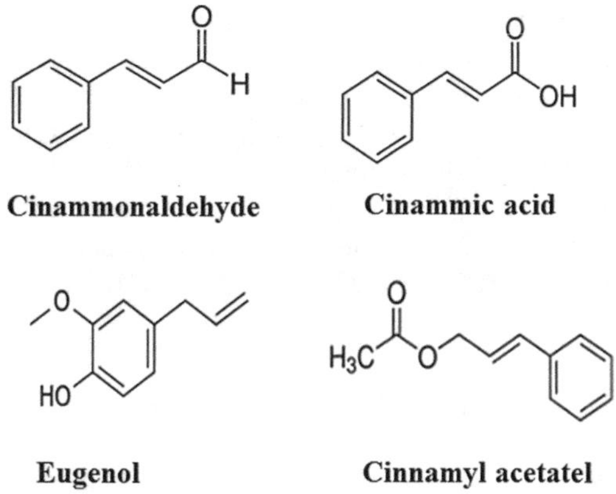

Fig. 1 Chemical
composition of cinnamon

Cinammonaldehyde   **Cinammic acid**

Eugenol   **Cinnamyl acetatel**

or true cinnamon (*Cinnamon zeylanicum* Blume), mostly grown in Sri Lanka and
Southern India, and the other one is cassia (*Cinnamom aromaticum* Ness), grown in
China, Indonesia, and Vietnam. Approximately 21 species of cinnamon have been
recognized in Peninsular Malaysia [29]. Cinnamon is one of the oldest spices known to
the world [30] and is obtained from the inner bark of cinnamon trees. The bark when
dried rolls into a tubular form known as a quill or cinnamon stick [26, 31].

2.2 Chemical and Phytochemical Composition of Cinnamon

Data about proximate composition of cinnamon is scanty, only few studies have been
done in this regard. The moisture content varies from 5.1 to 9.45 mg/100 g depending
on the species. Likewise, crude protein content varied from 3.5 to 5.0, crude fat from
3.5 to 5.0, and ash content from 2.4 to 3.7 mg/100 g. Cinnamon contains crude fiber
as 22.0 to 33.0 mg per 100 g [32, 33] (Fig. 1).

Cinnamon also contains variety of compounds such as mucilage, tannin, sugar, resin,
and essential oil, among which essential oil is the most important constituent [34]. As
cinnamon ages, it darkens in color and the resinous compounds rises [35]. The presence
of a wide range of essential oils, such as *trans*-cinnamaldehyde, cinnamyl acetate,
eugenol, L-borneol, caryophyllene oxide, β-caryophyllene, L-bornyl acetate, E-nerolidol,
α-cubebene, α-terpineol, terpinolene, and α-thujene, has been reported [36, 37].
Cinnamon oil is widely used in the food processing, cosmetic, flavorings, confectionaries,
and pharmaceutical industries [30].

The composition of essential oil varies within plant, viz. in leaves, bark, fruit,
and root. It also varies from species to species and geographical locations. The
essential oils from *Cinnamon cassia* contain 80.90% cinnamaldehyde with little
or no eugenol, while *Cinnamon zeylanicum* contains 60.80% cinnamaldehyde
and approximately 2% eugenol, however, essential oils from its leaves were found
to be rich in eugenol, 70.8% [25]. The principle volatile constituent cinnamaldehyde is responsible for the spicy flavor, aroma, and fragrance of cinnamon [25].

The crude extracts of cinnamon stick also contain high levels of nonvolatile compounds mainly condensed tannins, which consist of 23.2% proanthocyanidins and 3.6% catechins [25].

Cinnamaldehyde is the only unsaturated aldehyde which is approved by the Food and Drug Administration (FDA) (21CFR § 182.60) as seasoning, spice, and flavoring agent and has classified it in the category of foods as "Generally Recognized as Safe (GRAS)" by the "Flavor and Extract Manufacturers Association" (FEMA) in the United States (FEMA no. 2286, 2201) [38].

2.3   Medical Uses of Cinnamon

2.3.1   Cinnamon in Disease and Infection Prevention

Cinnamon is used as a spice in food preparation, both sweet and savory. It has been used in traditional medicine in India, Egypt, and China since ancient times, for various applications such as adenopathy, rheumatism, dermatosis, dyspepsia, stroke, tumors, elephantiasis, trichomonas, yeast, and virus infections [39, 40]. It possesses strong antioxidant, antibacterial, antipyretic, and anti-inflammatory properties, which play an important role in tissue repair [41, 42]. Cinnamon is also used as herbal remedy for the treatment of common colds, cardiovascular diseases, and chronic gastrointestinal and gynecological disorders [43]. Besides, cinnamon is used for treating sore throats, cough, indigestion, abdominal cramps, intestinal spasms, nausea, flatulence, and diarrhea [26]. It has also been found that cinnamon slows down food spoilage and exhibits antifungal properties [44]. Cinnamon is effective for antiulcer, probably by potentiating the defensive factors through the improvement of the circulatory disorder and gastric cytoprotection. Akira et al. [45] found that the intraperitoneal administration of an aqueous extract of cinnamon to rats prevented the occurrence of stress ulcers under exposure to a cold atmosphere 3–5 °C or on restraint in water 22–24 °C.

2.3.2   Cinnamon and Cancer Treatment

Cinnamon extract potently inhibit various tumor cell growths in vitro and suppressed in vivo melanoma progression [16]. Several studies have found that cinnamon extract (CE) displays anticancer activity and inhibits angiogenesis by blocking vascular endothelial growth factor (VEGF) 2 signaling [46, 47]. This may be due to the presence of bioactive and the polyphenolic compounds in cinnamon [43]. The anticancer effect of cinnamaldehyde and eugenol against breast (T47D) and lung (NCI-H322) cancer cell lines was reported by Sharma et al. [46]. Cinnamaldehyde has also been shown to inhibit cyclin-dependent kinases (CDKs), which are involved in cell cycle regulation [48].

Cinnamon extracts can inhibit proliferation of lymphoma, melanoma, hepatocellular cancer, cervix cancer and colon cancer cells in vitro and melanoma in vivo conditions and suppress angiogenesis [5, 26, 47, 49]. A major bioactive compound found in cinnamon, known as 2′-hydroxycinnamicaldehyde (2′-HCA), specifically inhibits the growth of human erythroleukemia or squamous epidermoid carcinoma cells by inducing apoptosis and Pim-1. Pim-1 (proto oncogene) is a kinase that is primarily involved in transcriptional activation and cellular signal transduction pathways related to cell cycle progression and apoptosis [50]. The overexpression of Pim-1 has been observed in many types of cancer, including leukemia, squamous cell carcinoma, prostate cancer, gastric carcinoma, and bladder cancer [51]. 2′-HCA potently suppressed the growth of mouse xenografts representing human leukemia or skin cancer, showing that 2′-HCA as a potent anticancer principle targeting of the Pim-1 kinase [52].

Cinnamon extract plays a therapeutic role in cervical cancer cells by depolarization of the mitochondrial membrane potential, resulting in cellular apoptosis [47]. It also can significantly reduce the migration of cancer cells, indicating its potential use as an anticancer drug in cervical cancer [47]. Cinnamon extract was shown to inhibit the growth of hematologic tumor cells. Moreover, the treatment of melanoma cell lines with CE also induced a decrease in Cox-2 and HIF-1a expression in the tumor tissues that mediate the potent antitumor activity of cinnamon. Both Cox-2 and HIF-1a are established cancer progression regulators and aggravate angiogenesis and metastasis [16]. Cuminaldehyde has the ability to generate vacuolation associated increased volume of the acidic compartment which is further responsible for apoptotic or necrotic cell. Since apoptotic cell death is a well-ordered process, an upregulated volume of acidic compartment may cause the self-digestion during cell death [53].

Cuminaldehyde suppressed the growth of human colorectal COLO 205 cells in a concentration as well as time-dependent manner. It caused apoptotic cell death, by loss of mitochondrial membrane potential, increase of caspase-3 and -9, along with morphological features of apoptosis, including apoptotic body formation, fragmentation, and nuclear condensation as demonstrated in different staining as well as comet assay [54].

Anticancer effect of cinnamon extracts is also associated with modulation of angiogenesis and effector function of CD8+ T cells. In fact, the antitumor effect of cinnamon extracts is linked with their enhanced pro-apoptotic activity by inhibiting the activities of NF-κB and AP1 in mouse melanoma model [16]. The essential oil of cinnamon exhibited significant anticancer activity against HNSCC cells in vitro through suppression of EGFR-TK [55]. Numerous in vitro studies have shown that cinnamon extract exert has an anticancer effect via attenuating NF-kB, AP1 and their target genes such as Bcl-2, BcL-xL and survive and inhibit angiogenesis by blocking vascular endothelial growth factor (VEGF) 2 signaling [5, 56]. The extract of cinnamon exhibits potent antiproliferative effect in vitro and induces active death of tumor cells by upregulating proapoptotic molecules.

Oral administration of cinnamon extracts can suppress azoxymethane-induced colon carcinogenesis in a mouse model [57]. As a matter of fact, the potent antioxidant properties of cinnamon can lessen lipid peroxidation that lead to cancer. According to Schoene et al. [58], the water extract of cinnamon can promote apoptosis of tumor cells and stop the cell cycle at the G1 phase. The extract also inhibits proliferation of HL-60 cells, and it was suggested that the antitumor effect of the extract of cinnamon is associated with the concentration and time of treatment [59]. Furthermore, the water extract of cinnamon also demonstrated antitumor effects in cervical cancer by altering the growth kinetics of the human cervical carcinoma cell line (SiHa cells), and the mechanism may be attributable to the loss of mitochondrial membrane potential, which induced apoptosis, or lower expression of cervical trans-membrane receptor protein Her-2 via inhibition of the metastasis of malignant cells [47].

2.4 Mechanism of Action of Cinnamon Against Cancer

The underlying mechanisms of cinnamon may be responsible for potent anticancerous property. It can be attributed to the antioxidant property, decreased inflammation, antimicrobial, anti-lipid peroxidation, and insulin-potentiating properties. Tumor cells are generally resistant to apoptosis; hence selective killing of tumor cells by promoting apoptosis pathway is an attractive and effective way for development of anticancer agents. Although anticancer drugs may act differently, apoptosis is the most common and preferred mechanism through which many anticancer agents kill and eradicate cancer cells [60].

2.4.1 Antioxidant Property

Many active components of herbs and spices can prevent lipid peroxidation through quenching free radicals or through activation of antioxidant enzymes like superoxide dismutase, catalase, glutathione peroxidase, and glutathione reductase [61]. Oxidative stress initiates numerous disease processes in human body. Under normal metabolic conditions about 2–5% of O2 used up by mitochondria is converted to ROS (reactive oxygen species). ROS along with RNS permanently modify the genetic material leading to numerous degenerative or chronic diseases [62]. RNS are produced from the nitric oxide (NO) and its metabolites.

Cinnamon has been listed as one of the top seven antioxidants in the world with an ORAC value of 267,536 μmol TE/100 g [63]. Cinnamon exhibited higher antioxidant activities compared to the other dessert spices [64]. The antioxidant activities of cinnamon have been elucidated by many scientists and researchers. The aqueous and alcoholic extract (1: 1) of cinnamon significantly inhibits fatty acid oxidation and lipid peroxidation in vitro that leads to cancer [65]. Different flavonoid compounds present in cinnamon have shown free-radical-scavenging activities [66]. Additionally, cinnamaldehyde and other compounds of cinnamon possess potential activity against the production of nitric oxide as well as the expression of inducible nitric oxide. The ethanolic extract of cinnamon exhibited significant inhibition (96.3%) compared to the natural antioxidant α-tocopherol (93.74%) [67].

2.4.2 Anti-inflammatory Activity

Inflammation is a part of body's immune response. It is responsible for pain and chronic diseases such as diabetes, heart diseases, allergies, neurodegenerative diseases, and cancer. Cinnamon has been reported to have anti-inflammatory activity through the potent inhibition of nitric oxide (NO) and cyclooxygenase. One of the most common features of inflammation is increased oxygenation of arachidonic acid, which is metabolized by two enzymic pathways—the cyclooxygenase (CO) and the 5-lipoxygenase (5-LO) leading to the production of prostaglandins and leukotrienes, respectively. Among the CO products, PGE2 and among the 5-LO products, LTB_4 are considered important mediators of inflammation [68]. The ethanolic extract of cinnamon showed significant anti-inflammatory effects by reducing the activation of Src/spleen-tyrosine-kinase- (Src/Syk-) mediated NF-κB [69, 70]. Cinnamon oil significantly inhibits the production of several protein biomarkers that are involved in inflammation and tissue remodeling [71].

2.4.3 Antimicrobial Activity

The antimicrobial activity of cinnamon is primarily due to its essential oil content. Though, the exact antimicrobial action of herbs and spices in vivo conditions is hard to evaluate, because of the very complex and balanced microbial populations in gastrointestinal tract and the interaction of active components from herbs and spices with other nutrients [72]. Cinnamon is a powerful antibacterial and makes a great natural disinfectant. Many gastric ailments such as antral gastritis, duodenal ulcer, and gastric lymphoma are frequently associated with *Helicobacter pylori* infection. So, eradication of *Helicobacter pylori* may be favorable to these diseases. Cinnamon oil has been found by researchers to be one of the most effective inhibitors of *Helicobacter pylori* that facilitate the invasion and progression of cancer. Researchers have also found that cinnamon extract has the ability to kill or inhibit the growth of gram positive as well as gram negative bacteria. Additionally, the methanolic extract of cinnamon bark significantly inhibit the growth of *Aspergillus niger* and *Candida albicans* compared to aqueous and chloroform extracts and was comparable with that of standard drug amphotericin [73]. Aspergillus niger and Candida albicans are fungus and at times can become pathogenic in immunocompromised individuals.

2.4.4 Insulin Potentiating Activity

Compounds found in cinnamon have insulin-potentiating properties and may be involved in the alleviation of the signs and symptoms of diabetes and cardiovascular diseases related to insulin resistance and metabolic syndrome [74]. The aqueous extract of cinnamon increases insulin sensitivity and less insulin is required to have larger insulin effects. It seems that more of the aqueous extract of cinnamon is similar to adding more insulin. People with metabolic syndrome have adequate amounts of insulin but not efficient enough to perform body functions. Studies have suggested that the components of cinnamon make insulin more efficient [75, 76]. Even the aqueous extract of "spent cinnamon" (product that is left when cinnamon oil is removed) has the same in vitro insulin-potentiating activity as extracts from the cinnamon before the cinnamon oil is removed. Cinnamaldehyde has also been observed reducing glucose levels and normalizing responses in circulating blood in animal models [77]. The cinnamic acid improves glucose tolerance and potentially stimulates insulin production [78].

2.5 Toxicity of Overdose

High amount of coumarin present in cinnamon can damage liver tissues although no such report has been published. High levels of coumarin did trigger cancer in experimental rodents [15], though most of the valuable constituents of cinnamon are water-soluble, but certain oil-soluble compounds, particularly the anticoagulant coumarin, are potentially harmful if taken in large quantities. This is why supplemental cinnamon should be taken only as a water-soluble extract.

3 Conclusion

Many diseases, which were a challenge for the mankind and considered incurable, have been successfully treated now, but the absolute and sustainable treatment of cancer has yet to come. A variety of treatments of cancer are available with their merits and demerits. Plant-derived products have always been a part of traditional folk medicine and food additives. Recently their medicinal properties are under extensive investigation and become a major part of complementary and alternative medicines. Plant-based medicines are good as they are green, clean, and safe, and mostly they don't produce any side effect. Cinnamon is an evergreen plant, grown worldwide from Asia to Africa and America to Australia. The inner bark of the plants is known as cinnamon stick and is used as a spice in food preparation, both sweet and savory. It has exceptional culinary and pharmaceutical properties. Cinnamon and its components possess strong antioxidant, antibacterial, antipyretic, and anti-inflammatory properties, which play an important role in tissue repair. Tumor cells are generally resistant to apoptosis; cinnamon can promote apoptosis of tumor cells and stop the cell cycle at the G1 phase. Anticancer effect of cinnamon extract is mediated by apoptosis induction and blockade of NFB and AP1. Hence it can be summarized that cinnamon and its components can be explored to develop potent antitumor drugs for the treatment of diverse cancers.

References

1. Sudhakar A. History of cancer, ancient and modern treatment methods. J Cancer Sci Ther. 2009;1:i–iv.
2. Esmonde L, Long AF. Complementary therapy use by persons with multiple sclerosis: benefits and research priorities. Complement Ther Clin Pract. 2008;14(3):176–84.
3. Längler A, Kaatsch P, Spix C, et al. Complementary and alternative treatment methods in children with cancer. A population based retrospective survey on the prevalence of use in Germany. Eur J Integr Med. 2008;1(Suppl. 1):10–4.
4. Miller JL, Binns HJ, Brickman WJ. Complementary and alternative medicine use in children with type 1 diabetes: a pilot survey of parents. EXPLORE J Sci Healing. 2008;4(5):311–4.
5. Kwon HK, Hwang JS, So JS, et al. Cinnamon extract induces tumor cell death through inhibition of NFkappaB and AP1. BMC Cancer. 2010;10:392.
6. Cravotto G, Boffa L, Genzini L, et al. Phytotherapeutics: an evaluation of the potential of 1000 plants. J Clin Pharm Ther. 2010;35:11–48.
7. Patel B, Das S, Prakash R, et al. Natural bioactive compound with anticancer potential. Int J Adv Pharm Sci. 2010;1:32–41.
8. Block G, Patterson B, Subar A. Fruit, vegetables, and cancer prevention: a review of the epidemiological evidence. Nutr Cancer. 1992;18:1–29.
9. Willett WC. Balancing life-style and genomics research for disease prevention. Science. 2002;296:695–8.

10. Middleton E Jr, Kandaswami C, Theoharides TC. The effects of plant flavonoids on mammalian cells: implications for inflammation, heart disease, and cancer. Pharmacol Rev. 2000;52:673–751.
11. Watson WH, Cai J, Jones DP. Diet and apoptosis. Annu Rev Nutr. 2000;20:485–505.
12. Yang CS, Landau JM, Huang MT, et al. Inhibition of carcinogenesis by dietary polyphenolic compounds. Annu Rev Nutr. 2001;21:381–406.
13. Priyadarsini RV, Nagini S. Cancer chemoprevention by dietary phytochemicals: promises and pitfalls. Curr Pharm Biotechnol. 2012;13:125–36.
14. Shukla S, Meeran SM, Katiyar SK. Epigenetic regulation by selected dietary phytochemicals in cancer chemoprevention. Cancer Lett. 2014;355:9–17.
15. Umadevi M, Kumar KPS, Bhowmik D. Traditionally used anticancer herbs in India. J Med Plants Stud. 2013;1(3):56–72.
16. Kwon H, Jeon WK, Hwang J, et al. Cinnamon extract suppresses tumor progression by modulating angiogenesis and the effecter function of CD8þ T cells. Cancer Lett. 2009;278:174–82.
17. Prakash O, Khan F. Cluster based SVR-QSAR modelling for HTS records: an implementation for anticancer leads against human breast cancer. Comb Chem High Throughput Screen. 2013;16:511–21.
18. Balachandran P, Govindarajan R. Cancer: an ayurvedic perspective. Pharmacol Res. 2005;51:19–30.
19. Singh IS, Ali W, Pathak RK. Effect of amalaki on experimental rats, with special reference to their nitrogen balance. J Res Indian Med. 1975;10:141–6.
20. Aggarwal BB, Ichikawa H, Garodia P, et al. From traditional Ayurvedic medicine to modern medicine: identification of therapeutic targets for suppression of inflammation and cancer. Expert Opin Ther Targets. 2006;10:87–118.
21. Chawla YK, Dubey P, Singh R, et al. Treatment of dyspepsia with Amalaki (Emblica officinalis Linn.)—an Ayurvedic drug. Indian J Med Res. 1982;76:95–8.
22. Mulabagal V, Subbaraju GV, Rao CV, et al. Withanolide sulfoxide from Aswagandha roots inhibits nuclear transcription factor-kappa-B, cyclooxygenase and tumor cell proliferation. Phytother Res. 2009;23:987–92.
23. Vyas P, Thakar AB, Baghel MS, et al. Efficacy of Rasayana Avaleha as adjuvant to radiotherapy and chemotherapy in reducing adverse effects. Ayu. 2010;31:417–23.
24. Baliga MS, Meera S, Vaishnav LK, et al. Rasayana drugs from the Ayurvedic system of medicine as possible radioprotective agents in cancer treatment. Integr Cancer Ther. 2013;12:455–63.
25. Shan B, Cai YZ, Brooks DJ, et al. Antibacterial properties and major bioactive component of cinnamon stick (Cinnamomum burmannii): activity against food has borne pathogenic bacteria. J Agric Food Chem. 2007;55:5484–90.
26. Vinitha M, Ballal M. In vitro anticandidal activity of *Cinnamomum verum*. J Med Sci. 2008;8:425–8.
27. Rana VS, Devi CB, Verdeguer N, et al. Variation of terpenoids constituents in natural population of Cinnamomum tamla (L.) leaves. J Essent Oil Res. 2009;21:531–4.
28. Wang R, Wang R, Yang B. Extraction of essential oils from five cinnamon leaves and identification of their volatile compound compositions. Innovative Food Sci Emerg Technol. 2009;10:289–92.
29. Kochummen KM. Family Lauraceae. In: Tree Flora of Malaya, vol. 4. Longmans: Kuala Lumpur; 1989. p. 124–32.
30. Jayatilaka A, Poole SK, Poole CF, et al. Simultaneous microsteam distillation/ solvent extraction for the isolation of semivolatile flavor compounds from Cinnamomum, their separation by series of coupled-column gas chromatography. Anal Chim Acta. 1995;302:147–62.
31. Ranasinghe P, Perera S, Gunatilake M, et al. Effects of *Cinnamomum zeylanicum* (Ceylon cinnamon) on blood glucose and lipids in a diabetic and healthy rat model. Pharm Res. 2012;4:73–9.
32. Al-Numair KS, Ahemed D, Ahemed SE et al. Nutritive value, levels of polyphenols and antinutritional factors in Sri Lankan cinnamon (*Cinnamomum Zeyalnicum*) and Chinese cinnamon (*Cinnamomum Cassia*). Res. Bult., No. (154), Food Sci. & Agric. Res. Center, King Saud Univ 5–21. 2007.
33. Gul S, Safdar M. Proximate composition and mineral analysis of cinnamon. Pak J Nutr. 2009;8(9):1456–60.

34. Senanayake UM, Lee TH, Wills RBH. Volatile constituents of cinnamon (*Cinnamomum zeylanicum*) oils. J Agric Food Chem. 1978;26(4):822–4.
35. Singh G, Maurya S, DeLampasona MP, et al. A comparison of chemical, antioxidant and antimicrobial studies of cinnamon leaf and bark volatile oils, oleoresins and their constituents. Food Chem Toxicol. 2007;45:1650–61.
36. Tung YT, Chua MT, Wang SY, et al. Antiinflammation activities of essential oil and its constituents from indigenous cinnamon (*Cinnamomum osmophloeum*) twigs. Bioresour Technol. 2008;99(9):3908–13.
37. Tung YT, Yen PL, Lin CY, et al. Antiinflammatory activities of essential oils and their constituents from different provenances of indigenous cinnamon (*Cinnamom umosmophloeum*) leaves. Pharm Biol. 2010;48(10):1130–6.
38. PROGRAM, NT. NTP Technical Report on the Toxicology and Carcinogenesis Studies of Trans-Cinnamaldehyde. Technical Report 514 NIH Publication No 04-4448. 2004.
39. Elshafie MM, Nawar IA, Algamal MA, et al. Evaluation of the biological effects for adding cinnamon volatile oil and TBHQ as antioxidant on rats'lipid profiles. Asian J Plant Sci. 2012;11:100–8.
40. Duke JA, Duke PAK, duCellier JL. Duke's handbook of medicinal plants of the bible. Boca Raton: CRC Press; 2008.
41. Lu J, Zhang K, Nam S, et al. Novel angiogenesis inhibitory activity in cinnamon extract blocks VEGFR2 kinase and downstream signaling. Carcinogenesis. 2010;31:481–8.
42. Molania T, Moghadamnia A, Aghel S, et al. The effect of cinnamaldehyde on mucositis and salivary antioxidant capacity in gamma-irradiated rats (a preliminary study). J Pharm Sci. 2012;20:89–95.
43. Hong JW, Yang GE, Kim YB, et al. Anti-inflammatory activity of cinnamon water extract in vivo and in vitro LPS-induced models. BMC Complement Altern Med. 2012;12:237–41.
44. Elahi RK. The effect of the cinnamon on dog's heart performance by focus on Korotkoff sounds. J Anim Vet Adv. 2012;11:3604–8.
45. Akira M, Tanaka S, Tabata M. Pharmacological studies on the antiulcerogenic activity of Chinese cinnamon. Planta Med. 1986;6:440–3.
46. Sharma UK, Sharma AK, Pandey AK. Medicinal attributes of major phenylpropanoids present in cinnamon. BMC Complement Altern Med. 2016;16:156.
47. Koppikar SJ, Choudhari AS, Suryavanshi SA, et al. Aqueous cinnamon extract (ACE-c) from the bark of Cinnamomum Cassia causes apoptosis in human cervical cancer cell line (SiHa) through loss of mitochondrial membrane potential. BMC Cancer. 2010;10:210.
48. Jeon CY, Haan MN, Cheng C, et al. Helicobacter pylori infection is associated with an increased rate of diabetes. Diabetes Care. 2012;35:520–5.
49. Choi J, Lee KT, Ka H, et al. Constituents of the essential oil of the cinnamon cassia stem bark and the biological properties. Arch Pharm Res. 2001;24(5):418–23.
50. Swords R, Kelly K, Carew J, et al. The Pim kinases: new targets for drug development. Curr Drug Targets. 2011;12(14):2059–66.
51. Blanco-Aparicio C, Carnero A. Pim kinases in cancer: diagnostic, prognostic and treatment opportunities. Biochem Pharmacol. 2013;85(5):629–43.
52. Kim JE, Son JE, Jeongc H, et al. A novel cinnamon-related natural product with Pim-1 inhibitory activity inhibits leukemia and skin cancer. Cancer Res. 2015;75(13):2716–28.
53. Ono K, Wang X, Han J. Resistance to tumor necrosis factor-induced cell death mediated by PMCA4 deficiency. Mol Cell Biol. 2001;21:8276–88.
54. Tsai KD, Liu YH, Chen TW, et al. Cuminaldehyde from *Cinnamomum verum* induces cell death through targeting topoisomerase 1 and 2 in human colorectal adenocarcinoma COLO 205 cells. Forum Nutr. 2016;8:318–25.
55. Yang S, Tsai K, Wong HY, et al. Molecular mechanism of Cinnamomum verum component cuminaldehyde inhibits cell growth and induces cell death in human lung squamous cell carcinoma NCI-H520 cells in vitro and in vivo. J Cancer. 2016;7:251–61.
56. Evdokimova OV, Neneleva EV, Tarrab I, et al. Comparison of lipophilic substances of the bark of Chinese (Cinnamomum cassia (L.) C. Presl.) and Ceylon cinnamon (Cinnamomum zeylanicum Blume). World Appl Sci J. 2013;27:70–3.

57. Bhattacharjee S, Rana T, Sengupta A. Inhibition of lipid peroxidation and enhancement of GST activity by cardamom and cinnamon during chemically induced colon carcinogenesis in Swiss albino mice. Asian Pac J Cancer Prev. 2007;8:578–82.
58. Schoene NW, Kelly MA, Polansky MM, et al. A polyphenol mixture from cinnamon targets p38MAP kinase-regulated signaling pathways to produce G2/M arrest. J Nutr Biochem. 2009;20:614–20.
59. Assadollahi V, Parivar K, Roudbari NH, et al. The effect of aqueous cinnamon extract on the apoptotic process in acute myeloid leukemia HL-60 cells. Adv Biomed Res. 2013;2:25–9.
60. Aleo E, Henderson CJ, Fontanini A, et al. Identification of new compounds that trigger apoptosome-independent caspase activation and apoptosis. Cancer Res. 2006;66:9235–44.
61. Niki E, Yoshida Y, Saito Y, et al. Lipid per-oxidation: mechanisms, inhibition, and biological effects. Biochem Biophys Res Commun. 2005;338:668–76.
62. Ames BM, Shigena MK, Hagen TM. Oxidants, antioxidants and the degenerative diseases of aging. Proc. Natl. Acad Sci. 1993;90:7915–22.
63. United Stated Department of Agriculture [USDA]. USDA Database for the Flavonoid Content of Selected Food s, Release 2.1. 2007. http://www.ars.usda.gov/SP2User Files/Place/12354500/Data/Flav/flav02–1.mdb. Accessed 21 June 21 2017.
64. Murcia MA, Egea I, Romojaro F, et al. Antioxidant evaluation in dessert spices compared with common food additives. Influence of irradiation procedure. J Agric Food Chem. 2004;52(2):1872–81.
65. Shobana S, Naidu KA. Antioxidant activity of selected Indian spices. Prostaglandins Leukot Essent Fatty Acids. 2000;62(2):107–10.
66. Okawa M, Kinjo J, Nohara T, et al. DPPH (1,1-diphenyl-2-Picrylhydrazyl) radical scavenging activity of flavonoids obtained fromsomemedicinal plants. Biol Pharm Bull. 2001;24(10):1202–5.
67. Lin CC, Wu SJ, Chang CH, et al. Antioxidant activity of *Cinnamomum cassia*. Phytother Res. 2003;17(7):726–30.
68. Grzanna R, Lindmark L, Frondoza CG. Gingeran herbal medicinal product with broad anti-inflammatory actions. J Med Food. 2005;8(2):125–32.
69. Youn HS, Lee JK, Choi YJ, et al. Cinnamaldehyde suppresses toll-like receptor 4 activation mediated through the inhibition of receptor oligomerization. Biochem Pharmacol. 2008;75(2):494–502.
70. Yu T, Lee S, Yang WS, et al. The ability of an ethanol extract of *Cinnamomum cassia* to inhibit Src and spleen tyrosine kinase activity contributes to its anti-inflammatory action. J Ethnopharmacol. 2012;139(2):566–73.
71. Han X, Parker TL. Antiinflammatory activity of cinnamon (*Cinnamomum zeylanicum*) bark essential oil in a human skin disease model. Phytother Res. 2017;31:1034–8.
72. Bhatt N. Herbs and herbal supplements a novel nutritional approach in animal nutrition. Iran J Appl Anim Sci. 2015;5(3):497–516.
73. Varalakshmi B, Vijaya Anand A, Karpagam T, et al. In vitro antimicrobial and anticancer activity of Cinnamomum zeylanicum linn bark extracts. Int J Pharm Pharm Sci. 2014;6(1):12–8.
74. Khan A, Bryden NA, Polansky MM, et al. Insulin potentiating factor and chromium content of selected foods and spices. Biol Trace Elem Res. 1990;24(3):183–8.
75. Anderson RA, Broadhurst CL, Polansky MM, et al. Isolation and characterization of polyphenol type-A polymers from cinnamon with insulin-like biological activity. J Agric Food Chem. 2004;52:65–70.
76. Wang JM, Xu B, Rao JY, et al. Diet habits, alcohol drinking, tobacco smoking, green tea drinking, and the risk of esophageal squamous cell carcinoma in the Chinese population. Eur J Gastroenterol Hepatol. 2007;19:171–6.
77. Subash Babu P, Prabuseenivasan S, Ignacimuthu S. Cinnamaldehyde—a potential antidiabetic agent. Phytomedicine. 2007;14(1):15–22.
78. Hafizur RM, Hameed A, Shukrana M, et al. Cinnamic acid exerts anti-diabetic activity by improving glucose tolerance in vivo and by stimulating insulin secretion in vitro. Phytomedicine. 2015;22(2):297–300.

Broccoli (*Brassica oleracea*) as a Preventive Biomaterial for Cancer

Sithara Suresh, Mostafa I. Waly, and Mohammad Shafiur Rahman

1 Introduction

Human life is greatly influenced by the quality and optimum quantity of food consumed. One of the most important requirements for ensuring a healthy population is to ensure balance diet. Broccoli (*Brassica oleracea*) is a member of Brassicaceae family comes in the genus Brassica. The family involves a group of vegetables, such as cauliflower, brussels sprouts, cabbage, and mustard [1]. The word broccoli means "the flowering crest of a cabbage." It has a large green flower head arranged in a tree-like structure branched out from a thick edible stalk. Broccoli, the "Crown Jewel of Nutrition," is a winter season vegetable crop found along the Mediterranean region and has been deemed as anti-cancerous food by the American Cancer Society [2, 3]. It is a low-carb and highly valued vegetable which is quite popular among the world for their edible inflorescences and fleshy stems [4]. The demand for broccoli is increasing globally due to their potential health boosting components, such as vitamins, minerals, dietary fiber, flavonol glycosides, hydroxycinnamic acids, and sulfur-containing compounds (such as glucosinolates) [5, 6].

Epidemiological studies have shown that a high intake of vegetables and fruits are correlated with a low risk of fatal diseases, like cancer due to their antioxidants [7–9]. Cancer is the second leading cause of death and is becoming common irrespective of age or gender. The process of cancer development is a consequence of genetic alterations which is a multi-step process that leads to disruption of basic biological functions and then to invasive carcinoma. It has been estimated that the number of new cancer cases will be increased by 70% worldwide in the year 2030 [10–12]. As per the World Health Organization estimate, around 17.5 million cancer

S. Suresh (✉) · M. I. Waly · M. S. Rahman
Department of Food Science and Nutrition, College of Agricultural and Marine Sciences, Sultan Qaboos University, Muscat, Oman

© Springer International Publishing AG, part of Springer Nature 2018
M. I. Waly, M. S. Rahman (eds.), *Bioactive Components, Diet and Medical Treatment in Cancer Prevention*, https://doi.org/10.1007/978-3-319-75693-6_5

deaths are expected to increase in the world by 2050 [13]. The main types of cancer include lung, stomach, colorectal, liver, and breast.

More than 30% of cancers are caused by behavioral, diet, and environmental risks that have potential to modify and prevent. Currently, the interest in natural antioxidants present in vegetables and fruits has been raised due to their reported chemotherapeutic property. Epidemiological studies have also shown that consumption of broccoli would help to decrease the risk of certain types of cancer. This is generally attributed to its high content of beneficial phytochemicals [1, 6, 14, 15]. The aim of this chapter is to discuss the multiple biological activities of broccoli and its potential chemopreventive and anticancer properties.

2   Nutritional Composition of Broccoli

The crown jewel of nutrition possesses most of the nutrients, such as vitamins, fiber, minerals, pectin, and secondary metabolites [14, 16, 17]. The nutritional composition depends on the vegetable's developmental stages, variety, soil type, storage conditions, and processing techniques. The edible portion of broccoli has high moisture content (89.3 g/100 g broccoli). Broccoli is a low-carb vegetable (2.3 g/100 g fresh broccoli) with total sugars 1.9 g/100 g fresh broccoli, whereas the observed levels of carbohydrate and total sugars in cooked or boiled broccoli were observed as 1.7 and 1.6 g/100 g, respectively. The other constituents include protein (4.4 g/100 g fresh broccoli), fat (0.6 g/100 g fresh broccoli), and fiber (4 g/100 g fresh broccoli). In boiled broccoli, the observed amounts of protein, fat, and fiber were 3.3, 0.5, and 2.8 g/100 g, whereas the amounts in steamed broccoli showed similar to that of fresh broccoli which were observed as 4.1, 0.5, and 3.8 g/100 g, respectively. The amounts of reducing sugars, fructose and glucose were measured as 1.2 and 0.7 g/100 g fresh broccoli [18, 19]. Broccoli also contains small amounts of polysaccharides, such as pectin, hemicellulose, and starch [20]. Some of the vitamins found are vitamin K (101.6 μg/100 g fresh broccoli) along with a low amount of riboflavin (0.35 mg/100 g fresh broccoli), thiamine (0.15 mg/100 g fresh broccoli), pantothenic acid (0.61 mg/100 g fresh broccoli), and vitamin B6 (0.21 mg/100 g fresh broccoli). In boiled broccoli, the measured amounts of vitamin K, riboflavin, thiamine, pantothenic acid, and vitamin B6 were observed as 141.1 μg/100 g, 0.3 mg/100 g, 0.04 mg/100 g, 0.28 mg/100 g, and 0.19 mg/100 g, respectively. Potassium and phosphorus are the two main minerals and the measured amounts were 487 and 104 mg/100 g fresh broccoli [19]. The quantities of potassium and phosphorus present in the boiled broccoli were found as 341 and 81 mg/100 g, respectively.

3 Phytochemicals in Broccoli

Plant products are valuable sources of natural phytochemicals, antioxidants, vitamins, and phenolic compounds which have been reported to give a promising and positive impact on human health [21–23]. All these reasons, as identified, have led to an increase in the recommended dietary intake of fruits and vegetables [24]. The major phytochemicals present in broccoli are glucosinolates, phenolic compounds, antioxidants, vitamins, and dietary essential minerals, which provide health benefits beyond basic nutrition content [6, 15]. Tiveron et al. [25] reported the antioxidant activity in broccoli by DPPH method and ABTS^{+}, and reported values were 33.4 and 43 μmol Trolox/g dry-solids, respectively.

Total phenolic content was measured as 198.6 mg/100 g broccoli and it was particularly high for raw broccoli, whereas it was low for boiled or cooked broccoli. The glucosinolate content of raw and boiled broccoli were measured as 61.7 mg/100 g and 37.2 mg/100 g, respectively [19]. The prominent glucosinolates in broccoli are glucoraphanin, glucoerucin, and glucobrassicin. Glucosinolates are glycoside compounds stored in the intracellular vacuoles within plant cells. Idioblasts within the plant cells contain the enzyme myrosinase. Upon broccoli cutting, chewing or damages, myrosinase is released from the broccoli cells to hydrolyze glucosinolates. Some of the hydrolyzed products are sulforaphane (SFN), erucin, and iberin [26]. SFN and erucin have attracted many researchers due to its promising chemopreventive property [26–30]. The range of SFN in different cultivar of broccoli florets, stem, and leaves was 63–982, 18–274, and 7–257 mg/kg dry-solids, respectively [31]. The SFN and erucin of broccoli seeds were measured as 62–1576 and 60–107 mg/kg, respectively [32]. Luteolin (8.6 mg/100 g broccoli) and kaempferol (4.01 mg/100 g broccoli) were the main flavonoids as reported in raw broccoli. The range of other bioactive nutrients reported in broccoli was β-carotene (0.37–2.42 mg/100 g broccoli), α-tocopherol (0.46–4.29 mg/100 g broccoli), glucoraphanin (0.8–21.7 μmol/g dry weight), and indolyl glucosinolates (0.4–6.2 μmol/g dry weight) [33]. Broccoli contains sufficient levels of vitamins A, C, and folate to meet the recommended dietary intake (RDI). The total vitamin A, C, and total folate in raw broccoli were 68 μg/100 g, 57 mg/100 g, and 75 μg/100 g, whereas in cooked broccoli the levels were 62 μg/100 g, 58 mg/100 g, and 53 μg/100 g, respectively [19].

4 Anticancer Effects as Evidenced from Cell Line Studies

Various types of human cancers are characterized by an uncontrolled cell growth. The control of cell cycle progression and cell proliferation are maintained by a balance between cyclins (proteins), cyclin-dependent kinases (Cdks) and phosphatases (enzymes). One of the mechanisms involved in uncontrolled cell growth is caused by cancer-associated mutations, overexpression of cell cycle-regulated protein, and loss of Cdk inhibitor expression [34].

Most chemopreventive agents are antioxidant in nature. Experimental evidences of broccoli are promising since broad spectrum of genes and proteins causing cancer growth and progression are suppressed. Extensive studies were performed to assess the anticancer activity of broccoli and its therapeutic potential in various experimental models. Hwang and Lim [35] studied the antioxidant and anticancer activities of broccoli by-products from different cultivars and maturity stages at harvest. The anticancer activities of 80% methanol extracts from different by-products were assessed against NCI-H1299 (i.e., human non-small lung carcinoma) cell lines using the 3-(4,5-dimethylthiazol-2-yl)-2,5-diphenyltetrazolium bromide (MTT) assay. The result showed that the inhibition activity of cell NCI-H1299 growth was highest in 80% methanol extracts (2 mg/ml) of florets, leaf stems, and stems from Kyoyoshi (early-maturing crop) than those of Myeongil 96 (middle-maturing crop) and SK3-085 (late-maturing crop). The cell growth inhibitory activity was observed as 15.6, 9.9, and 8.6%, respectively. On the other hand, the extract of leaves from Myeongil 96 showed the highest cell growth inhibition activity as compared to other by-products against NCI-H1299 cell lines. The inhibitory activity of 80% methanol leaf extract in Myeongil 96 was observed as 32.5%. The anticancer activities of 80% methanol extracts (2 mg/mL) of different by-products from different cultivars were also measured against HT-29 (human colon adenocarcinoma) cell lines. The leaves from all cultivars showed the inhibition of HT-29 growth. The cell growth inhibitory activity in Kyoyoshi, Myeongil 96, and SK3–085 was observed as 11.6, 9.2, and 6.6%, respectively. This study concluded that the major factor that is correlated with the anticarcinogenic activity against NCI-H1299 and HT-29 cell lines was total phenolic components rather than SFN content.

The SFN treatment caused an irreversible arrest in the G2/M phase of the PC-3 cell (i.e., human prostate cancer cell lines) cycle [36]. This study noticed that cell cycle arrest induced by SFN (20 µM) was accompanied by a significant decrease in the protein levels of cyclin B1, Cdc25B, and Cdc25C. Cdc25 is a dual-specificity protein tyrosine phosphatase, which catalyzes dephosphorylation and activation of cyclin-Cdk complexes through the removal of inhibitory phosphates. In prostate cancer, Cdc25A, Cdc25B, and Cdc25C were increased in cancerous lesions as compared to noncancerous lesions, and the levels were increased in higher Gleason grade tumors. The decreased levels of protein and enzymes led to the accumulation of Tyr-15-phosphorylated (inactive) cyclin-dependent kinase 1. SFN treatment also resulted in a rapid and sustained phosphorylation of Cdc25C at Ser-216, which led to its translocation from the nucleus to the cytoplasm because of increased binding with 14-3-3β. Increased Ser-216 phosphorylation of Cdc25C upon treatment with SFN was a result of activation of checkpoint kinase 2 (Chk2). Chk1 and Chk2 kinases can phosphorylate and inactivate the various Cdc25 isoforms. Therefore, Chk2 inactivates Cdc25 and cyclinB/CDK complex leading to the arrest of cells in G2/M phase. This same Chk2-dependent G2/M arrest was seen in the HCT116 human colon cancer cell line. These findings indicated that Chk2-mediated phosphorylation of Cdc25C played the major role in irreversible G2/M arrest by SFN.

Qazi et al. [37] studied the anticancer activity of SFN in Barrett esophageal adenocarcinoma cells (BEAC). Their study reported that SFN-induced both time- and dose-dependent decline in cell survival, cell cycle arrest, and apoptosis. Exposure to 7 μM SFN led to a complete cell death in BEAC cell lines tested, in a period of 3–5 days. A significant reduction in tumor volume was observed by SFN in a subcutaneous tumor model of BEAC. Exposure to SFN at 5 μM showed antiproliferative activity, which killed 100% of OE33 cells in 3 days and 83% of FLO-1 cells in 5 days. The treatment with 3 μM SFN on FLO-1 cells led to 74% cell death in 5 days. At a concentration of 1 μM SFN, the activity was less effective and killed 54% of OE33 cells in 3 days and 39% of FLO-1 cells in 5 days. This anticancer activity could be attributed to the induction of caspase 8 and p21 and downregulation of hsp90, a molecular chaperon required for activity of several proliferation-associated proteins. These data indicated that SFN, a natural product with antioxidant properties from broccoli has great potential to be used in chemoprevention and treatment of BEAC. Pledgie-Tracy et al. [38] examined the clinical potential of SFN in human breast cancer cell lines. They showed that SFN treatment inhibited cell growth, induced a G2-M cell cycle block, increased expression of cyclin B1, and induced oligonucleosomal DNA fragmentation in four human breast cancer cell lines examined (MDA-MB- 231, MDA-MB-468, MCF-7, and T47D cells). Activation of apoptosis by SFN in MDA-MB-231 cells seemed to be initiated through induction of Fas ligand, which resulted in activation of caspase-8, caspase-3, and poly (ADPribose) polymerase, whereas apoptosis in the other breast cancer cell lines was initiated by decreased Bcl-2 expression, release of cytochrome c into the cytosol, activation of caspase-9 and caspase-3. SFN also inhibited the HDAC activity and decreased expression of estrogen receptor-A, epidermal growth factor receptor, and human epidermal growth factor receptor-2 in each cell line. Shivale et al. [39] studied the antitumor activity of broccoli extract against two prolific cancer cell lines, HeLa (i.e., human epithelial cervix carcinoma), and MCF-7 (i.e., human breast carcinoma). A decrease of fast growing cells with exposure to broccoli extract showed a potential activity against tumors. Ullah [40] also mentioned the positive effect of 25 μM dose of SFN treatment on the enzymatic activities of GST, NQO1, aldo-keto reductase (AKR), and glutathione reductase (GR) through the induction of phase II enzyme in several mammalian cancer cell lines: HepG2, MCF7, MDA-MB-231, LNCaP, HeLa, and HT-29.

The ability of SFN to inhibit histone deacetylase (HDACs) enzymes could be another mechanism by which it acts as a chemoprevention agent. HDACs and histone acetyltransferase (HAT) enzymes have many crucial parts in the regulation of gene expression, cell proliferation, cell migration, cell death, and angiogenesis. The mechanism of histone acetylation depends on a balance between the enzymes with histone acetyltransferase (HAT) activity and enzymes that deacetylate histones (HDACs). The factors influencing this balance can contribute to cancer development [40, 41]. Clarke et al. [42] showed that SFN treatment in prostate cellular models (LnCap and PC3) reduced HDAC activity. Their study revealed that 15 μM SFN selectively induced cell cycle arrest and apoptosis in BPH1 (benign hyperplasia), LnCap, and PC3 cells. SFN treatment also decreased HDAC proteins followed by an increase in the acetylation of histone H3 at the p21 promoter and increased tubulin acetylation in prostate cancer cells (specifically in hyperplastic and cancer cells) which caused cell death.

The positive effect of SFN on HT29 human colon cancer cells was observed by cell cycle arrest and apoptosis [43]. The SFN ranging from 5 to 50 μM inhibited fetal calf serum induced cell growth and promoted cell cycle arrest in a dose-dependent manner, followed by cell death. This cell cycle arrest was correlated with an increased expression of cyclins A and B1. It was also demonstrated that SFN induced cell death through apoptotic process. Pappa et al. [44] compared the cell growth inhibitory potential of SFN, β-phenethyl isothiocyanate (PEITC), indole-3-carbinol, and 3,3'-diindolylmethane on the p53 wild-type human colon cancer cell line 40–16 (p53+/+) and its p53 knockout derivative 379.2 (p53−/−) (both derived from HCT116). Incubation with SFN, PEITC, indole-3-carbinol, or 3,3'-diindolylmethane at a concentration range of 0.4–50 μM led to a dose-dependent inhibition of cell proliferation. The cell death program induced by all four compounds could be attributed to caspase-9 activation and changes in the ratios of pro- and anti-apoptotic Bcl-2-family proteins. Khoobchandani et al. [45] coated gold nanoparticles with the phytochemicals of broccoli and studied in vitro anticancer activities against prostrate (PC-3), breast (triple negative MDA-MB-231, T47D, and SkBr3), and multiple myeloma (U266) cancer cell lines. They showed that B-AuNPs (Broccoli gold nanoparticles) inhibited maximum cell growth against cancer cell lines. Broccoli phytochemicals based gold nanoparticles showed synergistic effect and excellent internalization of prostate (PC-3) and breast (MDA-MB-231 and T47D) cancer cells when used at concentration of 25 and 50 μg/mL, respectively, with incubation time 18 h. It showed potent antiproliferative action.

5   Anticancer Effects as Evidence from Animal Trial

The term "preventive medicine" is seeking attraction based on the concept that an improvement in dietary pattern prevents diseases under stressful conditions. There are various studies investigating the potential anticancer components in broccoli and have developed a variety of products to contribute to preventive medicine. Isothiocyanates (ITC), a breakdown product of glucosinolates, have been demonstrated to inhibit certain types of cancer in animal studies. In that, SFN is one of the main targeted ITC found in broccoli that has been found to prevent carcinogenesis in animal by inducing detoxification enzymes. Zhang et al. [46] observed the inhibitory effects of SFN and three types of norbornyl-ITC on rat mammary cancer induced by 9,10-dimethyl-1, 2-benzanthracene (DMBA). They showed that the incidence of cancer (i.e., tumor multiplicity) was markedly reduced in rats treated with 150 μmol of SFN to 0.26 (i.e., total number of tumors/number of animals at risk) compared with 1.56 in the control. Norbornyl-ITC 2 showed potent activity comparable to that of SFN, whereas norbornyl-ITC 3 and -4 showed lower activity.

Suzuki et al. [47] studied the inhibitory effect of broccoli sprouts powder on azoxymethane (AOM) induced colonic aberrant crypt foci (ACF). They showed that broccoli sprout powder at a dose of 20 or 100 ppm for 4 weeks inhibited the development of AOM-induced rat ACF. The number of ACF lesions in the treatment groups administrated with broccoli sprout powder was significantly ($p < 0.001$) lowered as compared to the group administrated with AOM alone. They have concluded that SFN might have induced phase II detoxification enzymes thereby inhibiting the production of free radicals, thus inhibited the carcinogenesis in the colon. Similar result was also reported by Chung et al. [48]. Another study showed that pretreatment of A/J mice with phenethyl isothiocyanate for 96 h at a daily dose of 5 or 25 μmol inhibited lung tumor multiplicity induced by a single 10 μmol dose of 4-(methylnitrosamino)-1-(3-pyridyl)-1-butanone (NNK) by approximately 70 or 97%, respectively [49]. Keum et al. [50] studied the prostate chemopreventive activity of broccoli sprouts. They showed that transgenic adenocarcinoma of mouse prostate mice fed with 240 mg broccoli sprouts/mouse/day demonstrated a significant retardation of prostate tumor growth. The western blot analysis revealed that expression levels of Nrf2, *HO-1*, cleaved-Caspase-3, cleaved-PARP, and Bax proteins were increased. Finley et al. [51] studied the protective ability of high-selenium (Se) broccoli or high-Se broccoli sprouts against chemically induced mammary or colon cancer. Sprague-Dawley rats that consumed high-Se broccoli (3 μg of Se/g) had significantly reduced mammary tumors than rats fed with 0.1 μg of Se as selenite with or without the addition of regular broccoli. Fisher F-344 rats fed with 2.0 μg of Se/g of diet supplied as either high-Se broccoli florets or high-Se broccoli sprouts had significantly lower aberrant colon crypts than rats fed with 0.1 or 2 μg of Se/g of diet supplied as selenite with or without the addition of low-Se broccoli.

Qazi et al. [37] studied the anticancer activity of broccoli derivative, SFN in Barrett adenocarcinoma. This study showed that the mice treated with SFN (0.75 mg) significantly reduced the tumor size as compared to control mice. Another study showed that mice treated with a single oral dose of 10 μmol SFN significantly inhibited HDAC activity in the colonic mucosa and suppression of tumor development in APC^{min} mice (i.e., mouse model of multiple intestinal neoplasia with APC gene mutation) [52]. Smith et al. [53] showed the inhibition of dimethylhydrazine (DMH)-induced ACF and induction of apoptosis in rat colon followed by the oral administration of the glucosinolate sinigrin. The level of apoptosis was significantly higher in DMH-treated rats administrated with sinigrin (400 μg/g diet) as compared to control ($P < 0.05$), and the numbers of ACF were significantly lower in sinigrin-treated rats ($p < 0.001$). Balansky et al. [54] studied the prevention of cigarette smoke-induced lung tumors in mice by PEITC and N-acetylcysteine. Exposure to cigarette smoke resulted in a high incidence and multiplicity of benign lung tumors and significantly increased malignant lung tumors and other histopathological alterations in neonatal mice. The treatment with

PEITC (1000 mg/kg diet) and N-acetylcysteine (1000 mg/kg body weight) considerably decreased both the incidence and multiplicity of lung tumors. Conaway et al. [55] showed the chemopreventive activity of PEITC, sulforaphane, and their N-acetylcysteine conjugates during progression of lung adenomas to malignant tumors in A/J mice. The incidence of lung adenocarcinoma in the 3 µmol/g diet PEITC group and 8 µmol/g diet PEITC-N-acetylcysteine groups was reduced from 19 to 13%, respectively, when compared to carcinogen-treated control group (42%). The lung tumor incidences in groups treated with SFN-N-acetylcysteine (i.e., 4 and 8 µmol/g diet) were also significantly reduced to 11 or 16%. Furthermore, the malignant lung tumor multiplicity was significantly reduced from 1.0 tumor/mouse in the carcinogen-treated control group to 0.3 in the SFN low-dose group (1.5 µmol/g), 0.3 and 0.4 in the two SFN-N-acetylcysteine groups (4 and 8 µmol/g), and 0.4 in the PEITC high-dose group (3 µmol/g). The malignant tumor multiplicities in other treatment groups (PEITC-N-acetylcysteine, 4 and 8 µmol/g and sulforaphane, 3 µmol/g) were also reduced (0.5–0.8 tumors/mouse), but not significantly. Gills et al. [56] showed that SFN (1, 5, 10 µmol/mouse) significantly inhibited 7,12-dimethylbenz(a)anthracene/12-O-tetradecanoylphorbol 13-acetate (TPA)-induced mouse skin tumorigenesis. Another study showed that 6-phenylhexyl isothiocyanate (640 mg/kg diet) inhibited AOM induced colon tumors in male F344 rats. The apoptotic index in colonic mucosa of rats fed with 6-phenylhexyl isothiocyanate diet was 7.0%, when compared to control rats (8.3%) [57]. Izzotti et al. [58] showed that dietary PEITC (i.e., 500 mg/kg diet) significantly reduced tobacco smoke-induced DNA adducts in BAL cells, tracheal epithelium, lung, and heart; oxidative DNA damage (8-hydroxy-2′-deoxyguanosine [8-OH-dG]) in lung; hemoglobin adducts; and cytogenetic damage in alveolar macrophages and polychromatic erythrocytes from bone marrow of Sprague-Dawley rats exposed to a mixture of mainstream and side stream tobacco smoke for 28 days.

Munday et al. [59] studied the inhibition of urinary bladder carcinogenesis by broccoli sprouts. They observed that there was a significant and dose-dependent inhibition of bladder cancer development by the administration of freeze-dried aqueous extract of broccoli sprouts. They also showed that the extract inhibited the incidence, multiplicity, size, and progression of bladder cancer. The extract caused the induction of glutathione S-transferase and NAD(P)H:quinine oxidoreductase 1 in the bladder, which are protectants against oxidants and carcinogens. Cornblatt et al. [60] studied the chemopreventive action of SFN in 10-week-old female Sprague-Dawley rat mammary gland. They showed that a single oral dose (i.e., 150 µmol) of SFN showed a threefold increase in the NQO1 enzymatic activity and 4-fold elevated immune staining of HO-1 in the rat mammary epithelium, which provided a strong evidence of pharmacodynamics action of SFN. Another study reported by Chen et al. [61] showed that dietary broccoli diminished the development of fatty liver and liver cancer in 4 weeks old male B6C3F1 mice induced with diethylnitrosamine. The mice fed with broccoli exhibited low hepatic triglycerides, non-alcoholic fatty liver disease (NAFLD) scores, decreased plasma alanine aminotransferase, suppressed activation of hepatic CD68+ macrophages ($P < 0.0001$), and reduced the initiation and progression of hepatic neoplasm.

6 Clinical Trials

The clinical trials on the positive effects of SFN or isothiocyanates against cancer are very limited due to lack of suitably formulated agents for oral administration, regulatory issues requiring investigational new drug application submission and approval from the Federal Drug Administration. The complexities associated with primary prevention clinical trials requiring thousands of subjects and years of follow-up to draw meaningful conclusions [62]. However, a few pilot and phase 1 human SFN trials have been examined. Experimental studies have shown that SFN and its metabolites act as HDAC inhibitors. Clinical trials are pointed at demonstrating the chemotherapeutic efficacy of HDAC inhibitors, based on evidence that cancer cells undergo cell cycle arrest, differentiation and apoptosis in vitro, and tumor volume and/or tumor numbers may be reduced in animal models.

Kensler et al. [63] conducted a placebo-controlled, randomized chemoprevention trial in 200 healthy adults, and consumed hot drinking water infused with 3-day old sprout extracts with defined concentrations of glucosinolates (400 or <3 μmol glucoraphanin) for 2 weeks. Administration of broccoli sprouts containing glucosinolates led to a non-significant reduction in urinary excretion of aflatoxin-*N*-guanine. An insignificant reduction in *trans, anti*-phenanthrene tetraol, a metabolite of the combustion product phenanthrene, was also observed in the urinary excretion. This study concluded that reduction in the excretion of *trans, anti*-phenanthrene tetraol supports the action of sulforaphane on inducing phase 2 enzymes in the study participants. Cornblatt et al. [60] studied the clinical observation of SFN for chemoprevention in the breast cancer. A single oral dose of broccoli sprouts containing 200 μmol of SFN to eight healthy women undergoing reduction mammoplasty showed the presence of dithiocarbamate (DTCs, SFN metabolites) in the breast tissue. The DTCs concentration was observed as 1.45 pmol/mg in the right breast and 2.00 pmol/mg in the left, approximately 100 min after ingestion. They also measured the detoxification genes, *NQO1* and heme *oxygenase*-1 (*HO-1*) transcripts, as well as *NQO1* enzymatic activity in human breast tissue. This study concluded the pharmacodynamics action of SFN in the breast tissue. Cipolla et al. [64] studied a double-blinded, randomized, placebo-controlled multicenter trial with SFN in 78 patients (i.e., mean age, 69 ± 6 years) with increasing prostate-specific antigen (PSA) levels after radical prostatectomy. This study was designed to detect a 0.012 log (ng/mL)/month decrease in the log PSA slope in the sulforaphane group from baseline to 6 months (M0 to M6). The mean changes in PSA levels between M6 and M0 were significantly lower in the SFN group ($+0.099 \pm 0.341$ ng/mL) than in placebo ($+0.620 \pm 1.417$ ng/mL; $p = 0.0433$). This study confirmed that daily administration of SFN promised in managing biochemical recurrences in prostate cancer after radical prostatectomy.

7 Conclusion

Cancer is a multifaceted disease spreading across the world that impacts morbidity and mortality. Lifestyle changes can potentially eliminate or control the occurrence of types of cancer. In this chapter, we have summarized and discussed the potential role of broccoli and its phytochemical components in cancer chemoprevention. Collective data from various epidemiological, in vitro, in vivo animal models and clinical studies demonstrated an inverse relationship between broccoli intake and cancer risk. The bioactive components especially SFN and other isothiocyanates present in broccoli have shown to inhibit cancer initiation and progression by interfering with multiple cellular targets and mechanisms. However, further clinical studies are required to confirm the cancer preventing and treating efficacy of phytochemicals present in broccoli. Consumption of broccoli as such may be difficult and hence extraction of bioactive components from broccoli and conversion into various formulations is the alternative and challenging since the extract is hygroscopic in nature. Hence, proper care should be taken for a longer shelf life. Formulations of pure isothiocyanates for clinical investigations are limited. Advances in genotyping and biomarker technologies, combined with maturing large studies of diet and biomarkers in humans would be fundamental in moving the field of diet and cancer further. SFN itself may not be the only important bioactive component to protect against tumor formation. Hence, further investigation is needed to explore the mechanisms of broccoli and its active components in the protection against cancer. In summary, broccoli derived bioactive components is a promising agent for supplemented chemopreventive product.

References

1. Latte KP, Appel KE, Lampen A. Health benefits and possible risks of broccoli—an overview. Food Chem Toxicol. 2011;49:3287–309.
2. Lee SG, Kim JH, Son MJ, Lee EJ, Park WD, Kim JB, Lee SP, Lee IS. Influence of extraction method on quality and functionality of broccoli juice. Prev Nutr Food Sci. 2013;18(2):133–8.
3. El-Magd MMA. Evaluation of some broccoli cultivars growth, head yield and quality under different planting dates. J Appl Sci Res. 2013;9(11):5730–6.
4. Rybarczyk-Plonska A. Health-related compounds in broccoli (*Brassica oleracea* L. var. italica) as affected by postharvest temperature, light and UV-B irradiation, Ph.D. thesis. 2016. ISBN 978–82–575-1334-4.
5. Suresh S, Al-Habsi N, Guizani N, Rahman MS. Thermal characteristics and state diagram of freeze-dried broccoli: freezing curve, maximal-freeze-concentration condition, glass line and solids-melting. Thermochim Acta. 2017;655:129–36.
6. Ares AM, Nozal MJ, Bernal J. Extraction, chemical characterization and biological activity determination of broccoli health promoting compounds. J Chromatogr A. 2013;1313:78–95.
7. Yu D, Zhang X, Gao YT, Li H, Yang G, Huang J, Zheng W, Xiang YB, Shu XO. Fruit and vegetable intake and risk of coronary heart disease: results from prospective cohort studies of Chinese adults in Shanghai. Br J Nutr. 2014;111:353–62.

8. Wootten-Beard PC, Ryan L. Improving public health?: the role of antioxidant-rich fruit and vegetable beverages. Food Res Int. 2011;44:3135–48.
9. Bergquist SAM, Gertsson UE, Olsson ME. Influence of growth stage and postharvest storage on ascorbic acid and carotenoid content and visual quality of baby spinach (Spinacia oleracea L.). J Sci Food Agric. 2006;86:346–55.
10. Turrini E, Ferruzzi L, Fimognari C. Potential effects of pomegranate polyphenols in cancer prevention and therapy. Oxidative Med Cell Longev. 2015;2015:938475.
11. Sestili P, Fimognari C. Cytotoxic and antitumor activity of sulforaphane: the role of reactive oxygen species. Biomed Res Int. 2015;2015:1–9.
12. Thun MJ, DeLancey JO, Center MM, Jemal A, Ward EM. The global burden of cancer: priorities for prevention. Carcinogenesis. 2010;31:100–10.
13. Marrett LD, De P, Airia P, Dryer D. Cancer in Canada in 2008. CMAJ. 2008;179:1163–70.
14. Rybarczyk-Plonska A, Hansen MK, Wold AB, Hagen SF, Borge GIA, Bengtsson GB. Vitamin C in broccoli (Brassica oleracea L. var. italica) flower buds as affected by postharvest light, UV-B irradiation and temperature. Postharvest Biol Technol. 2014;98:82–9.
15. Moreno DA, Carvajal M, Lopez-Berenguer C, García-Viguera C. Chemical and biological characterisation of nutraceutical compounds of broccoli. J Pharm Biomed Anal. 2006;41:1508–22.
16. Madhu KA. Proximate composition, available carbohydrates, dietary fibre and anti-nutritional factors of broccoli (Brassica oleracea l var. Italica plenca) leaf and floret powder. Biosci Discov. 2014;5(1):45–9.
17. Porter Y. Antioxidant properties of green broccoli and purple-sprouting broccoli under different cooking conditions. Biosci Horiz. 2012;5:1–11.
18. Roe M, Church S, Pinchen H, Finglas P. Nutrient analysis of fruit and vegetables. 2013. www.gov.uk/government/publications/nutrient-analysis-of-fruit-and-vegetables. Accessed December 2016.
19. Campbell B, Han DY, Triggs CM, Fraser AG, Ferguson LR. Brassicaceae: nutrient analysis and investigation of tolerability in people with Crohn's disease in a New Zealand study. Func Foods Health Dis. 2012;2:460–86.
20. Houben K, Jolie RP, Fraeye I, Loey AMV, Hendrickx ME. Comparative study of the cell wall composition of broccoli, carrot, and tomato: structural characterization of the extractable pectins and hemicelluloses. Carbohydr Res. 2011;346:1105–11.
21. Allaith AAA. Antioxidant activity of Bahraini date palm (Phoenix dactylifera L.) fruit of various cultivars. Int J Food Sci Technol. 2008;43:1033–40.
22. Rice-Evans C, Miller N, Paganga G. Antioxidant properties of phenolic compounds. Trends Plant Sci. 1997;2:152–9.
23. Arts ICW, Hollman PCH. Polyphenols and disease risk in epidemiologic studies. Am J Clin Nutr. 2005;81:317–25.
24. WHO. Measuring intake of fruits and vegetables. 2005. http://apps.who.int/iris/bitstream/10665/43144/1/9241592826_eng.pdf. Accessed 8 Aug 2017.
25. Tiveron AP, Melo PS, Bergamaschi KB, Vieira TMFS, Regitano-d' Arce MAB, Alencar SM. Antioxidant activity of Brazilian vegetables and its relation with phenolic composition. Int J Mol Sci. 2012;13:8943–57.
26. Han D, Row KH. Separation and purification of sulforaphane from broccoli by solid phase extraction. Int J Mol Sci. 2011;12:1854–61.
27. Liang H, Yuan QP, Dong HR, Liu YM. Determination of sulforaphane in broccoli and cabbage by high-performance liquid chromatography. J Food Compos Anal. 2006;19:473–6.
28. Geurrero-Beltran CE, Calderon-Oliver M, Pedraza-Chaverri J, Chirino YI. Protective effect of sulforaphane against oxidative stress: recent advances. Exp Toxicol Pathol. 2012;64:503–8.
29. Guo Q, Guo L, Wang Z, Zhuang Y, Gu Z. Response surface optimization and identification of isothiocyanates produced from broccoli sprouts. Food Chem. 2013;141:1580–6.
30. Melchini A, Traka MH. Biological profile of erucin: a new promising anticancer agent from cruciferous vegetables. Toxins. 2010;2:593–612.

31. Li Z, Liu Y, Fang Z, Yang L, Zhuang M, Zhang Y, Sun P. Development and verification of sulforaphane extraction method in cabbage (Brassica oleracea L. var. capitata) and broccoli (Brassica oleracea L. var. italic planch.). J Med Plants Res. 2012;6:4796–803.
32. You Y, Wu Y, Mao J, Zou L, Liu S. Screening of Chinese Brassica species for anti-cancer sulforaphane and erucin. Afr J Biotechnol. 2008;7:147–52.
33. Jeffery EH, Brown AF, Kurilich AC, Keck AS, Matusheski N, Klein BP, Juvik JA. Variation in content of bioactive components in broccoli. J Food Compos Anal. 2003;16:323–30.
34. Nemoto K. G2/M accumulation in prostate cancer cell line PC-3 is induced by Cdc25 inhibitor 7-chloro-6-(2-morpholin-4-ylethylamino) quinoline-5, 8-dione (DA 3003-2). Exp Ther Med. 2010;1:647–50.
35. Hwang JH, Lim SB. Antioxidant and anticancer activities of broccoli by-products from different cultivars and maturity stages at harvest. Prev Nutr Food Sci. 2015;20:8–14.
36. Singh SV, Herman-Antosiewicz A, Singh AV, Lew KL, Srivastava SK, Kamath R, Brown KD, Zhang L, Baskaran R. Sulforaphane-induced G2/M phase cell cycle arrest involves checkpoint kinase 2-mediated phosphorylation of cell division cycle 25C. J Biol Chem. 2004;279:25813–22.
37. Qazi A, Pal J, Maitah M, Fulciniti M, Pelluru D, Nanjappa P, Lee S, Batchu RB, Prasad M, Bryant CS, Rajput S, Gryaznov S, Beer DG, Weaver DW, Munshi NC, Goyal RK, Shammas MA. Anticancer activity of a broccoli derivative, sulforaphane, in barrett adenocarcinoma: potential use in chemoprevention and as adjuvant in chemotherapy. Transl Oncol. 2010;3:389–99.
38. Pledgie-Tracy A, Sobolewski MD, Davidson NE. Sulforaphane induces cell type-specific apoptosis in human breast cancer cell lines. Mol Cancer Ther. 2007;6:1013–21.
39. Shivale N, Shah S, Sampat K, Deshpande K. Broad range activity of sulforaphane extracted from broccoli. Bionano Frontier. 2014;7:82–5.
40. Ullah MF. Sulforaphane (SFN): an isothiocyanate in a cancer chemoprevention paradigm. Medicines. 2015;2:141–56.
41. Legube G, Trouche D. Regulating histone acetyltransferases and deacetylases. EMBO Rep. 2003;4:944–7.
42. Clarke JD, Hsu A, Yu Z, Dashwood RH, Ho E. Differential effects of sulforaphane on histone deacetylases, cell cycle arrest and apoptosis in normal prostate cells versus hyperplastic and cancerous prostate cells. Mol Nutr Food Res. 2011;55:999–1009.
43. Gamet-Payrastre L, Li P, Lumeau S, Cassar G, Dupont MA, Chevolleau S, Gasc N, Tulliez J, Tercé F. Sulforaphane, a naturally occurring isothiocyanate, induces cell cycle arrest and apoptosis in HT29 human colon cancer cells. Cancer Res. 2000;60:1426–33.
44. Pappa G, Lichtenberg M, Iori R, Barillari J, Bartsch H, Gerhäuser C. Comparison of growth inhibition profiles and mechanisms of apoptosis induction in human colon cancer cell lines by isothiocyanates and indoles from Brassicaceae. Mutat Res. 2006;599:76–87.
45. Khoobchandani M, Zambre A, Katti K, Lin CH, Katti KV. Green nanotechnology from Brassicaceae: development of broccoli phytochemicals-encapsulated gold nanoparticles and their applications in nanomedicine. Int J Green Nanotechnol. 2013;1:1–15.
46. Zhang Y, Kensler TW, Cho CG, Posner GH, Talalay P. Anticarcinogenic activities of sulforaphane and structurally related synthetic norbornyl isothiocyanates. Proc Natl Acad Sci. 1994;91:3147–50.
47. Suzuki R, Kohno H, Sugie S, Okada T, Tanaka T. Suzuki et al. (2004) studied the inhibitory effect of broccoli sprouts powder on azoxymethane (AOM) induced colonic aberrant crypt foci (ACF). J Toxicol Pathol. 2004;17:119–26.
48. Chung FL, Conaway CC, Rao CV, Reddy BS. Chemoprevention of colonic aberrant crypt foci in Fischer rats by sulforaphane and phenethyl isothiocyanate. Carcinogenesis. 2000;21:2287–91.
49. Morse MA, Amin SG, Hecht SS, Chung FL. Effects of aromatic isothiocyanates on tumorigenicity, 06-methylguanine formation, and metabolism of the tobacco-specific nitrosamine 4-(methylnitrosamino)-l-(3-pyridyl)-l-butanone in A/J mouse lung. Cancer Res. 1989;49:2894–7.

50. Keum YS, Khor TO, Lin W, Shen G, Kwon KH, Barve A, Li W, Kong AN. Pharmacokinetics and pharmacodynamics of broccoli sprouts on the suppression of prostate cancer in transgenic adenocarcinoma of mouse prostate (TRAMP) mice: implication of induction of Nrf2, HO-1 and apoptosis and the suppression of Akt-dependent kinase pathway. Pharm Res. 2009;26:2324–31.
51. Finley JW, Ip C, Lisk DJ, Davis CD, Hintze KJ, Whanger PD. Cancer-protective properties of high-selenium broccoli. J Agric Food Chem. 2001;49:2679–83.
52. Myzak MC, Dashwood WM, Orner GA, Ho E, Dashwood RH. Sulforaphane inhibits histone deacetylase *in vivo* and suppresses tumorigenesis in apc-minus mice. FASEB J. 2006;20:506–8.
53. Smith TK, Lund EK, Johnson IT. Inhibition of dimethylhydrazine-induced aberrant crypt foci and induction of apoptosis in rat colon following oral administration of the glucosinolate sinigrin. Carcinogenesis. 1998;19:267–73.
54. Balansky R, Ganchev G, Iltcheva M, Steele VE, Flora SD. Prevention of cigarette smoke–induced lung tumors in mice by budesonide, phenethyl isothiocyanate, and *N*-acetylcysteine. Int J Cancer. 2010;126:1047–54.
55. Conaway CC, Wang CX, Pittman B, Yang YM, Schwartz JE, Tian D, McIntee EJ, Hecht SS, Chung FL. Phenethyl isothiocyanate and sulforaphane and their *N*-acetylcysteine conjugates inhibit malignant progression of lung adenomas induced by tobacco carcinogens in A/J mice. Cancer Res. 2005;65:8548–57.
56. Gills JJ, Jeffery EH, Matusheski NV, Moon RC, Lantvit DD, Pezzuto J m. Sulforaphane prevents mouse skin tumorigenesis during the stage of promotion. Cancer Lett. 2006;236:72–9.
57. Samaha HS, Kelloff GJ, Steele V, Rao CV, Reddy BS. Modulation of apoptosis by sulindac, curcumin, phenylethyl-3-methylcaffeate, and 6-phenylhexyl isothiocyanate: apoptotic index as a biomarker in colon cancer chemoprevention and promotion. Cancer Res. 1997;57:1301–5.
58. Izzotti A, Balansky RM, Agostini FD, Bennicelli C, Myers SR, Grubbs CJ, Lubet RA, Kelloff GJ, Flora SD. Modulation of biomarkers by chemopreventive agents in smoke-exposed rats. Cancer Res. 2001;61:2472–9.
59. Munday R, Mhawech-Fauceglia P, Munday CM, Paonessa JD, Tang L, Munday JS, Lister C, Wilson P, Fahey JW, Davis W, Zhang Y. Inhibition of urinary bladder carcinogenesis by broccoli sprouts. Cancer Res. 2008;68:1593–600.
60. Cornblatt BS, Ye L, Dinkova-Kostova AT, Erb M, Fahey JW, Singh NK, Chen MA, Stierer T, Garrett-Mayer E, Argani P, Davidson NE, Talalay P, Kensler TW, Visvanathan K. Preclinical and clinical evaluation of sulforaphane for chemoprevention in the breast. Carcinogenesis. 2007;28:1485–90.
61. Chen YJ, Walliq MA, Jeffery EH. Dietary broccoli lessens development of fatty liver and liver cancer in mice given diethylnitrosamine and fed a western or control diet. J Nutr. 2016;146:542–50.
62. Singh S, Singh K. Cancer chemoprevention with dietary isothiocyanates mature for clinical translational research. Carcinogenesis. 2012;33:1833–42.
63. Kensler WT, Chen JG, Egner PA, Fahey JW, Jacobson LP, Stephenson KK, Ye L, Coady JL, Wang JB, Wu Y, Sun Y, Zhang QN, Zang BC, Zhu YR, Qian GS, Carmella SG, Hecht SS, Benning L, Gange SJ, Groopman JD, Talalay P. Effects of glucosinolate-rich broccoli sprouts on urinary levels of aflatoxin-DNA adducts and phenanthrene tetraols in a randomized clinical trial in He Zuo township, Qidong, People's Republic of China. Cancer Epidemiol Biomark Prev. 2005;14:2605–13.
64. Cipolla BG, Mandron E, Lefort JM, Coadou Y, Negra ED, Corbel L, Scodan RL, Azzouzi AR, Mottet N. Effect of sulforaphane in men with biochemical recurrence after radical prostatectomy. Cancer Prev Res. 2015;8:712–9.

Garlic Preventive Effect on Cancer Development

Mostafa I. Waly and Mohammad Shafiur Rahman

1 Introduction

Today, millions of people are living with cancer or have had cancer. The risk of developing most types of cancer can be reduced by changes in a person's lifestyle or by adopting primary intervention strategies. Often, the sooner a cancer is found and treatment begins, the better are the chances for living for many years. Cancer is a disorder of cell proliferation and it is the leading global cause of death. Cancer research has traditionally focused on allocating bioactive components for the cancer prevention by eliminating cancerous cells and cellular carcinogenesis metabolites. Carcinogenesis is a multistage process that is distinguished with two steps; the first step is called initiation that occurs when cells are exposed to cancer-producing agents, which damage the cell's deoxynucleic acid. The second step is called promotion which occurs when the cancerous cells divided subsequently, and this post ignition step is characterized by neoplasia and DNA adducts formation. Cancer morbidity and mortality afflicts both genders, and at a global level, there are about 945,000 new cancer cases and 620,000 death cases annualy.

The field of complementary and alternative medicine has focused on the use of botanical medicines and nutritional therapies, such as antitumor bioactive agents in food and other natural products. Garlic is a commonly worldwide used food, and it is known for its antibacterial, anticarcinogenic, hypolipidemic, hypoglycemic, anti-fungal, and anti-atherosclerotic properties. Increasing evidence suggests that garlic consumption constituents are significantly decreasing cancer risk. Recently, garlic supplements protect against chemically induced carcinogenesis and oxidative stress in human-based clinical trials. This chapter provides in-depth molecular

M. I. Waly (✉) · M. S. Rahman
Department of Food Science and Nutrition, College of Agricultural and Marine Sciences,
Sultan Qaboos University, Muscat, Oman
e-mail: shafiur@squ.edu.om

© Springer International Publishing AG, part of Springer Nature 2018
M. I. Waly, M. S. Rahman (eds.), *Bioactive Components, Diet and Medical Treatment in Cancer Prevention*, https://doi.org/10.1007/978-3-319-75693-6_6

understanding of the specific mechanisms by which garlic acts as an effective dietary intervention for cancer prevention and therapy.

2 Medicinal Aspects of Allium Foods

Garlic (*Allium sativum* L.) along with onions, leeks, and chives represent the major allium foods that are known for centuries for their medicinal properties and have been used in many different centuries for human chronic disease treatment. Garlic is among the oldest of all cultivated plants being used as a food, having a unique taste and odor along with some medicinal qualities [1]. Folk medicine has continued to advocate garlic as an immune-stimulating dietary bioactive agent. Epidemiological studies have reported that high intake of allium vegetables were associated with a lower risk of stomach cancer [2]. It was observed that stomach cancer mortality was 13 times lower among cancer patients who consumed 20 g garlic per day than those who consumed 1 g garlic per day [3]. The Iowa Women's Health Study including 41,837 women showed the link between a high intake of garlic and a 3% reduced risk of colon cancer [4]. It was observed that a study of male health professionals in Shanghai, China, had lower risk of colon cancer with a consumption of garlic (two servings per week) as compared with that of nonconsumers of garlic [5]. A recent study reported that a diet rich in allium vegetables (10 g per day) reduced the risk of prostate cancer as compared with those men who consumed less than 2 g allium vegetables/day [6]. However, the data for other types of cancers were inconsistent and inconclusive.

3 Anticancer Effects of Garlic

Garlic (*Allium sativum*) and its organosulfur components have been shown to have anticancer properties. Human clinical studies have documented that the risk of stomach, colon, and prostate cancer has been decreased with garlic consumption [7]. Experimental models of cancer provided strong evidence that garlic and its organosulfur components are effectively inhibiting cancer development in human cultures cancer cells, including breast, colon, skin, and lung cancers [8–10]. Garlic contain 33 different organosulfur compounds in addition to 17 amino acids, vitamins, and micronutrients [11]. The allyl sulfur compounds formed by alliinase enzymatic activity when garlic is minced or crushed, such as allicin, water-soluble S-allylmercaptocysteine (SAMC) and S-allylcysteine (SAC), oil-soluble diallyl sulfide, (DAS), diallyl disulfide (DADS), and diallyl trisulfide (DATS), are accountable for the anticancer effects of garlic [12]. The characteristic odor of garlic is mainly from allicin and other oil-sulfur components which also contribute to cancer prevention by inhibiting the proliferation of human breast and gastric cancer cells [13, 14].

Yang et al. [15] reviewed the beneficial effects of the supplement of hydrogen sulfite in great significance for the treatment of diseases, such as cancer, glycometabolic disorders, and diabetes. They identified different methods including garlic as a source. Garlic is rich in sulfur-containing compounds and can be considered as an active hydrogen sulfite pool. Allicin (diallyl thiosulfinate) is commonly characterized in garlic. In aqueous solutions allicin decomposes to a number of reactive sulfur-containing compounds, including diallyl sulfide (DAS), diallyl disulfide (DADS), diallyl trisulfide (DATS), S-allylmercaptocysteine (SAMC), and S-allylcysteine (SAC), and these can release hydrogen sulfite in different manners [1, 16]. Inactivation of alliinase by heating prevented the formation of allyl sulfur compounds in garlic and blocking the garlic ability to inhibit carcinogenesis.

Previous studies have shown that SAMC inhibits growth, arrest cells at G2/M phase of the cell cycle, and induces apoptosis in a variety of cancer cell lines [17]. Further studies revealed that SAMC and SAC are associated with microtubule depolymerization and induce cleavage of pro-caspase-3 and poly(ADP-ribose) polymerase associated with inhibition of cancer cells growth, indicating their efficiency in chemoprevention of cancer [18]. A high concentration of SAC inhibited the proliferation of melanoma cells [19]. Pretreatment of cancer cells with SAC significantly reduced the incidence of cancer by increasing cyclooxygenase-2 inhibition, heme oxygenase-1 induction, and histone deacetylation inhibition [20]. SAC protect against carcinogenic-induced DNA adducts in a mechanism that involves the activation of phase II drug-metabolizing enzymes, glutathione-S-transferase and UDP-glucuronosyltransferase [21]. SAC prevents the formation of DNA adduct, which is a reliable marker for carcinogenesis based on the fact that cancer patients have significantly high level of DNA adduct as compared to negative controls [22].

Recent studies indicate that SAMC is a substrate for mitochondrial aspartyl aminotransferase; this reaction liberates pyruvate with the apparent concomitant formation of allyl mercaptan metabolites which might play a positive role in the antiproliferative properties of SAMC [23]. Other mechanisms might also be involved in the anticancer effects of SAMC and SAC which include the activation of extracellular signal related kinase phosphorylation during the entry of cells into the M phase with subsequent arrest of cells in this phase [24]. Also SAMC and SAC inhibit p34cdc2 kinase activity which is required for the G2/M phase of cell cycle progression [25]. The esophageal-gastric junction adenocarcinoma (AEG) is an aggressive tumor with high incidence and dismal prognosis, and 5-year survival rate still remains low. Yin et al. [10] demonstrated that DADS inhibited cell viability of OE19 cells and nontoxic doses of DADS were ≤ 10 μg/mL for a 24-h treatment. They observed that nontoxic doses blocked the metastasis of OE19 cells by suppressing MMPs, increasing u-PA and TIMPs, as well as altering the balance of MMPs/TIMPs. This was the result of suppressing NF-κB and PI3K/AKT signaling pathways.

Jurkowska et al. [26] observed the inhibition of proliferation of cancer cells (U87MG and SH-SY5Y U87MG cells) by DATS. They suggested that DATS can function as a donor of sulfane sulfur atom, transferred by sulfurtransferases, to sulfhydryl groups of cysteine residues of Bcl-2 and reduced the active form of Bcl-2 by

S-sulfuration. In addition, DATS acts as an antioxidant protein. It was observed that DATS regulates multiple cancer hallmark pathways including cell cycle, apoptosis, angiogenesis, invasion, and metastasis and suggested that it could be used as a cancer chemopreventive agent.

Zhu et al. [17] observed that S-allylmercaptocysteine (SAMC) (i.e., water-soluble organosulfur garlic derivative) suppressed tumors. They observed that SAMC suppressed human gastric cancer SGC-7901 cells when inoculated subcutaneously in BALB/c nude mice. The mice were treated with SAMC for 30 days when tumor was grown a specific size. It was observed that the growth was delayed and suggested that this activity may arise from its effects on the caspase activation and modulation of MAPK and PI3K/Akt signaling pathways.

Talib [27] studied the combined effects of garlic and lemon extract on the cancer-tumor (EMT6/P breast cancer cells). They observed that both extracts act synergistically against breast cancer in mice and 80% treated mice was cured. The inhibition was due to the angiogenesis, induced apoptosis, and systemic activation in the immune system. Wei et al. [28] observed that DATS dose-dependently inhibited HIF-1α transcriptional activity and hypoxia-induced hematogenous metastasis of MDA-MB-231 cells; thus efficient inhibition of HIF-1α expression was required for DATS to resist breast cancer. In another study, a total of 22 stabilized thiosulfinate derivatives were synthesized and screened for their in vitro antiproliferative activities against drug-sensitive (MCF-7) and multidrug-resistant (MCF-7/Dx) human adenocarcinoma breast cancer cells [13]. Seven compounds showed greater antiproliferative activity against MCF-7/Dx cells than allicin as observed from cell death, apoptosis, cell cycle progression, and mitochondrial bioenergetic function assays. These compounds were also selective towards multidrug-resistant (MDR) cells, altered cellular morphology and arrested the cell cycle at the G2/M phase.

4   Bioavailability of Garlic-Derived Compounds

Garlic-derived compounds are promising in the field of cancer prevention; however, their use in dietary intervention needs to clearly identify their bioavailability and pharmacokinetic. Allicin is rapidly metabolized both in vivo and in vitro, and could not be detected in human serum or urine [29]. Similarly, SAMC was not detected in human fluids (urine and blood) even after a large oral dose, but its sulfate metabolites were detected in the liver tissue [30]. The pharmacokinetic of SAC was well known, as it was rapidly absorbed in the intestine and was distributed mainly in blood, liver, and kidney [29].

5   Garlic as a Phytochemical Agent

Phytochemicals are nonnutritive components in plants that have beneficial health to human. Organosulfur compounds (such as allyl sulfides) in garlic are among these phytochemicals, and numerous cell culture and experimental studies revealed the protective effect of organosulfur compounds against the initiation and progression phases of carcinogenesis [31]. It is well documented that allyl sulfur compounds inhibited Phase I drug-metabolizing enzymes and suppressed carcinogen bioactivation [32]. In addition, these compounds exert their antiproliferative effects in cancer cells through impairing cell cycle progression, induction of apoptosis, modulation of signal transduction pathways, and altering profiles of gene expression [33]. Allyl sulfides act as antioxidants and scavenge free radicals, and thereby protecting DNA from oxidative damage and maintain genomic stability [34]. Taken all together, these effects contribute positively for the primary prevention of cancer specifically by preventing the formation of mutant cells and blocking the initiation stage of carcinogenesis, as well as eliminating damaged or mutated cells by induction of apoptosis.

6   Conclusion

The most important evidence that garlic is reducing the risk of cancer is based on epidemiological studies. Garlic is with potent antioxidant and anticancer properties; this synergistic effect was effective in reducing the risk of different types of cancers even though it was most effective in gastrointestinal tract cancers. The mechanism of cancer prevention has not been determined, although there is a possibility for induction of liver detoxification enzymes, suppressing mechanisms of cancerous cells growth, or DNA repair mechanisms.

References

1. Sultana S, Asif HM, Nazar HMI, Akhtar N, Rehman JU, Rehman RU. Medicinal plants combating against cancer—a green anticancer approach. Asian Pac J Cancer Prev. 2014;15(11):4385–94.
2. Turati F, Pelucchi C, Guercio V, La Vecchia C, Galeone C. Allium vegetable intake and gastric cancer: a case-control study and meta-analysis. Mol Nutr Food Res. 2015;59(1):171–9.
3. Lazarevic K, Nagorni A, Rancic N, Milutinovic S, Stosic L, Ilijev I. Dietary factors and gastric cancer risk: hospital-based case control study. J BUON. 2010;15(1):89–93.
4. Steinmetz KA, Kushi LH, Bostick RM, Folsom AR, Potter JD. Vegetables, fruit, and colon cancer in the Iowa Women's Health Study. Am J Epidemiol. 1994;139(1):1–15.
5. Nelson SM, Gao YT, Nogueira LM, Shen MC, Wang B, Rashid A, Hsing AW, Koshiol J. Diet and biliary tract cancer risk in Shanghai, China. PLoS One. 2017;12(3):e0173935.

6. Zhou XF, Ding ZS, Liu NB. Allium vegetables and risk of prostate cancer: evidence from 132,192 subjects. Asian Pac J Cancer Prev. 2013;14(7):4131–4.
7. Kim JY, Kwon O. Garlic intake and cancer risk: an analysis using the Food and Drug Administration's evidence-based review system for the scientific evaluation of health claims. Am J Clin Nutr. 2009;89(1):257–64.
8. Li X, Meng Y, Xie C, Zhu J, Wang X, Li Y, Geng S, Wu J, Zhong C, Li M. Diallyl trisulfide inhibits breast cancer stem cells via suppression of Wnt/β-catenin pathway. J Cell Biochem. 2017. https://doi.org/10.1002/jcb.26613.
9. Saini V, Manral A, Arora R, Meena P, Gusain S, Saluja D, Tiwari M. Novel synthetic analogs of diallyl disulfide triggers cell cycle arrest and apoptosis via ROS generation in MIA PaCa-2 cells. Pharmacol Rep. 2017;69(4):813–21.
10. Yin X, Feng C, Han L, Zhang Y, Zhang J. Diallyl disulfide inhibits the metastasis of type II esophageal-gastric junction adenocarcinoma cells via NF-κB and PI3K/AKT signaling pathways in vitro. Oncol Rep. 2018;39(2):784–94.
11. Tsubura A, Lai YC, Kuwata M, Uehara N, Yoshizawa K. Anticancer effects of garlic and garlic-derived compounds for breast cancer control. Anti Cancer Agents Med Chem. 2011;11(3):249–53.
12. Petropoulos S, Di Gioia F, Vegetable Organosulfur NG. Compounds and their health promoting effects. Curr Pharm Des. 2017;23(19):2850–75.
13. Roseblade A, Ung A, Bebawy M. Synthesis and in vitro biological evaluation of thiosulfinate derivatives for the treatment of human multidrug-resistant breast cancer. Acta Pharmacol Sin. 2017;38(10):1353–68.
14. Zhang X, Zhu Y, Duan W, Feng C, He X. Allicin induces apoptosis of the MGC-803 human gastric carcinoma cell line through the p38 mitogen-activated protein kinase/caspase-3 signaling pathway. Mol Med Rep. 2015;11(4):2755–60.
15. Yang C, Chen L, Xu S, Day JJ, Li X, Xian M. Recent development of hydrogen sulfide releasing/stimulating reagents and their potential applications in cancer and glycometabolic disorders. Front Pharmacol. 2017;8:664.
16. Amagase H. Clarifying the real bioactive constituents of garlic. J Nutr. 2006;136(Suppl. 3):716S–25S.
17. Zhu X, Jiang X, Li A, Sun Y, Liu Y, Sun X, Feng X, Li S, Zhao Z. S-allylmercaptocysteine suppresses the growth of human gastric cancer xenografts through induction of apoptosis and regulation of MAPK and PI3K/Akt signaling pathways. Biochem Biophys Res Commun. 2017;491(3):821–6.
18. Xiao D, Pinto JT, Gundersen GG, Weinstein IB. Effects of a series of organosulfur compounds on mitotic arrest and induction of apoptosis in colon cancer cells. Mol Cancer Ther. 2005;4(9):1388–98.
19. Xiao D, Pinto JT, Soh JW, Deguchi A, Gundersen GG, Palazzo AF, Yoon JT, Shirin H, Weinstein IB. Induction of apoptosis by the garlic-derived compound S-allylmercaptocysteine (SAMC) is associated with microtubule depolymerization and c-Jun NH(2)-terminal kinase 1 activation. Cancer Res. 2003;63(20):6825–37.
20. Park JM, Han YM, Kangwan N, Lee SY, Jung MK, Kim EH, Hahm KB. S-allyl cysteine alleviates nonsteroidal anti-inflammatory drug-induced gastric mucosal damages by increasing cyclooxygenase-2 inhibition, heme oxygenase-1 induction, and histonedeacetylation inhibition. J Gastroenterol Hepatol. 2014;29(Suppl 4):80–92.
21. Cho O, Hwang HS, Lee BS, Oh YT, Kim CH, Chun M. Met inactivation by S-allylcysteine suppresses the migration and invasion of nasopharyngeal cancer cells induced by hepatocyte growth factor. Radiat Oncol J. 2015;33(4):328–36.
22. Xu YS, Feng JG, Zhang D, Zhang B, Luo M, Su D, Lin NM. S-allylcysteine, a garlic derivative, suppresses proliferation and induces apoptosis in human ovarian cancer cells in vitro. Acta Pharmacol Sin. 2014;35(2):267–74.

23. Shirin H, Pinto JT, Kawabata Y, Soh JW, Delohery T, Moss SF, Murty V, Rivlin RS, Holt PR, Weinstein IB. Antiproliferative effects of S-allylmercaptocysteine on colon cancer cells when tested alone or in combination with sulindac sulfide. Cancer Res. 2001;61(2):725–31.

24. Liu Y, Yan J, Han X, Hu W. Garlic-derived compound S-allylmercaptocysteine (SAMC) is active against anaplastic thyroid cancer cell line 8305C (HPACC). Technol Health Care. 2015;23(Suppl 1):S89–93.

25. Yan JY, Tian FM, Hu WN, Zhang JH, Cai HF, Li N. Apoptosis of human gastric cancer cells line SGC 7901 induced by garlic-derived compound S-allylmercaptocysteine (SAMC). Eur Rev Med Pharmacol Sci. 2013;17(6):745–51.

26. Jurkowska H, Wrobel M, Kaczor-Kaminska M, Jasek-Gajda E. A possible mechanism of inhibition of U87MG and SH-SY5Y cancer cell proliferation by diallyl trisulfide and other aspects of its activity. Amino Acids. 2017;49:1855–66.

27. Talib WH. Consumption of garlic and lemon aqueous extracts combination reduces tumor burden by angiogenesis inhibition, apoptosis induction, and immune system modulation. Nutrition. 2017;43–44:89–97.

28. Wei Z, Shan Y, Tao L, Liu Y, Zhu Z, Liu Z, Wu Y, Chen W, Wang A, Lu Y. Diallyl trisulfides, a natural histone deacetylase inhibitor, attenuate HIF-1α synthesis, and decreases breast cancer metastasis. Mol Carcinog. 2017;56:2317–31.

29. Borlinghaus J, Albrecht F, Gruhlke MC, Nwachukwu ID, Slusarenko AJ. Allicin: chemistry and biological properties. Molecules. 2014;19(8):12591–618.

30. Majewski M. Allium sativum: facts and myths regarding human health. Rocz Panstw Zakl Hig. 2014;65(1):1–8.

31. Chen LY, Chen Q, Zhu XJ, Kong DS, Wu L, Shao JJ, Zheng SZ. Diallyl trisulfide protects against ethanol-induced oxidative stress and apoptosis via a hydrogen sulfide-mediated mechanism. Int Immunopharmacol. 2016;36:23–30.

32. Locatelli DA, Nazareno MA, Fusari CM, Camargo AB. Cooked garlic and antioxidant activity: correlation with organosulfur compound composition. Food Chem. 2017;220:219–24.

33. Zeng Y, Li Y, Yang J, Pu X, Du J, Yang X, Yang T, Yang S. Therapeutic role of functional components in alliums for preventive chronic disease in human being. Evid Based Complement Alternat Med. 2017;2017:9402849.

34. Beretta HV, Bannoud F, Insani M, Berli F, Hirschegger P, Galmarini CR, Cavagnaro PF. Relationships between bioactive compound content and the antiplatelet and antioxidant activities of six allium vegetable species. Food Technol Biotechnol. 2017;55(2):266–75.

Antioxidant and Health Properties of Beehive Products Against Oxidative Stress-Mediated Carcinogenesis

Hassan Talib Al-Lawati, Hajar Ibrahim Salim Al-Ajmi, and Mostafa I. Waly

1 Introduction

Environmental toxins and oxidizing agents are the common causes of oxidative stress in different biological systems. Oxidative stress is a common etiological factor of cancer in different human organs, and the oxidative stress-mediated carcinogenesis includes activation of oncogenic transcription factors, inhibition of antioxidant enzymes (catalase, glutathione-S-transferase, glutathione peroxidase, and superoxide dismutase), and depletion of glutathione, the major cellular antioxidant. Clinical studies continue to support the notion that different beehive products (honey, pollen, propolis, royal jelly, and venom) supplementation combats cancer development based on their antioxidant and health properties.

2 Beehive Products and Cancer

Apitherapy is known as the use of bee products in the treatment and prevention of diseases. The use of natural products and their active compounds in the treatment of various ailments is based majorly on traditional medical experiences in various ethnic communities in addition to epidemiological observations [1]. Beehive products have been used in traditional medicine from ancient time. Bioactive compounds found in raw content, crude extracts and purified bioactive substances found in them have been seen to exhibit several biological activities, such as

H. T. Al-Lawati (✉)
Department for Honey Bee Research, Ministry of Agriculture and Fisheries, Muscat, Oman

H. I. S. Al-Ajmi · M. I. Waly
Department of Food Science and Nutrition, College of Agricultural and Marine Sciences, Sultan Qaboos University, Muscat, Oman

© Springer International Publishing AG, part of Springer Nature 2018   97
M. I. Waly, M. S. Rahman (eds.), *Bioactive Components, Diet and Medical Treatment in Cancer Prevention*, https://doi.org/10.1007/978-3-319-75693-6_7

antioxidant, anti-inflammatory, and antimicrobial activities [2]. Bees have thrived worldwide in various localities, for more than 125 million years. The success in the use of bee products as a treatment is due to the different chemical compounds which they synthesize by themselves, such as honey, beeswax, royal jelly, propolis, bee venom, and pollen [3].

Apitherapy in which apis referred as a Latin word meaning bee is the treatment by using bee products including bee venom, propolis, and honey for disease treatment or prevention. Also, it can be defined as the science of using honeybee products, in maintaining health and assisting the person health. Beehives' products are currently used as dietary natural products and traditional medicine in the files of cancer [4].

2.1   Honey

Honey is a natural product made by honeybees (*Apis mellifera*) from secretions of plants and the nectar of blossoms or a combination of both. It has both enzymatic and non-enzymatic antioxidant activities [5]. It is commonly used as sweetener. It contains about 181 compounds and is primarily a mixture of sugars, the fructose (38%) and glucose (31%) are the most important and the moisture content is about 17.7%, total acidity 0.08%, and ashes constitute 0.18% [6]. It is well recognized as a supersaturated solution that in addition to sugar it also contains little amount of other compounds such as proteins, vitamins, organic acids, minerals, phenolic compounds, flavonoids, and enzymes (catalase, glucose oxidase, peroxides).

According to climatic and geographical conditions, different types of honey contain variety range of phytochemicals involving phenolic acids and polyphenols, which play a role as antioxidants. Modern studies have relived that the biological activities of honey are due to its polyphenolic contents, which are antiproliferative, antimicrobial, anti-inflammatory, and antioxidant activities [6]. There is a variation in the color of the honey collected by the bees due to the geographical origin and the mineral content, which often ranges from dark amber to water white. Honey flavor is dependent upon its color, commonly honey darkness is referred to the stronger quality and flavor [7].

Honey health advantage in the treatment of various diseases is related to its diverse phytochemically active compounds, specifically phenolic and flavonoids compounds. Several phenolic and flavonoids compounds have been found in honey, among them are caffeic acid, kaempferol, ferulic acid, pinobanksin, naringenin, pinocembrin, apigenin, genistein, vanillic, hesperetin, quercetin, gallic acid, ellagic acid, *p*-coumaric acid, luteolin, chrysin, and syringic acid. These compounds found in honey are commonly known to induce antitumor, anti-inflammatory, antiproliferative, antioxidant, anticancer, and antimetastatic biological effects. Thus, the inhibition role of honey against cancer cells and tumors can be attributed to the occurrence of these phenolic acids and flavonoids [8].

For centuries, honey has been used for its health and medicinal properties. It is rich in different types of phytochemicals with higher content of flavonoid and phenolic compounds which is related to its high antioxidant activity. Substances that induce strong antioxidant properties may have a preventive effect against the development of cancer as oxidative stress and free radicals help in inducing the formation of cancers. The phytochemicals in honey can be referred to as polyphenols and phenolic acids. Varity of polyphenols present in honey are known to have antiproliferative action against different types of cancer [9]. Researches about the effectiveness of crude honey in cancer are few. New researches have been conducted that illustrate the honey possesses apoptosis inducing capability.

Honey is used to induce apoptosis in patient colon cancer cells by stopping the cells at G1 phase. It was shown that honey having higher tryptophan and phenolic quantity was more powerful in the inhibition of the colon cancer cell proliferation. It was also illustrated that honey induced apoptosis was aid with PARP cleavage and Caspase-3 activation [10]. Honey has an antitumor activity similar to the chemotherapeutic drugs such as 5-fluorouracil and cyclophosphamide. Reports about anticancer effectiveness of honey range starting from tissue cultures and animal models to clinical trials. Polyphenols present in honey are proved as the major factors responsible for the anticancer action [8].

2.2 Pollen

Bee pollen grains are known as the male reproductive section of seed-bearing plants which consist of variety of nutrients and phytochemicals. Since ancient times, individuals around the world consume pollens to treat premature aging, anemia, flu, colds, colitis, and ulcers. It is now well reported that many bee pollen secondary metabolites have an effective health benefits [9]. Bee pollen is considered as apicultural product made for human diet because of its nutritional content. Its main content involves carbohydrates, fats, lipids, ashes, minerals, and vitamins, and flavonoids, which is known for its protection properties [10]. For bee survival, pollen grains are important as a major source of proteins. At the time of collecting trips, bees pack pollen grains from the flowers into pollen pellets on their hind legs with the support of many hairs and combs. Then, the pollen is stored inside the hive individually away from the nectar cells [11]. The antioxidant properties of bee pollen are very high and corresponded with the phenylpropanoid level; this notion is supported by a study in which different species of bee pollen have been investigated that showed great differences in the hydroxyl radical-scavenging activity and in the radical-scavenging activity [12].

2.3 Propolis

Propolis is defined as a resinous substance gathered by bees from the bark of trees especially conifer trees and the leaf buds. Propolis is used by bees in addition to bees wax to build their hives and in the defense of the bee community, strengthening and coating the inner walls of the hive [13]. Moreover it is used in covering cracks and holes and to repair combs, reducing the microbial growth on the walls of the hive, avoiding insect invasions, and preventing water and wind from going inside [14]. It is constructed as a gum secretion collected by bees from different plants, and can differ in color depending on the origin of plant species [15]. The process of collection of propolis from reddish resinous exudates of *D. ecastophyllum* by Africanized *Apis mellifera* involves first secretion of reddish exudates from a hole in a branch of the tree, collecting the reddish exudates and passing the collected exudates to the hind leg to make propolis [16]. Propolis resinous bee product is used recently worldwide, and a number of biological actions have been investigated, involving antioxidant, anti-inflammatory, anticancer, antifungal, and antibiotic activities (please see your whatsapp). This biological action of propolis is related to the natural active chemical compounds, such as phenolic acid and their esters, flavonoid, aglycones, polyphenols, caffeic acid and their esters and phenolic ketones and aldehydes [17]. In fact, the major constituents of propolis are fatty, aromatic, and aliphatic acids, sugars, terpenes, alcohols, esters, and flavonoids [18].

Clearly, propolis resulted by the water extraction consists of carbohydrates, organic matter, and amino acids that do not exist in the ethanol extraction. Propolis obtained by water extraction is commonly used as a cosmetics or food additive, because there is lower olfactory stimulation. Its main components are cinnamic acid derivatives and caffeoylquinic acid derivatives, and regarding on how the quality is, antibacterial activity can be established in variety of samples [19]. In nature, propolis consists of 50% resin and vegetable balsam, 30% wax, 10% essential and aromatic oils, 5% pollen, and other constituents [20].

Propolis helps in decreasing the chance and multiplicity of mammary carcinomas, suppressing tumor growth in a malignant tumor cell line, showing antitumor impact in mature mice-bearing Ehrlich carcinoma and preventing renal carcinogenesis enhanced by ferric nitrilotriacetate in mice. The major important components of propolis are flavonoids and phenolic acid, cinnamic derivatives involving caffeic acid phenyl esters (CAPE), as propolis and CAPE have similar pharmacological properties involving anticancer impact against liver, mammary, and renal carcinogenesis. Moreover, CAPE have a chemopreventive impact on human colon adenocarcinoma cell growth, induces carcinogen biochemical alterations, and preneoplastic lesions in rat colons [21].

Propolis has an antioxidant capacity that is related to its biological roles, involving chemoprevention. The main active compounds of water-extracted propolis were ranked in order caffeic acid, artepillin C, drupanin. The scavenging impact of caffeic acid was as effective as those of trolox, but stronger than those of vitamin C or *N*-acetyl cysteine [22]. There are synergistic and cooperative mechanisms between propolis and its polyphenolic compounds in the protection against reactive oxygen species-induced damage [23]. The effect of water-soluble propolis on tumor growth has concluded that the orally administered water-soluble propolis is significantly inhibiting the growth of transplanted tumors in animal models [24].

In vivo studies show that propolis can enhance antioxidant capacity in humans and animals, resulting in decrease of lipid peroxidation, which is highly linked with the risk of cancer, and the propolis antioxidant activity was attributed to its content of phenolic acids, flavonoids, amino acids, steroids, terpenes, ketones, and alde-hydes [25]. The flavonoids found in propolis are potential antioxidants, have the ability of scavenging free radicals and thereby have the ability in protecting the cell membrane versus lipid peroxidation. Cellular reactive oxygen species results in cel-lular damage and cancer development, and different compounds found in propolis have been suggested to have a potential inhibition ability against various reactive oxygen species [26]. Even though there is high variation in the composition of prop-olis, one of its main components, CAPE, helps in blocking reactive oxygen species production in many systems.

2.4   Royal Jelly

Royal jelly is a viscous and white jelly-like structure form of mandibular and hypopharyngeal gland secretion from the bee's worker. It is commonly referred as a "superfood" that is known to be consumed by the queen bee. Royal jelly is also consumed by the honeybee larvae upon hatching and helps to nurture the brood. Royal jelly is known to be used as a dietary nutritional mixture and its benefit to help combat different chronic health conditions. Moreover, many pharmacologi-cal actions such as antitumor, antibacterial, immunomodulatory, anti-inflamma-tory, and anti-allergy effects have also been established [19]. The exclusive food of the queen honeybee (Apis mellifera) larva is royal jelly. The chemical composi-tions of royal jelly consist of (50–60%) water, (18%) proteins, (15%) carbohy-drates, (3–6%) lipids, (1.5%) mineral salts, and vitamins in addition to a large number of bioactive compounds including 10-hydroxyl-2-decenoic acid with immunomodulation properties, antibacterial fatty acids, protein, and peptides. Also, the royal jelly showed significant enhancement in the recovery from 5-fluo-rouracil-induced damage [6]. Royal jelly has shown remarkable antioxidant prop-erties against different cancer cell lines such as colorectal (Caco-2), liver (HeP-G2), and breast (MCF-7) cancer cell lines [26].

2.5   Venom

Recent pharmacological reports suggested that bee venom has antitumor impacts by improving tumor cell apoptosis, inhibiting angiogenesis and migration, and block-ing tumor cell growth. Bee venom is known as a complex mixture of substances that help the bee colony in defending against a wide variety of predators involving arthropods and vertebrates. It is produced from the venom gland presented in the abdominal cavity and it consists of many biologically active peptides, involving mast cell degranulating peptide, adolapin, melittin, apamin, and several other enzymes, in addition to non-peptide constituents, such as dopamine, phospholipase A_2 (PLA$_2$), norepinephrine, and histamine. Traditionally, bee venom has been con-sumed by patients as a nonsteroidal anti-inflammatory drug for relieving their pain and for treating many chronic inflammatory diseases, including multiple sclerosis and rheumatoid arthritis, in addition to the treatment of tumors [27]. Bee venom therapy is known as applied therapeutic method of honeybee venom for treating different diseases. It has been applied as a traditional medicine in the treatment of various health conditions, such as cancerous tumors, back pain, skin diseases, rheumatism, and arthritis. Bee venom consists of nearly 18 active compounds, involving peptides, biogenic amines, and enzymes, which have various pharmaceutical benefits. It might alter the immune system work in the body and is related to the enhanced production of cortisol [27].

The neurotoxic and vasoactive constitutes of the venom, show a local reaction including tenderness, redness, swelling and pain at the location of the sting. Most people of the general population (20.7%) shows a hypersensitivity reaction of type 1, and sensitization can result in a wide range of medical signs, including a life-threatening systemic anaphylactic shock and a local edematic swelling of the skin [28].

The use of bee venom (api-toxin) in the treatment of several immune-related diseases, in addition to the treatment of tumors. Many cancer cells, involving lung, bladder, prostate, renal, mammary, and liver cancer cells in addition to leukemia cells, can be blocked by bee venom peptides such as phospholipase A and melittin [29]. Bee venom (BV) has been applied in the treatment of different disorders, and the major component of BV is melittin which is composed of 26 amino acids long chain peptide [30].

3 Conclusion

Beehive products are a good source of phytochemical constituents; therefore, it is recommended to be used as a dietary supplementation to enhance the antioxidant cellular capacity against oxidative stress. Long-term supplementation of beehives is needed to be developed as it has a synergistic and effective antioxidant and health properties against chronic diseases, including cancer.

References

1. Gajski G, Garaj-Vrhovac V. Melittin: a lytic peptide with anticancer properties. Environ Toxicol Pharmacol. 2013;36(2):697–705.
2. Premratanachai P, Chanchao C. Review of the anticancer activities of bee products. Asian Pac J Trop Biomed. 2014;4(5):337–44.
3. Inoue K, Saito M, Kanai T, Kawata T, Shigematsu N. Anti-tumor effects of water-soluble propolis on a mouse sarcoma cell line in vivo and in vitro. Am J Chin Med. 2008;36(03):625–34.
4. Badria F, Fathy H, Fatehe A, Elimam D, Ghazy M. Evaluate the cytotoxic activity of honey, propolis, and bee venom from different localities in Egypt against liver, breast, and colorectal cancer. J Apither. 2017;2(1):1–4.
5. Mouhoubi-Tafinine Z, Ouchemoukh S, Tamendjari A. Antioxydant activity of some algerian honey and propolis. Ind Crop Prod. 2016;88:85–90.

6. Viuda-Martos M, Ruiz-Navajas Y, Fernández-López J, Pérez-Álvarez J. Functional properties of honey, propolis, and royal jelly. J Food Sci. 2008;73(9):R117–24.
7. Jaganathan S, Mandal M. Antiproliferative effects of honey and of its polyphenols: a review. J Biomed Biotechnol. 2009;2:1–13.
8. Ahmed S, Othman N. Honey as a potential natural anticancer agent: a review of its mechanisms. Evid Based Complement Alternat Med. 2013;3:1–7.
9. Jannesar M, Shoushtari MS, Ahmad M, Pourpak Z. Bee pollen flavonoids as a therapeutic agent in allergic and immunological disorders. Iran J Allergy Asthma Immunol. 2017;16(3):171–8.
10. Erejuwa O, Sulaiman S, Wahab M. Effects of honey and its mechanisms of action on the development and progression of cancer. Molecules. 2014;19(2):2497–522.
11. Šarić A, Balog T, Sobočanec S, Kušić B, Šverko V. Antioxidant effects of flavonoid from Croatian Cystusincanus L. rich bee pollen. Food Chem Toxicol. 2009;47(3):547–54.
12. Ramadan MF, Al-Ghamdi A. Bioactive compounds and health-promoting properties of royal jelly: a review. J Funct Foods. 2012;4(1):39–52.
13. Leja M, Mareczek A, Wyżgolik G, Klepacz-Baniak J, Czekońska K. Antioxidative properties of bee pollen in selected plant species. Food Chem. 2007;100(1):237–40.
14. Najafi MF, Vahedy F, Seyyedin M, Jomehzadeh HR, Bozary K. Effect of the water extracts of propolis on stimulation and inhibition of different cells. Cytotechnology. 2007;54(1):49–56.
15. López BGC, Schmidt EM, Eberlin MN, Sawaya AC. Phytochemical markers of different types of red propolis. Food Chem. 2014;146:174–80.
16. Popova M, Dimitrova R, Al-Lawati H, Tsvetkova I, Najdenski H. Omani propolis: chemical profiling, antibacterial activity and new propolis plant sources. Chem Cent J. 2013;7(1):158–64.
17. Da Rocha A. Natural products in anticancer therapy. Curr Opin Pharmacol. 2001;1(4):364–9.
18. Carvalho A, Finger D, Machado C, Schmidt E, Costa P. In vivo antitumoural activity and composition of an oil extract of Brazilian propolis. Food Chem. 2011;126(3):1239–45.
19. Sawicka D, Car H, Borawska MH, Nikliński J. The anticancer activity of propolis. Folia Histochem Cytobiol. 2012;50(1):25–37.
20. Pasupuleti V, Sammugam L, Ramesh N, Gan S. Honey, propolis, and royal jelly: a comprehensive review of their biological actions and health benefits. Oxidative Med Cell Longev. 2017;7:1–21.
21. Borrelli F, Izzo A, Di Carlo G, Maffia P, Russo A. Effect of a propolis extract and caffeic acid phenethyl ester on formation of aberrant crypt foci and tumors in the rat colon. Fitoterapia. 2002;73:S38–43.
22. Nakajima Y, Tsuruma K, Shimazawa M, Mishima S, Hara H. Comparison of bee products based on assays of antioxidant capacities. BMC Complement Altern Med. 2009;9(1):4–8.
23. Oršolić N. Bee venom in cancer therapy. Cancer Metastasis Rev. 2012;31(1):173–94.
24. Waly MI, Al-Ajimi H, Al-Lawati HT, Guizani N, Rahman MS. In vivo and in vitro evidence of anticancer effects of Omani propolis against colon cancer. FASEB J. 2017;31(1):Supplement 790.22.
25. Vit P, Huq F, Barth O, Campo M, Pérez-Pérez E. Use of propolis in cancer research. Br J Med Med Res. 2015;8(2):88–109.
26. Aruoma OI. Free radicals, oxidative stress, and antioxidants in human health and disease. J Am Oil Chem Soc. 1998;75(2):199–212.
27. Stan SD, Kar S, Stoner GD, Singh SV. Bioactive food components and cancer risk reduction. J Cell Biochem. 2008;104(1):339–56.
28. Son D, Lee J, Lee Y, Song H, Lee C. Therapeutic application of anti-arthritis, pain-releasing, and anti-cancer effects of bee venom and its constituent compounds. Pharmacol Ther. 2007;115(2):246–70.
29. Peiren N, Vanrobaeys F, de Graaf D, Devreese B, Van Beeumen J, Jacobs F. The protein composition of honeybee venom reconsidered by a proteomic approach. Biochim Biophys Acta. 2005;1752(1):1–5.
30. Rady I, Siddiqui IA, Rady M, Mukhtar H. Melittin, a major peptide component of bee venom, and its conjugates in cancer therapy. Cancer Lett. 2017;28(402):16–31.

Chemopreventive Effect of Date Pit Extract

Mostafa I. Waly, Nejib Guizani, Ahmed Al Alawi,
and Mohammad Shafiur Rahman

1 Introduction

Clinical studies have claimed in general to show a correlation between high consumption of phenolic antioxidants and reduced risks of certain types of cancer. The main antioxidant activity that has been associated with polyphenols is the ability to scavenge free radicals. Prevention of cancer may be accomplished through primary prevention, secondary prevention, or a combination of these approaches. The objective of primary prevention is to prohibit effective contact of a carcinogenic agent with a susceptible target in the human body, so that the sequence of events that culminates in the occurrence of clinical cancer does not begin or is aborted at the start. Primary prevention of cancer might be implemented by fortifying the human diet with an effective dietary chemoprevention, among this approach is the date pit extract.

Phenolic compounds of date pit, mainly phenolic and flavonoids compounds, have been shown to possess antioxidant, antimutagenic, and anticarcinogenic properties. Pits of date palm are a waste product of many date-processing industries, after transformation of the date fruits into different products, and are used mainly for animal feeds in the cattle, sheep, and camel and poultry industries. Therefore, utilization of such waste is very important to develop value-added products, as a functional food of medicinal and therapeutic applications in special context to cancer. This chapter represents an attempt to identify the date plant pit extract on the basis of herbal medicine, coherent scientific reasoning, and inferences.

M. I. Waly (✉) · N. Guizani · A. Al Alawi · M. S. Rahman
Department of Food Science and Nutrition, College of Agricultural and Marine Sciences,
Sultan Qaboos University, Muscat, Oman
e-mail: guizani@squ.edu.om; shafiur@squ.edu.om

© Springer International Publishing AG, part of Springer Nature 2018
M. I. Waly, M. S. Rahman (eds.), *Bioactive Components, Diet and Medical Treatment in Cancer Prevention*, https://doi.org/10.1007/978-3-319-75693-6_8

2   Composition of Date Pit

Date palm is grown in many regions of the world, resulting in a surplus production of dates [1]. The date has been an important crop in arid and semiarid regions of the world. Main parts of date palm tree are: stems, leaves, flowers, fruits, and pits. Preclinical studies have shown that the date fruits possess free radical scavenging, antioxidant, antimutagenic, anti-inflammatory, gastroprotective, hepatoprotective, nephroprotective, anticancer, and immunostimulant activities [2]. It was stated that potent antioxidant and antimutagenic activities of dates implicate free radical scavenging activity [3]. In addition, Guo et al. [4] reported that dates had the second highest antioxidant value of 28 fruits commonly consumed in China. The observed antioxidant activity of dates has been attributed to phenolic compounds, anthocyanins, flavonoid glycosides, and procyanidins present in it [5, 6].

The date fruit is composed of a fleshy pericarp and seed which constitutes between 10 and 15% of date fruit weight [7]. Chemical and nutritional constituents of date pits were reported to have functional health properties [8]. Their reported composition was 3.10–7.10% moisture, 2.30–6.40% protein, 5.00–13.20% fat, 0.90–1.80% ash, and 22.50–80.20% dietary fiber. Also date pits contain high levels of phenolics, 3102–4430 mg gallic acid equivalents/100 g, antioxidants, 580–929 μm trolox equivalents/g, and dietary fiber 78–80 g/100 g [8]. Phenolic compounds in date pits are mainly phenolic acids and flavonids, which show to possess antioxidant, anticarcinogenic, antimutagenic, and anti-inflammatory activities [9, 10]. Phenolic acids and flavonoids in date palm fruit-extract was found to be useful for the prevention of oxidative stress induced hepatotoxicity [11]. Recent studies have indicated that the aqueous extracts of dates have potent antioxidant and antimutagenic activity [3, 6, 8, 12–14].

3   Polyphenolic Content of Date Pit

Over the past 10 years, researchers and food manufacturers have become increasingly interested in polyphenols. The main reason for this interest is the recognition of the antioxidant properties of polyphenols. They are widely found in natural products; nowadays they are extensively used in food and beverage industry and in pharmaceutical and nutraceutical industry for their positive effects on human health [15]. Polyphenols are a large and diverse class of compounds, many of which occur naturally in a range of food plants. Phenols (hydroxybenzenes) and especially polyphenols (containing two or more phenol groups) are ubiquitous in plant foods eaten within human and animal diets and, apart from known vitamins and minerals, may be one of the widest marketed groups of dietary supplement. This class of plant metabolites contains more than 8000 known compounds, ranging from simple phenols such as phenol itself to materials of complex and variable composition such as tannins [16].

Polyphenols may be further classified into four groups, according to the number of phenol rings they contain: flavonoids, phenolic acids, stilbenes, and lignans. The flavonoids may themselves be classified into the following subgroups: flavonols, flavones, isoflavones, flavanones, flavanols, and anthocyanidins [17]. Phenolic compounds, especially phenolic acids and flavonoids, are ubiquitously present in vegetables, fruits, seeds, tea, wines, and juices; thus, they are an integral part of the human diet [18].

Polyphenol contents in date pits varied from 21 to 62 mg gallic acid equivalents (GAE)/g date pits when acetone–water, ethanol–water, methanol–water, and water alone were used as solvents for extraction at temperatures 22, 45, and 60 °C [19]. Phenolic compounds of date pits, mainly phenolic acids and flavonoids, have been shown to possess antioxidant, anticarcinogenic, antimicrobial, antimutagenic, and anti-inflammatory activities [9, 10], as well as reduction of cardiovascular diseases. Thus, it is considered important to increase the antioxidant intake in the human diet and one way to achieve this by enriching food with phenolics. In acute toxicity experiment of date pits coffee, no mortality was recorded among groups of experimental rats given up to 42 mg/g rat body weight [20].

4   Antioxidant Effects of Date Pit

Polyphenols in date pit induce antioxidant enzymes such as glutathione transferase that will enhance the excretion of oxidizing species, and metallothionein, a metal-binding protein with antioxidant property [21]. It also inhibits cytochrome P450s or enzymes such as cyclooxygenase or lipoxygenase that have oxidant activities [16]. A significant consequence of oxidative stress is DNA damage, and it has been estimated that in tumor cells, the phenolic compounds of date pit combat oxidative stress and prevent oxidative stress-mediated DNA damage that might generate more mutations; activation of growth-promoting transcription factors and modulation of genes involved in carcinogenesis and uncontrolled cells proliferation [22, 23].

Interest has recently grown in the role and usage of natural antioxidants as a strategy to prevent oxidative damage in various health disorders with oxidative stress as a factor in their pathophysiology [24–27]. Dietary antioxidants in date pit increased the cellular antioxidant status, which is a major determinant to oxidative damage, and is usually altered in response to oxidative stress [28–30]. Increased oxidative stress and lipid peroxidation are being implicated in different types of human cancers [31].

Several studies indicated that the use of synthetic antioxidants has begun to be restricted because of their health risks and toxicity. Therefore, the importance of replacing synthetic antioxidants with natural ingredients from plant materials has greatly increased. Different components isolated from fruits and vegetable have been proven in model systems, being effective as antioxidants as synthetic antioxidants [27]. The extraction and purification of antioxidants from natural sources is desired, since these bioactive substances are often used in functional foods, food additives, nutraceuticals, pharmaceuticals, and cosmetic industries [32].

In order to neutralizing the threat of free radicals to the tissues and cells, a wide variety of antioxidant and repair systems have been evolved. Defense mechanisms against oxidative stress can be divided into: antioxidant, preventative and repair mechanisms, and physical defenses. Many enzymes that participate in free radical neutralizing processes include glutathione peroxidase, superoxide dismutase, and catalase. The non-enzymatic antioxidants that participate in oxidative stress defense include vitamin C, vitamin E, glutathione, carotenoids, and flavonoids. In the normal and healthy cells, there is a precise balance between free radicals production and the level of antioxidant molecules, but under oxidative stress condition, the balance has been tilted towards excessive of oxidative radicals [33].

The notion that prevention of any disease is preferable over treatment is widely accepted, and in this context, several studies suggest that regular consumption of fruits, vegetables, and spices has health benefits including risk reduction of developing a cancer [34]. Much of the protective effects have been attributed to phytochemicals such as polyphenols, terpenes, and alkaloids, present in low levels in plants [35]. Polyphenols in date pit include several hundreds of compounds and are the most studied groups [17].

Prevention of DNA damage by date pit is one of the cellular mechanisms that may prevent cancer, and this protective effect observed in many studies is due to the presence of phenolic constituents that have ability to act as antioxidant by free radical scavenging and chelating metal ions. Also, date pit modulates the antioxidant/oxidant balance by increasing levels of intracellular antioxidants such as glutathione, and by increasing the activity of antioxidant enzymes such as catalase, glutathione peroxidase, and superoxide dismutase [36–38].

5 Conclusion

Cancer treatment is costly; therefore, prevention strategies are crucial for primary prevention of this chronic disease. Date pits serve as a rich source of total phenolics and antioxidant activity that could potentially be considered as inexpensive source of natural antioxidants. The antioxidant function of date pit acted as a potent radical scavenger and efficiently improved the redox status of cells. In this chapter, date pit was found to function as an antioxidant as well as displaying anticarcinogenic potential by reducing in vivo oxidation effect mediated by oxidizing agents in different tissues. Therefore, date pits can be used as a functional food ingredient to increase the antioxidant intake in the human food chain diet by enriching food products with date pit. There is a need for further investigation to validate date pit efficacy as a phytonutrient against cancer and to its safety doses as a supplement.

References

1. Hamada JS, Hashim IB, Sharif FA. Preliminary analysis and potential uses of date pits in foods. Food Chem. 2002;76(2):135–7.
2. Baliga BRV, Baliga MS, Kandathil SM, Bhat HP, Vayalil PK. A review of the chemistry and pharmacology of the date fruits (*Phoenix dactylifera* L.). Food Res Int. 2011;44(7):1812–22.
3. Vayalil PK. Antioxidant and anti-mutagenic properties of aqueous extract of date fruit (*Phoenix dactylifera* L.). J Agric Food Chem. 2002;50:610–7.
4. Guo C, Yang J, Wei J, Li Y, Xu J, Jiang Y. Antioxidant activities of peel, pulp and seed fractions of common fruits as determined by FRAP assay. Nutr Res. 2003;23:1719–26.
5. Abdul A, Allaith A. Antioxidant activity of Bahraini date palm (Phoenix dactylifera L.) fruit of various cultivars. Int J Food Sci Technol. 2008;43:1033–1040.
6. Al Farsi M, Alasalvar C, Morris A, Baron M, Shahidi F. Compositional and sensory characteristics of three native sun-dried date (*Phoenix dactylifera* L.) varieties grown in Oman. J Agric Food Chem. 2005;53:7586–91.
7. Hussein AS, Alhadrami GA, Khalil YH. The use of dates and dates pits in broiler starter and finisher diets. Bioresour Technol. 1998;66:219–23.
8. Al-Farsi M, Alasalvar C, Al-Abid M, Al-Shoaily K, Al-Amry M, Al-Rawahy F. Compositional and functional characteristics of dates, syrups, and their by-products. Food Chem. 2007;104:943–7.
9. Diplock A, Charleux J, Wilii G, Koko K, Rice-Evans C, Roberfroid M. Functional food sciences and defense against reactive oxidative species. Br J Nutr. 1998;80:77–82.
10. Halliwell B. Antioxidants and human disease: a general introduction. Nutr Rev. 1997;55:44–52.
11. Saafi EB, Louedi M, Elfeki A, Zakhama A, Najjar MF, Hammami M, Achour L. Protective effect of date palm fruit extract (Phoenix dactylifera L.) on dimethoate induced oxidative stress in rat liver. Exp Toxicol Pathol. 2011;63:433–41.
12. Allaith AAA. Antioxidant activity of Bahraini date palm (*Phoenix dactylifera* L.) fruit of variouscultivars. Int J Food Sci Technol. 2007;19:119–28.
13. Biglari F, AlKarkhi AFM, Easa AM. Antioxidant activity and phenolic content of various date palm (Phoenix dactylifera) fruits from Iran. Food Chem. 2008;107:1636–41.
14. Saafi E, El Arem A, Issaoui M, Hammami M, Achour L. Phenolic content and antioxidant activity of four date palm (Phoenix dactylifera L.) fruit varieties grown inTunisia. Int J Food Sci Technol. 2009;44:2314–49.
15. Manach C, Scalbert A, Morand C, Remesy C, Jimenez L. Polyphenols: food sources and bioavailability. Am J Clin Nutr. 2004;79(5):727–47.
16. Ferguson L. Role of plant polyphenols in genomic stability. Mutat Res. 2001;475(1–2):89–111.
17. Ross JA, Kasum CM. Dietary flavonoids: bioavailability, metabolic effects, and safety. Annu Rev Nutr. 2002;22:19–34.
18. Kaur CH, Kapoor HC. Antioxidants in fruits and vegetables— the millennium's health. Int J Food Sci Technol. 2001;36:703–25.
19. Suresh S, Guizani N, Al-Ruzeiki M, Al-Hadhrami A, Al-Dohani H, Al-Kindi I, Rahman MS. Thermal characteristics, chemical composition and polyphenol contents of date-pits powder. J Food Eng. 2013;119(3):668–79.
20. Hussein MA, Abdullah MAE, Guinena AH, Abdel-Megeid SF, El Emary N. Adulteration of coffee by similarly treated seeds of dates (*Phoenix Dactylifera* L.). In: First symposium on date palm, Egypt, 1983. p. 560–2.
21. Aherne SA, Kerry JP, O'Brien NM. Effects of plant extracts on antioxidant status and oxidant-induced stress in Caco-2 cells. Br J Nutr. 2007;97:321–8.
22. Allen RG, Tresini M. Oxidative stress and gene regulation. Free Radic Biol Med. 2000;28:463–99.
23. Karihtala P, Soini Y. Reactive oxygen species and antioxidant mechanisms in human tissues and their relation to malignancies. APMIS. 2007;115:81–103.

24. Khan SM, Sobti RC, Kataria L. Pesticide-induced alteration in mice hepato- oxidative status and protective effects of black tea extract. Clin Chim Acta. 2005;358:131–8.
25. Koechlin-Ramonatxo C. Oxygen, stress oxidant supplementations anti-oxydantes ou un aspect different de la nutrition dans les maladies respiratoires. Nutr Clin Metab. 2006;20:165–77.
26. Mehmetcik G, Ozdemirler G, Koc-ak-Toker N, Cevikbas U, Uysal M. Effect of pretreatment with artichoke extract on carbon tetrachloride-induced liver injury andoxidativestress. Exp Toxicol Pathol. 2008;60:475–80.
27. Shireen KF, Pace RD, Mahboob M, Khan AT. Effects of dietary vitamin E, C and soybean oil supplementation on antioxidant enzyme activities in liver and muscles of rats. Food Chem Toxicol. 2008;46:3290–4.
28. Kiefer I, Prock P, Lawrence C, Wise J, Bieger W, Bayer P, et al. Supplementation with mixed fruit and vegetable juice concentrates increased serum antioxidants and folate in healthy adults. J Am Coll Nutr. 2004;23:205–11.
29. Pincemail J, Bonjean K, Cayeux K, Defraigne JO. Mecanismes physiologiques de la defense antioxidant. Nutr Clin Metab. 2002;16:233–9.
30. Prior RL, Cao G. Antioxidant phytochemicals in fruits and vegetables; diet and health implications. Hortic Sci. 2000;35:588–92.
31. Bartsch H, Nair J. New DNA-based biomarkers for oxidative stress and cancer chemoprevention studies. Eur J Cancer (Oxford, England: 1990). 2000;36(10):1229–34.
32. Shahidi F, Naczk M. Phenolics in food and nutraceuticals. Boca Raton: CRC Press; 2004. p. 1–80.
33. Conner EM, Grisham MB. Inflammation, free radicals, and antioxidants. Nutrition. 1996;12(4):274–7.
34. Terry P, Giovannucci E, Michels KB, Bergkvist L, Hansen H, Holmberg L, Wolk A. Fruit, vegetables, dietary fiber, and risk of colorectal cancer. J Natl Cancer Inst. 2001;93:525–33.
35. Adami H, Day NE, Trichopoulos D, Willett WC. Primary and secondary prevention in the reduction of cancer morbidity and mortality. Eur J Cancer. 2001;37:118–27.
36. Alia M, Ramos S, Mateos R, Bravo L, Goya L. Response of the antioxidant defense system to tert-butyl hydroperoxide and hydrogen peroxide in a human hepatoma cell line (HepG2). J Biochem Mol Toxicol. 2005;19:119–28.
37. Lima CF, Fernandes-Ferreira M, Pereira-Wilson C. Phenolic compounds protect HepG2 cells from oxidative damage: relevance of glutathione levels. Life Sci. 2006;79:2056–68.
38. Waly MI, Al-Ghafri BR, Guizani N, Rahman MS. Phytonutrient effects of date pit extract against azoxymethane—induced oxidative stress in the rat colon. Asian Pac J Cancer Prev. 2015;16(8):3473–7.

Nutrition and Colorectal Cancer Pathogenesis

Mostafa I. Waly and Amanat Ali

1 Introduction

The common etiological factors for cancer are obesity, nutritional deficiencies, smoking, radiation, environmental toxins, sedentary lifestyle, and aging. These factors cause cancer by damaging genes in combination with existing genetic mutation within cells. Epidemiological studies have shown that diet containing fruits and vegetables reduce the risk of several types of cancer. High intake of fruits and vegetables has an active role in the prevention of chronic disease associated with oxidative stress-mediated carcinogenesis. World Health Organization projects 10,000,000 cases of cancer per year worldwide and 6,000,000 mortality from cancer per year worldwide. It also projected 15 million cases/year in 2020. Cancers vary on the basis of age, gender, race, and genetic predisposition.

Despite the continuous advances in cancer treatment and early diagnosis, yet colorectal cancer (CRC) is still worldwide afflicting large numbers of people of all social classes. The CRC incidence is increasing rapidly in many countries where previous rates were low in the past years, indicating the existence of a common etiological factor as being the trigger for CRC occurrence in susceptible subjects. CRC is one of the commonest cancers and the third leading cause of cancer death. CRC incidence has decreased as a result of effective intervention and lifestyle changes in the West. The risk of CRC increases with age as 91% of cases are diagnosed in individuals aged 50 and older. Several modifiable factors are associated with increased risk of colorectal cancer; among these are obesity, physical inactivity, a diet high in red or processed meat, heavy alcohol consumption, and possibly smoking and inadequate intake of fruits and vegetables.

M. I. Waly (✉) · A. Ali
Department of Food Science and Nutrition, College of Agricultural and Marine Sciences,
Sultan Qaboos University, Muscat, Oman

© Springer International Publishing AG, part of Springer Nature 2018   111
M. I. Waly, M. S. Rahman (eds.), *Bioactive Components, Diet and Medical
Treatment in Cancer Prevention*, https://doi.org/10.1007/978-3-319-75693-6_9

Prevention of CRC remains a theoretic possibility and ought to be pursued, especially for patients whose family histories place them at high risk. Identifying genetic predisposition, dietary modifications, cessation of alcohol and tobacco use, and chemoprevention represent the spectrum of primary preventive measures. The role of genetic predisposition in CRC is most prominent for patients with familial polyposis, inflammatory bowel disease, a family history of colon cancer, and a family history of adenomatous polyps. The first two categories require aggressive and regular surveillance to identify the development and removal of early adenomas up to and including total colectomy. This chapter addresses different aspects of cancer pathogenesis and the role of nutrition in colorectal cancer prevention.

2   Cancer Pathogenesis and Stages

Cancers represent a heterogeneous group of diseases characterized by uncontrolled growth and spread of abnormal cells in the body. Cancer may affect people at all ages, even fetuses, but the risk for most varieties increases with age. The disruptive behaviors of cancer cells reflect dynamic changes in their genomes and in genes that result in disruption of normal regulatory signaling circuits. Cancers vary on the basis of both the biologic features of the disease and the characteristics of the affected organism. The process by which normal cells are transformed into cancer cells is known as carcinogenesis. Cancers are multifactorial diseases, with environmental and endogenous factors contributing at a different level in determining cancer risk [1, 2]. Cancer begins when cells in a part of the body start to grow out of control. There are many kinds of cancer, but they all start because of out-of-control growth of abnormal cells [3]. There are many different forms of cancer. Their manifestation is a growth of cells and tissues, which differ in various aspects from the surrounding tissue. Cancers occur in all living things. All life forms share similar deoxyribonucleic acid (DNA) and ribonucleic acid (RNA) blueprints and cell physiology. Therefore, the mechanisms for cancer development and methods for cancer treatment are similar [4].

Normal body cells grow, divide, and die in an orderly fashion. During the early years of a person's life, normal cells divide faster to allow the person to grow. After the person becomes an adult, most cells divide only to replace worn-out or dying cells or to repair injuries [3]. Nearly all cancers are caused by abnormalities in the genetic material of the transformed cells. These abnormalities may be due to the effects of carcinogens, such as tobacco smoke, radiation, chemicals, or infectious agents. Other cancer-promoting genetic abnormalities may be randomly acquired through errors in DNA replication, or are inherited, and thus present in all cells from birth. The heritability of cancers are usually affected by complex interactions between carcinogens and the host's genome. New aspects of the genetics of cancer pathogenesis, such as DNA methylation, and microRNAs are increasingly recognized as important. Genetic abnormalities found in cancer typically affect two general classes of genes. Cancer-promoting oncogenes are typically activated in cancer cells, giving those cells new properties, such as hyperactive growth and division, protection against programmed cell death, loss of respect for normal tissue boundaries, and the ability to become established in diverse tissue environments [5].

Cancer cells are formed from normal cells due to a modification, mutation of DNA and/or RNA. These modifications/mutations can occur spontaneously or they may be induced by other factors such as nuclear radiation, electromagnetic radiation (microwaves, X-rays, Gamma-rays, Ultraviolet-rays), viruses, bacteria and fungi, parasites (due to tissue inflammation/ irritation), heat, chemicals in the air, water, and food, mechanical cell-level injury, free radicals, evolution and aging of DNA and RNA, plus poor diet, stress, lack of proper exercise, and lack of sufficient rest and sleep. All these can produce mutations that may start cancer. Cancer can be called therefore "Entropic Disease" since it is associated with the increase of entropy of the organism to the point where the organism cannot correct this itself. External intervention is required to allow the organism to return to a stable entropic state [6]. Although the relatively small risks associated with low-level exposure to carcinogens in air, food, or water are difficult to detect in epidemiological studies, scientific and regulatory bodies throughout the world have accepted the principle that it is reasonable and prudent to reduce human exposure to substances shown to be carcinogenic at higher levels of exposure [6].

The transformation of a normal cell to a cancer cell occurs through three distinct phases, initiation, promotion, and progression. Initiation of cancer occurs in the normal cells due to exposure of carcinogenic and mutagenic agents. The initiated cells are irreversibly altered and are at greater risk of neoplastic transformation. However, initiation alone is not sufficient for tumor formation [7]. In promotion phase, tumor promoters convert the initiated cells into neoplastic cells [8]. Progression involves a stepwise evolution of neoplastic cells into higher degree of malignancy [7, 8]. In clinical practice, cancer is divided into five stages: stage 0, 1, 2, 3, and 4. In stage 0 cancer cells are found in one tissue area and have not invaded normal surrounding tissue, whereas in stage 1 and 2, cancer is found only in the organ where it started to grow. Stage 3 is also known as regional and here cancer cells start to spread to the surrounding tissues or lymph nodes, metastasis [9]. Eventually it moves to other organs and systems of the body in stage 4, the last stage of cancer [9].

3   Colorectal Cancer

Cancer of the large bowel is a major health problem. Worldwide each year, over 900,000 new cases are diagnosed, and almost 500,000 people die from the disease [3]. About two-thirds of the incident cases occur in developed countries, where colorectal cancer is the third most common cancer in men and second most common in women [8]. Relatively few colorectal cancers occur in persons younger than 40. Rates increase rapidly with age thereafter, more markedly for colon than for rectal cancer [9]. The burden of colorectal cancer is, therefore, expected to increase in the future as a result of population aging and increased life expectancy. This is particularly true for developing countries [3]. Colorectal cancer ranks second in terms of incidence and mortality in more developed countries. There is a significant geographical variation in age-standardized incidence rates that vary approximately 20-fold around the world with high rates occurring in countries of Europe, North America, Australia, and Japan. Although the colon and rectum have different etiological background, they are usually considered together. Migrants groups from low incidence countries rapidly reach the higher level of adopted country, suggesting that environmental factors play an important role in etiology [10].

Large bowel cancer is predominant in affluent societies and most frequent in North America, Western Europe, Australia, New Zealand, and the southern part of South America. CRC is the third most commonly diagnosed cancer and the third leading cause of cancer death in both men and women in the USA [11]. Colon cancer is cancer that starts in the large intestine or the rectum. Such cancer is sometimes referred to as "colorectal cancer." Other types of colon cancer such as lymphoma, carcinoid tumors, melanoma, and sarcomas are rare. The term "colon cancer" refers to colon carcinoma and not these rare types of colon cancer. CRC ranks second in terms of incidence and mortality in more developed countries. There is a significant geographical variation in age-standardized incidence rates that vary approximately 20-fold around the world with high rates occurring in countries of Europe, North America, Australia, and Japan. Although the colon and rectum have different etiological background, they are usually considered together. Migrants groups from low incidence countries rapidly reach the higher level of adopted country, suggesting that environmental factors play an important role in etiology.

Many epidemiologic studies have indicated that the risks of CRC include genetic predisposition, modern lifestyle, environmental toxins, high consumption of red meat, alcohol, and low intakes of vegetables and fruits [12]. Among all of these etiological factors, the role of diet remains an effective approach for primary intervention for CRC. Recent case-control studies have shown that low or moderate intake of folate and B_{12} results in impairment of methylation reactions, including DNA hypomethylation which is thought to be the trigger of tumorigenesis in human cells [13]. In addition, low intakes of folate and vitamin B_{12} decrease the antioxidant capacity of human cells with a consequent reduction in glutathione, the major intracellular antioxidant. Oxidative stress has been associated with different types of cancers [14]. In developing countries, CRC account for just 2.5% of all cancers. Almost all colorectal cancers are adenocarcinomas. The incidence rate is a little higher in North Africa than in sub-Saharan Africa [15].

Environmental factors such as diet and alcohol intake also differ in their role in the development of tumors in the three segments, proximal colon, distal colon, and rectum. Proximal shift of colon cancer has been known for some time, and survival rates of colorectal cancer are higher when rectal cancers are excluded, both of which emphasize the three different segments of colorectal cancer and their different properties [16]. Meanwhile, colonic and rectal cancers are distinctive therapeutic entities. The concept of three entities of colorectal cancer may be important in designing clinical trials or therapeutic strategies [17]. CRC is malignant cells found in the colon or rectum. Because colon cancer and rectal cancer have many features in common, they are sometimes referred to together as colorectal cancer. Colon cancer is cancer that starts in the large intestine (colon) or the rectum (end of the colon). Other types of colon cancer such as lymphoma, carcinoid tumors, melanoma, and sarcomas are rare [17].

CRC is a disease in which cancerous growths (tumors) are found in the tissues of the colon and/or rectum. The colon is the upper five to six feet of the large intestine; the rectum is the last 15 inches of the colon [7, 8]. It usually develops slowly over a period of many years, and usually begins as a noncancerous polyp, which may eventually change into cancer. A polyp is a growth of tissue that develops on the lining of the colon or rectum. Certain kinds of polyps, called adenomatous polyps or adenomas, are most likely to become cancers, although most adenomas do not become cancerous. More than half of all individuals will eventually develop one or more adenomas. About 96% of colorectal cancers are adenocarcinomas, which evolve from glandular tissue. The great majority of colon and rectum cancers arise from an adenomatous polyp, which is visible through a scope or on an X-ray [18].

Globally CRC is one of the commonest cancers and the third leading cause of cancer death. CRC incidence has decreased as a result of effective intervention and lifestyle changes in the West. The risk of colorectal cancer increases with age; 91% of cases are diagnosed in individuals aged 50 years and older. Several modifiable factors are associated with increased risk of colorectal cancer. Among these are obesity, physical inactivity, a diet high in red or processed meat, heavy alcohol consumption, and possibly smoking and inadequate intake of fruits and vegetables. Studies indicate that compared to healthy-weight individuals, men and women who are overweight are more likely to develop and die from colorectal cancer. Colorectal cancer risk is also increased by certain inherited genetic mutations [familial adenomatous polyposis (FAP) and hereditary non-polyposis colorectal cancer (HNPCC), also known as Lynch syndrome], a personal or family history of colorectal cancer and/or polyps, or a personal history of chronic inflammatory bowel disease [19].

The exact cause of most colorectal cancer is unknown, but the known risk factors are the most likely causes. Less than 10% of CRC are caused by inherited gene mutations. People with a family history of colorectal cancer may wish to consider genetic testing. The American Cancer Society suggests that anyone undergoing such tests have access to a physician or geneticist qualified to explain the significance of these test results. According to the American Cancer Society, colorectal cancer is one of the leading causes of cancer-related deaths in the United States (however, early diagnosis often leads to a complete cure). There is no single cause for colon cancer. Nearly all colon cancers begin as noncancerous (benign) polyps, which slowly develop into cancer [18, 19].

4   Nutrition and Colorectal Cancer

It has been estimated that 30–40% of all CRC tumors can be prevented with a correct lifestyle and diet [20]. CRC is a preventable disease. When people migrate from low incidence countries, such as Japan or Africa, to a high incidence country such as the United States, the rates of disease among their offspring increase to those of their adopted country. This indicates that there is something in the environment that is responsible. There is about a ninefold difference in the incidence of colorectal cancer in the highest risk countries compared to the lowest risk countries. Based on these differences in incidence and the experience of migrants, experts have estimated that as much as 80% of colorectal cancer might be explained by environmental factors. The term "environment" in this instance does not refer to air or water pollution, but rather to dietary and lifestyle factors that are part of our environment. Although the environment is central to the etiology of most colorectal cancers, individual genetically determined susceptibility is also important, as well as to understand gene-environment interaction as it relates to colorectal cancer risk. The implications of an environmental cause of colon cancer are clear. If we could identify and modify the relevant environmental factors, we could prevent most colorectal cancer.

Diet has received the greatest attention for obvious reasons—diet is a factor that changes markedly with migration and acculturation. Moreover, what we eat ends up in our colon, in one form or another. There have been a large number of studies of diet and colon cancer. It was summarized that the information on dietary and lifestyle factors that have been linked with colorectal cancer were qualitative and subjective [10, 20]. The comparison of CRC incidence in various countries strongly suggests that sedentarily, high caloric intake, and perhaps a diet high in meat (red or processed) could increase the risk of colorectal cancer. In contrast, a healthy body weight, physical fitness, and good nutrition decreases cancer risk in general. Accordingly, lifestyle changes could decrease the risk of colorectal cancer as much as 60–80% [21]. Fruits and vegetables have received much interest because they contain numerous substances (vitamins, minerals and fiber) with anticarcinogenic activity. Case-control studies concluded that diets high in fruits and vegetables were consistently associated with lower risk of some, but not all, cancers [22]. In addition, the world cancer research fund (WCRF) panel concluded that the consumption of fruits and vegetables has been consistently associated with a reduced risk of human cancers at many sites, reduced risk of adenomas and especially of colon cancer [23].

Consumption of diets rich in cruciferous vegetables (broccoli, cabbage, and cauliflower) appears to be associated with a reduction in the risk of cancer of the colon and rectum. These vegetables are rich in isothiocyanate compounds. Animal studies have shown that diets rich in these substances are chemopreventive, when provided before chemical carcinogens, but when they are administered after the carcinogen they increase tumorigenesis [24]. Fruits and vegetables are rich in dietary antioxidants, vitamin C, and β-carotenoids. High consumption of foods rich in these antioxidants results in a decreased risk for many cancers, including colorectal and lung [25]. A high intake of dietary fiber (from eating fruits, vegetables, cereals, and other high-fiber food products) has, until recently, been thought to reduce the risk of colorectal cancer and adenoma; it has been found that a fiber-rich diet does not reduce the risk of colon cancer [12]. The Harvard School of Public Health states: "Health Effects of Eating Fiber: Long heralded as part of a healthy diet, fiber appears to reduce the risk of developing various conditions, including heart disease, diabetes, diverticular disease, and constipation [12]. Despite what many people may think, however, fiber probably has little, if any effect on colon cancer risk" [12, 26].

Cohort studies concluded that diets high in total fat increases the risk of lung, colorectal, breast, and prostate cancers. Fat intake, owing to its high caloric density, increased risk of obesity, an indirect risk factor for endometrial, postmenopausal breast and renal cancers [27]. Total fat intake includes saturated, monounsaturated, and polyunsaturated fats. Saturated fats are derived from animal fat and are associated with greater risk of cancer, meanwhile monounsaturated fat intake, and the primary source is olive oil, has been hypothesized as a protective measure against cancer. Polyunsaturated fats include the n-3 fatty acids, conjugated linolenic acids (CLA) that are derived largely from fatty fish, and *trans* fatty acids present in variable quantities in hydrogenated oils and fast foods [28, 29]. CLA polyunsaturated fatty acids are well documented in preventing chemical carcinogens and are found mainly in dairy fats, milk, and cheeses. The CLA amounts in foods are not well documented in food composition tables, so human exposures are difficult to quantify in epidemiological studies [30, 31].

5   Conclusion

Regular screening examinations by a health care professional can result in the detection and removal of precancerous growths, as well as the diagnosis of cancers at an early stage, when they are most treatable. CRC is among cancers that can be diagnosed early through screening and early detection; this approach has been proven to reduce CRC mortality. In the majority of people CRC can be prevented with proper lifestyle modifications which include low-entropy diet, exercise, sleep, and stress reduction. In most cases cancer develops slowly over many years. With a positive change of lifestyle and healthy environment this trend can be reversed in the majority of CRC diagnosed patients. CRC etiology is complex and involves both genetic and environmental factors. Among the environmental factors, the dietary habits play a major role. Low intake of fibers, fruit, and vegetables and high intake of fat have been linked with increased risk of CRC. Therefore, dietary recommendations have been established to encourage people to change their dietary habits. Dietary fat and protein strongly correlate with the incidence of CRC, while low-fat, high-fiber, high-calcium diets, and diets with a high vegetable content appeared to be protective.

Dietary factors that have been studied for their possible role in the cause of colon and rectum cancer include high intake of red meat, alcohol, refined sugar, saturated/animal fat, and processed meat. Meanwhile high intake of fruits and vegetables acts as a preventive factor against colon and rectum cancer occurrence. Molecular biology studies indicate that micronutrients deficiencies, particularly folate and vitamin B_{12}, induce carcinogenesis in susceptible persons, via mechanisms that involve cell signaling, cell division, and DNA methylamines. There is robust evidence from cross-sectional and longitudinal studies to support that an energy-dense, high fat diet and physical inactivity are independent risk factors for weight gain and obesity. Overweight and obesity are established risk factors for CRC, as supported by both animal studies and human epidemiologic studies.

Many studies have revealed that dietary fiber contributes quantitatively to colorectal cancer risk or prevention. The protective effect of high intake of dietary fiber against colorectal cancer is mainly due to two major's mechanisms; firstly fiber decreases fecal transit time so it diminishes the exposure time of stool with toxins to epithetical cells. Secondly dietary fiber adsorbs stool toxins thus protecting the colonic epithelial cells. In the west the primary preventive measures for CRC include maintaining a healthy body weight, being physically active, and minimizing consumption of red meat and alcohol. In addition, early screening of colorectal cancer in the west results in early detection of the disease and removal of colorectal polyps before they become cancerous; therefore, the mortality rate of CRC in the west is lower than that in the developing countries.

References

1. Dereu D, Savoldelli GL, Combescure C, Mathivon S, Rehberg B. Development of a simple preoperative risk score for persistent pain after breast cancer surgery: a prospective observational cohort study. Clin J Pain. 2017. https://doi.org/10.1097/AJP.0000000000000575.
2. Lee AYY. When can we stop anticoagulation in patients with cancer-associated thrombosis? Hematology. Am Soc Hematol Educ Program. 2017;2017(1):128–35.
3. Hughes LAE, Simons CCJM, van den Brandt PA, van Engeland M, Weijenberg MP. Lifestyle, diet, and colorectal cancer risk according to (epi)genetic instability: current evidence and future directions of molecular pathological epidemiology. Curr Colorectal Cancer Rep. 2017;13(6):455–69.
4. Fagunwa IO, Loughrey MB, Coleman HG. Alcohol, smoking and the risk of premalignant and malignant colorectal neoplasms. Best Pract Res Clin Gastroenterol. 2017;31(5):561–8.
5. Boscolo-Rizzo P, Furlan C, Lupato V, Polesel J, Fratta E. Novel insights into epigenetic drivers of oropharyngeal squamous cell carcinoma: role of HPV and lifestyle factors. Clin Epigenetics. 2017;9:124.
6. Yahyapour R, Motevaseli E, Rezaeyan A, Abdollahi H, Farhood B, Cheki M, Najafi M, Villa V. Mechanisms of radiation bystander and non-targeted effects: implications to radiation carcinogenesis and radiotherapy. Curr Radiopharm. 2017. https://doi.org/10.2174/1874471011666171229123130.
7. Vela CM, Grate LM, McBride A, Devine S, Andritsos LA. A retrospective review of fall risk factors in the bone marrow transplant inpatient service. J Oncol Pharm Pract. 2017. https://doi.org/10.1177/1078155217697485.

8. Kolak A, Kamińska M, Sygit K, Budny A, Surdyka D, Kukiełka-Budny B, Burdan F. Primary and secondary prevention of breast cancer. Ann Agric Environ Med. 2017;24(4):549–53.

9. Jabir NR, Anwar K, Firoz CK, Oves M, Kamal MA, Tabrez S. An overview on the current status of cancer nanomedicines. Curr Med Res Opin. 2017;26:1–22.

10. Gigic B, Boeing H, Toth R, Böhm J, Habermann N, Scherer D, Schrotz-King P, Abbenhardt-Martin C, Skender S, Brenner H, Chang-Claude J, Hoffmeister M, Syrjala K, Jacobsen PB, Schneider M, Ulrich A, Ulrich CM. Associations between dietary patterns and longitudinal quality of life changes in colorectal cancer patients: the colocare study. Nutr Cancer. 2018;70(1):51–60.

11. Hu Y, Ding M, Yuan C, Wu K, Smith-Warner SA, Hu FB, Chan AT, Meyerhardt JA, Ogino S, Fuchs CS, Giovannucci EL, Song M. Association between coffee intake after diagnosis of colorectal cancer and reduced mortality. Gastroenterology. 2017. pii: S0016-5085(17)36368-0. https://doi.org/10.1053/j.gastro.2017.11.010.

12. van Zutphen M, Kampman E, Giovannucci EL, van Duijnhoven FJB. Lifestyle after colorectal cancer diagnosis in relation to survival and recurrence: a review of the literature. Curr Colorectal Cancer Rep. 2017;13(5):370–401.

13. Beeken RJ, Croker H, Heinrich M, Obichere A, Finer N, Murphy N, Goldin R, Guppy NJ, Wilson R, Fisher A, Steptoe A, Gunter MJ, Wardle J. The impact of diet-induced weight loss on biomarkers for colorectal cancer: an exploratory study (INTERCEPT). Obesity (Silver Spring). 2017;25(Suppl 2):S95–S101.

14. de Vries E, Quintero DC, Henríquez-Mendoza G, Herrán OF. Population attributable fractions for colorectal cancer and red and processed meats in Colombia—a macro-simulation study. Colomb Med (Cali). 2017;48(2):64–9.

15. Asadi K, Ferguson LR, Philpott M, Karunasinghe N. Cancer-preventive properties of an anthocyanin-enriched sweet potato in the APC(MIN) mouse model. J Cancer Prev. 2017;22(3):135–46.

16. Mehra K, Berkowitz A, Sanft T. Diet, physical activity, and body weight in cancer survivorship. Med Clin North Am. 2017;101(6):1151–65.

17. Reblin M, Birmingham WC, Kohlmann W, Graff T. Support and negation of colorectal cancer risk prevention behaviors: analysis of spousal discussions. Psychol Health Med. 2017;6:1–7.

18. Fan Y, Jin X, Man C, Gao Z, Wang X. Meta-analysis of the association between the inflammatory potential of diet and colorectal cancer risk. Oncotarget. 2017;8(35):59592–600.

19. Egnell M, Fassier P, Lécuyer L, Gonzalez R, Zelek L, Vasson MP, Hercberg S, Latino-Martel P, Galan P, Druesne-Pecollo N, Deschasaux M, Touvier M. Antioxidant intake from diet and supplements and risk of digestive cancers in middle-aged adults: results from the prospective NutriNet-Santé cohort. Br J Nutr. 2017;118(7):541–9.

20. Donovan MG, Selmin OI, Doetschman TC, Romagnolo DF. Mediterranean diet: prevention of colorectal cancer. Front Nutr. 2017;4:59.

21. Akinyemiju T, Moore JX, Pisu M. Mediating effects of cancer risk factors on the association between race and cancer incidence: analysis of the NIH-AARP Diet and Health Study. Ann Epidemiol. 2017;17:S1047–2797.

22. Jain A, Tiwari A, Verma A, Jain SK. Vitamins for cancer prevention and treatment: an insight. Curr Mol Med. 2017;17(5):321–40. https://doi.org/10.2174/1566524018666171205113329.

23. Schwingshackl L, Schwedhelm C, Hoffmann G, Knüppel S, Laure Preterre A, Iqbal K, Bechthold A, De Henauw S, Michels N, Devleesschauwer B, Boeing H, Schlesinger S. Food groups and risk of colorectal cancer. Int J Cancer. 2017. https://doi.org/10.1002/ijc.31198.

24. Tollosa DN, Van Camp J, Huybrechts I, Huybregts L, Van Loco J, De Smet S, Sterck E, Rabâi C, Van Hecke T, Vanhaecke L, Vossen E, Peeters M, Lachat C. Validity and reproducibility of a food frequency questionnaire for dietary factors related to colorectal cancer. Forum Nutr. 2017;9(11):pii:E1257. https://doi.org/10.3390/nu9111257.

25. Zhao Z, Feng Q, Yin Z, Shuang J, Bai B, Yu P, Guo M, Zhao Q. Red and processed meat consumption and colorectal cancer risk: a systematic review and meta-analysis. Oncotarget. 2017;8(47):83306–14.

26. Song M, Wu K, Meyerhardt JA, Ogino S, Wang M, Fuchs CS, Giovannucci EL, Chan AT. Fiber intake and survival after colorectal cancer diagnosis. JAMA Oncol. 2018;4(1):71–9. https://doi.org/10.1001/jamaoncol.2017.3684.
27. Sasso A, Latella G. Dietary components that counteract the increased risk of colorectal cancer related to red meat consumption. Int J Food Sci Nutr. 2017;2:1–13.
28. Brandão D, Ribeiro L. Dietary fatty acids modulation of human colon cancer cells: mechanisms and future perspectives. Int J Food Sci Nutr. 2017:1–14.
29. Watson H, Mitra S, Croden FC, Taylor M, Wood HM, Perry SL, Spencer JA, Quirke P, Toogood GJ, Lawton CL, Dye L, Loadman PM, Hull MA. A randomised trial of the effect of omega-3 polyunsaturated fatty acid supplements on the human intestinal microbiota. Gut. 2017. pii: gutjnl-2017-314968. https://doi.org/10.1136/gutjnl-2017-314968.
30. Lee JY, Sim TB, Lee JE, Na HK. Chemopreventive and chemotherapeutic effects of fish oil derived omega-3 polyunsaturated fatty acids on colon carcinogenesis. Clin Nutr Res. 2017;6(3):147–60.
31. Zhang LJ, Chen B, Zhang JJ, Li J, Yang Q, Zhong QS, Zhan S, Liu H, Cai C. Serum polyunsaturated fatty acid metabolites as useful tool for screening potential biomarker of colorectal cancer. Prostaglandins Leukot Essent Fatty Acids. 2017;120:25–31.

Modifiable and Non-modifiable Risk Factors for Colon and Rectal Cancer

Smitha Padmanabhan, Mostafa I. Waly, Varna Taranikanti, Nejib Guizani, Mohammad S. Rahman, Amanat Ali, Zaher Al-Attabi, and Richard C. Deth

1 Introduction

Colorectal cancer (CRC) is the world's third most common cancer. Before the twentieth century, CRC was relatively uncommon; however, the incidence has risen dramatically especially in the last 50 years. Several risk factors have been proposed, including the adoption of westernized diet, obesity, and physical inactivity. The majority of colorectal cancer continues to occur in industrialized countries. According to the recent studies, CRC is associated with several modifiable and non-modifiable risk factors. These risk factors involve CRC history in first-degree relative, inflammatory bowel disease, consumption of red meat, fruit, and vegetables, cigarette smoking, body mass index to overall population, race, gender, personal habit of alcohol consumption and smoking, ethnicity diabetes, and physical activity. Here we review the key evidence for the role of different risk factors and their effect on CRC prevention and progression.

S. Padmanabhan (✉) · M. I. Waly · N. Guizani · M. S. Rahman · A. Ali · Z. Al-Attabi
Department of Food Science and Nutrition, College of Agricultural and Marine Sciences, Sultan Qaboos University, Muscat, Oman
e-mail: guizani@squ.edu.om; shafiur@squ.edu.om

V. Taranikanti
Department of Human and Clinical Anatomy, College of Medicine and Health Sciences, Sultan Qaboos University, Muscat, Oman

R. C. Deth
Department of Pharmaceutical Sciences, Nova Southeastern University, Fort Lauderdale, FL, USA

© Springer International Publishing AG, part of Springer Nature 2018
M. I. Waly, M. S. Rahman (eds.), *Bioactive Components, Diet and Medical Treatment in Cancer Prevention*, https://doi.org/10.1007/978-3-319-75693-6_10

2 Modifiable Risk Factors and Their Prevention

Most risk factors associated with CRC are modifiable, and they involve obesity and the consumption of food rich in saturated fats. They also involve low physical activity, increased body mass index, cigarette smoking, low fruit consumption, low vegetable consumption, low folate intake, high alcohol intake, disturbance in energy balance, and red meat intake, which are associated with moderately higher risk of CRC. As a result of these lifestyle risk factors, there is a significant differences in incidence and mortality rate from colorectal cancer across the world.

There is a strong association between colorectal cancer risk and alcohol: people drinking a lot of alcohol had 60% higher risk of colorectal cancer in comparison with none or light consumers. Obesity, smoking, high meat intakes, and diabetes all are associated with a 20% higher risk of colorectal cancer in comparison with people in the lowest categories for each. Protection against colorectal cancer is associated with physical activity. Public health strategies that enhance increased physical activity, moderate consumption of red and processed meat, modest alcohol consumption, smoking cessation, and weight loss in most of the times cause significant benefits at the population range for decreasing the chance of colorectal cancer.

2.1 Red Meat and Processed Meat Consumption

Several epidemiologic studies have shown that meat intake is significantly associated with an increased risk of colon cancer [1–3]. In 2007, the World Cancer Research Fund released a report stating that there was convincing evidence of a causal role for red and processed meat in CRC [4]. Also, a quantitative evaluation of 26 cohort studies reports with information about 15,057 people with CRC, examined the association between meat (red meat, processed meat, fish, and poultry) and CRC [5]. The evaluation concluded that compared with people having the lowest intake of processed meat, those having the highest intake experienced a 20% increased risk for developing CRC [5]. The authors did not observe any apparent association between risk of CRC and consumption of either fish or poultry [5]. Another meta-analysis published in 2013 also observed an elevated risk of colorectal adenoma with intake of red and processed meat [6]. Red meat might be related to the incidence of CRC either directly or indirectly. Frying, grilling, broiling, or cooking meat over coal at high temperatures can lead to the formation of mutagenic and carcinogenic heterocyclic amines through the interaction of muscle creatine with amino acids and to the formation of N-nitroso compounds [7]. Those substances can induce genetic alterations and form DNA adducts characteristic of colorectal tumors [7].

The heme iron content of meats might contribute to colorectal neoplasia by inducing oxidative DNA damage and by increasing endogenous formation of N-nitroso compounds, which are known to be powerful multisite carcinogens [8].

Thus, the greater abundance of heme in darker meats than in white meats could increase the risk of CRC. Many studies have observed a positive association between heme and the development of colonic polyps, adenomas, and CRC [9]. Fish and poultry are alternative sources of protein and have been shown to reduce the risk of colon cancer and adenoma. Mechanisms such as the presence of n-3 polyunsaturated fatty acids, especially in oily fish, and more efficient methylation because of the high methionine content in those foods have been proposed for the protective effect of white meats [10]. In this regard, a preventive diet might involve limitation or avoidance of red or processed meats and consumption of white meat and fish [11]. Although epidemiologic studies have observed a strong association between meat intake and an increased risk of CRC, it is important to mention that some components of meat are anticancer substances and essential for optimal human health (selenium; zinc; omega-3 fatty acids; vitamins B6, B12, D, and folic acid) [12].

2.2   Protective Role of Fruit and Vegetables

Dietary fiber varies significantly in physical properties and chemical composition, but can be classified according to water solubility, which affects its function in the body and might be relevant to the risk of CRC. Bran fiber is insoluble; fruit and vegetable fiber tends to be more soluble [13]. After observing the low incidence of CRC in African nations whose populations consume a high-fiber diet, the hypothesis that high fiber consumption might reduce the risk of CRC was proposed by Burkitt and colleagues in the 1970s [14]. Cellulose, hemicellulose, and pectin are plant materials that are defined as fiber [15]. Their protective effect against CRC could be explained by the fact that their presence in meals contributes to lower transit time through the gastrointestinal tract, reducing the concentrations of intestinal carcinogens because of increased stool mass, diluting colonic contents, and enhancing bacterial fermentation, which leads to increased production of short chain fatty acids (acetate, propionate, and butyrate). The latter substances were found to induce apoptosis in CRC cells in rats. Dietary fiber has also been proved to have an anti-inflammatory function, lowering the production of interleukin 6, tumor necrosis factor α, cyclooxygenase 2, and gene expression of inducible nitric oxide synthase.

In addition, in an animal model of CRC, short-chain fatty acids interfered with numerous regulators of cell-cycle proliferation and apoptosis such as the beta-catenin, p53, p21, Bax, and caspase 3 genes. Thus, diets high in wheat bran, fruit and vegetables, citrus fruits, cruciferous vegetables, dark green vegetables, onions, garlic, and tomatoes might have a protective effect against colorectal adenomas and subsequently CRC [16]. Fruits and vegetables also contain many potentially protective substances that affect various biochemical pathways. Their benefits can be observed in inhibitory action at early tumor stages or at advanced or metastatic tumor stages [17–20].

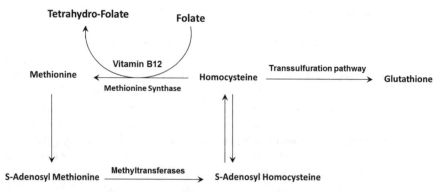

Fig. 1 Simplified schematic of the folate-dependent methionine cycle. Homocysteine is converted into methionine by methionine synthase, which utilizes vitamin B12 as a cofactor and acquires a methyl group from folate which is subsequently converted to tetrahydrofolate. Methionine is further converted to S-adenosylmethionine through the activity of methionine S-adenosyltransferase, the major methyl donor for all methyltransferases, which adds methyl groups to various acceptor molecules such as DNA, RNA, phospholipids, and proteins. S-adenosylmethionine is then converted to S-adenosylhomocysteine, which is reversibly converted to homocysteine in a reaction catalyzed by hydrolase. Homocysteine is remethylated back to methionine, or transsulfurated into glutathione biosynthesis pathway, based on the availability of folate and vitamin B12

2.3   Protective Role of B Vitamins (Folate, Vitamin B6, and Vitamin B12)

Folate deficiency results in genomic hypomethylation and defects in DNA synthesis, both of which can contribute to colonic carcinogenesis. Methionine and folate are required in the production of S-adenosylmethionine, the primary methyl donor, but when methionine levels are low, more folate is used as methyl tetrahydrofolate to form methionine (Fig. 1). The lower levels of methyl tetrahydrofolate might affect DNA synthesis, which could explain the protective effect associated with higher folate levels for those with low methionine intake [21, 22]. Interestingly, compared with people having a high methionine intake but low folate intake, those having high intakes of both methionine and folate were observed to have a significantly increased risk for CRC. The reduction in the CRC incidence in the United States and Canada might be a result of dietary folate supplementation that reduced the risk for colon adenoma development [23]. It was suggested that folate supplementation could be associated with a higher risk of adenoma recurrence and might even be harmful to patients with a prior history of colon cancer [23].

In a randomized clinical trial, it was found that folic acid supplementation at a dose of 1 mg daily is harmful, causing an increase, by a factor of 2.3, in the total number of colonic adenomas and an increased risk, by a factor of 1.7, for advanced colonic adenomas [24]. Physiologic levels of folic acid play a protective role and that intense supplementation could lead to progression of small preexisting adenomas. Moreover, especially in the elderly population, folic acid supplementation at high doses (1000 µg/day) appears to enhance the risk of neoplasms [24]. Vitamin B6 (pyridoxal phosphate) is an important protective anticancer nutrient that is found in numerous grains, fruits, and vegetables. In a meta-analysis of prospective studies, it was suggested that a 49% decrease in CRC risk for every 100 pmol/mL is assocaited with an increase in serum level of pyridoxal phosphate concentration [25]. To summarize, diets rich in folate, vitamin B6, and vitamin B12 might prevent colorectal carcinoma.

2.4 Role of Calcium and Vitamin D

Vitamin D, a fat-soluble vitamin, is synthesized mostly endogenously from skin exposure to ultraviolet sunlight. Some comes from the diet as the provitamin cholecalciferol (D3), which is found naturally in oily saltwater fish, liver, and egg yolk. The plant-derived provitamin ergocalciferol (D2) is found in foods such as mushrooms. Food fortification can provide an extra source of vitamin D. The active form of vitamin D, which is synthesized by hydroxylating provitamins in the liver and kidneys, is 1,25-dihydroxyvitamin D3 (calcitriol). The use of calcitriol in experimental studies has been shown to induce differentiation and inhibition of tumor cell proliferation in various types of cancer cells; however, because of the development of toxic hypercalcemia, such use is limited. For those reasons, calcitriol analogues are usually used [26]. Epidemiologic studies show that deaths from CRC are higher in areas with less sunlight. Also, populations consuming higher amounts of fresh fish, shellfish, calcium, and vitamin D have lower rates of CRC [27]. A meta-analysis suggested an inverse association between circulating levels of 25-hydroxyvitamin D3 and risk of CRC. In countries in which vitamin D-fortified foodstuffs are available (for example, the United States and some Scandinavian countries), the prevalence of vitamin D deficiency is between 1.6% and 14.8% in various age groups. In countries with an insufficient dietary supply of vitamin D or in which foodstuffs are not supplemented, dietary intake of vitamin D is generally low [28].

2.5 Sedentary Life Style and Obesity

In a meta-analysis of CRC risk factors, data from 2309 colon cancer patients and 66,199 CRC patients in 23 studies was used to investigate the relationship between body mass index and risk of CRC. Body mass index and CRC were found to be significantly associated (relative risk: 1.10 per 8 kg/m²) [29]. A meta-analysis used data from 5994 colon cancer patients and 5099 CRC patients in 21 studies to examine the relationship between physical activity and CRC. Without adjustment for any covariates, a significant negative correlation between CRC risk and physical activity was observed (relative risk: 0.88 per two standard score; 95% confidence interval: 0.86–0.91) [30]. In developed countries during the past few decades, physical activity levels for both adults and children have steadily declined. Those declines in physical activity level are suggested to be a result of more time spent watching television and playing computer games and of a decrease in opportunities for physical activity in schools and communities.

3 Non-modifiable Risk Factors for Colon and Rectum Cancer

Several risk factors are associated with the incidence of colorectal cancer. Those that an individual cannot control include age, inflammatory bowel disease, history of CRC in first-degree relatives, and hereditary factors. People with a family history of colorectal cancer have a significantly higher risk of having the disease compared with people without such a history. Risks increased in a number of cases including patients with relatives' diagnosed young, patients with relatives having colonic cancers, and those with more than one affected relatives. The incidence of CRC is low under the age of 45 years. The chance and the risk of this disease elevates with age, as it is well accepted that the diagnosis rate is higher in old people aged 65–84 years. Moreover the average lifetime risk of having CRC is two to three times more in people with a first-degree relative who has an adenomatous polyp or colon cancer than in the general population.

3.1 Hyperhomocysteinemia and Oxidative Stress

Oxidative stress is a condition under which the intracellular antioxidant (GSH), antioxidant enzymes (glutathione peroxidase, superoxide dismutase, and catalase), and dietary antioxidants are not counter balancing the reactive oxygen species-mediated cellular oxidative damages (lipid peroxidation, protein inactivation, and DNA breakdown), eventually leading to many chronic diseases such as CRC [31]. Oxidative stress as a consequence of increased production of nitrogen or oxygen reactive species has been demonstrated in inflammatory bowel disease and CRC. Major etiologic factor for the development of CRC is chronic inflammation of large intestine and rectum. Infectious agents or inflammatory bowel disease, an independent risk factor for CRC, may result in this inflammation. Another consequence if this inflammatory bowel disease might be the localized response to tissue stressors which may include premalignant lesions, adenomatous polyps. Metabolic conditions like nutritional deficiencies which promote systemic or localized inflammation could increase the inflammatory response within large intestine and rectum.

Hyperhomocysteinemia, possibly through inflammatory mechanisms is an established independent risk factor for vascular disease. It is not very clear whether hyperhomocysteinemia has a role in promoting the development of CRC. Hyperhomocysteinemia might be directly linked with inflammation and CRC. It may be due to decreased absorption or increased requirements for folate and other nutrients required for one-carbon and homocysteine metabolism. Homocysteine may induce an inflammatory response in cultures of human intestinal microvascular endothelial cells [32, 33]. There could be a link between CRC and folate through homocysteine.

Adequate consumption of folate and vitamin B_{12} is crucial for supporting several metabolic pathways, especially the methionine cycle, Fig. 1 [33]. Under conditions of low folate and vitamin B_{12}, methionine synthase (a key enzyme in the methionine cycle) becomes hypoactive leading to an accumulation of precursors, including homocysteine, and eventually to the impairment of homocysteine dependent-transsulfuration to GSH, the major intracellular antioxidant, and it has been proved that glutathione depletion is often associated with oxidative stress [33]. Folate and B12 are the dominant nutritional modifiable environmental risk factors in relation to CRC development.

Folate is involved in the transfer of one-carbon units in the de novo synthesis of thymidylate, purines, and methionine. Adequate folate consumption is therefore essential for the synthesis, stability, and repair of DNA and normal cell division. Vitamin B_{12} acts as a coenzyme for methionine synthase (MTR) in the conversion of homocysteine to methionine, a folate-dependent reaction that creates the substrates for de novo nucleotide synthesis and S-adenosyl-methionine, a universal methyl donor. A methyl group from 5-methyltetrahydrofolate, produced by the enzyme methylenetetrahydrofolate reductase (MTHFR), can be transferred to homocysteine by MTR to form methionine and tetrahydrofolate. Deficiency of folate and B_{12} could also result in hyperhomocysteinemia. Several studies suggested that elevated blood concentrations of homocysteine (hyperhomocysteinemia) are a pathological metabolite marker for oxidative stress and for CRC [33].

3.2 Genetic Risk Factors

Less than 10% of patients have an inherited predisposition to CRC, and these cases are subdivided according to whether or not colonic polyps are a major disease manifestation. The diseases with polyposis include familial adenomatous polyposis (FAP) and the hamartomata's polyposis syndromes (e.g., Peutz-Jeghers, juvenile polyposis) [4], while those without polyposis include hereditary non-polyposis colorectal cancer (HNPCC, Lynch syndrome I) and the cancer family syndrome (Lynch syndrome II) [34]. These conditions are associated with a high risk of developing CRC, and the genetic mutations underlying many of them have been identified. The third and least well understood pattern is known as "familial" CRC. Up to 25% of affected patients have a family history of CRC, but the pattern is not consistent with one of the inherited syndromes described above. Individuals from these families are at increased risk of developing CRC, although the risk is not as high as with the inherited syndromes. It was proposed that this group of patients represents individuals with genetic changes with an autosomal recessive pattern of inheritance. Indeed the discovery that biallelic mutations of the base excision repair gene, the MutY human homologue (MYH) resulted in an increased risk of colorectal adenomas and cancer led to the first description of an autosomal recessive cancer syndrome [35].

4 Conclusion

Colon and rectum cancers are one of the most common incident cancers and a common cause of cancer death worldwide. B vitamins (folate and vitamin B_{12}) status is a major determinant of serum homocysteine as it is elevated in CRC patients with folate or vitamin B_{12}. Although supplementation of B vitamins combats hyperhomocysteinemia, yet its etiologic relationship to hyperhomocysteinemia-mediated oxidative stress in relation to CRC remains poorly understood. Accumulated evidence suggests that aging is associated with increased production of free radicals, resulting in increased oxidation of lipids, proteins, and genetic material. Oxidative conditions cause progressive structural and functional alterations of cellular organelles and changes in redox-sensitive signaling processes, such cellular conditions contribute to increased susceptibility to a variety of diseases, including inflammation and cancer. Primary and secondary prevention, with attention to a healthy lifestyle, physical activity, and screening should be enhanced in the general population. Modifiable and non-modifiable risk factors for colon and rectum cancer synergize for the pathogenesis of colon and rectum cancer.

References

1. Zhao Z, Feng Q, Yin Z, Shuang J, Bai B, Yu P, et al. Red and processed meat consumption and colorectal cancer risk: a systematic review and meta-analysis. Oncotarget. 2017;8(47):83306–14.
2. Diallo A, Deschasaux M, Latino-Martel P, Hercberg S, Galan P, Fassier P, et al. Red and processed meat intake and cancer risk: results from the prospective NutriNet-Sante cohort study. Int J Cancer. 2018;142(2):230–7.
3. Carr PR, Jansen L, Bienert S, Roth W, Herpel E, Kloor M, et al. Associations of red and processed meat intake with major molecular pathological features of colorectal cancer. Eur J Epidemiol. 2017;32(5):409–18.
4. Hughes LAE, Simons CCJM, van den Brandt PA, van Engeland M, Weijenberg MP. Lifestyle, diet, and colorectal cancer risk according to (epi) genetic instability: current evidence and future directions of molecular pathological epidemiology. Curr Colorectal Cancer Rep. 2017;13(6):455–69.

5. Huxley RR, Ansary-Moghaddam A, Clifton P, Czernichow S, Parr CL, Woodward M. The impact of dietary and lifestyle risk factors on risk of colorectal cancer: a quantitative overview of the epidemiological evidence. Int J Cancer. 2009;125(1):171–80.
6. Powell JB, Ghotbaddini M. Cancer-promoting and inhibiting effects of dietary compounds: role of the aryl hydrocarbon receptor (AhR). Biochem Pharmacol (Los Angel). 2014;3(1):24–8.
7. Aykan NF. Red meat and colorectal cancer. Oncol Rev. 2015;9(1):288–93.
8. Santarelli RL, Pierre F, Corpet DE. Processed meat and colorectal cancer: a review of epidemiologic and experimental evidence. Nutr Cancer. 2008;60(2):131–44.
9. Baena R, Salinas P. Diet and colorectal cancer. Maturitas. 2015;80(3):258–64.
10. Song M, Garrett WS, Chan AT. Nutrients, foods, and colorectal cancer prevention. Gastroenterology. 2015;148(6):1244–60.
11. Burkitt DP, Walker AR, Painter NS. Dietary fiber and disease. JAMA. 1974;229(8):1068–74.
12. Yao Y, Suo T, Andersson R, Cao Y, Wang C, Lu J, et al. Dietary fibre for the prevention of recurrent colorectal adenomas and carcinomas. Cochrane Database Syst Rev. 2017;1:CD003430.
13. Asano T, McLeod RS. Dietary fibre for the prevention of colorectal adenomas and carcinomas. Cochrane Database Syst Rev. 2002;2:CD003430.
14. Bassett JK, Severi G, Hodge AM, Baglietto L, Hopper JL, English DR, et al. Dietary intake of B vitamins and methionine and colorectal cancer risk. Nutr Cancer. 2013;65(5):659–67.
15. Pericleous M, Mandair D, Caplin ME. Diet and supplements and their impact on colorectal cancer. J Gastrointest Oncol. 2013;4(4):409–23.
16. Wang TP, Hsu SH, Feng HC, Huang RF. Folate deprivation enhances invasiveness of human colon cancer cells mediated by activation of sonic hedgehog signaling through promoter hypomethylation and cross action with transcription nuclear factor-kappa B pathway. Carcinogenesis. 2012;33(6):1158–68.
17. Cole BF, Baron JA, Sandler RS, Haile RW, Ahnen DJ, Bresalier RS, et al. Folic acid for the prevention of colorectal adenomas: a randomized clinical trial. JAMA. 2007;297(21):2351–9.
18. Zhang X-H, Ma J, Smith-Warner SA, Lee JE, Giovannucci E. Vitamin B6 and colorectal cancer: current evidence and future directions. World J Gastroenterol: WJG. 2013;19(7):1005–10.
19. Zhang X, Giovannucci E. Calcium, vitamin D and colorectal cancer chemoprevention. Best Pract Res Clin Gastroenterol. 2011;25(4–5):485–94.
20. Hessami Arani S, Kerachian MA. Rising rates of colorectal cancer among younger Iranians: is diet to blame? Curr Oncol. 2017;24(2):e131–7.
21. Wei MY, Garland CF, Gorham ED, Mohr SB, Giovannucci E. Vitamin D and prevention of colorectal adenoma: a meta-analysis. Cancer Epidemiol Biomark Prev. 2008;17(11):2958–69.
22. Robsahm TE, Aagnes B, Hjartaker A, Langseth H, Bray FI, Larsen IK. Body mass index, physical activity, and colorectal cancer by anatomical subsites: a systematic review and meta-analysis of cohort studies. Eur J Cancer Prev. 2013;22(6):492–505.
23. Johnson CM, Wei C, Ensor JE, Smolenski DJ, Amos CI, Levin B, et al. Meta-analyses of colorectal cancer risk factors. Cancer Causes Control. 2013;24(6):1207–22.
24. Colditz GA, Peterson LL. Obesity and cancer: evidence, impact, and future directions. Clin Chem. 2018;64(1):154–62. pii: clinchem.2017.277376. https://doi.org/10.1373/clinchem.2017.277376.
25. Wang Z, Li S, Cao Y, Tian X, Zeng R, Liao DF, et al. Oxidative stress and carbonyl lesions in ulcerative colitis and associated colorectal cancer. Oxidative Med Cell Longev. 2016;2016:9875298.
26. Zhu S, Li J, Bing Y, Yan W, Zhu Y, Xia B, et al. Diet-induced hyperhomocysteinaemia increases intestinal inflammation in an animal model of colitis. J Crohns Colitis. 2015;9(9):708–19.
27. Keshteli AH, Baracos VE, Madsen KL. Hyperhomocysteinemia as a potential contributor of colorectal cancer development in inflammatory bowel diseases: a review. World J Gastroenterol. 2015;21(4):1081–90.
28. Al-Maskari MY, Waly MI, Ali A, Al-Shuaibi YS, Ouhtit A. Folate and vitamin B12 deficiency and hyperhomocysteinemia promote oxidative stress in adult type 2 diabetes. Nutrition. 2012;28(7–8):e23–6.

29. Waly MI, Ali A, Al-Nassri A, Al-Mukhaini M, Valliatte J, Al-Farsi Y. Low nourishment of B-vitamins is associated with hyperhomocysteinemia and oxidative stress in newly diagnosed cardiac patients. Exp Biol Med. 2016;241(1):46–51.
30. White MC, Holman DM, Boehm JE, Peipins LA, Grossman M, Henley SJ. Age and cancer risk: a potentially modifiable relationship. Am J Prev Med. 2014;46(3 Suppl 1):S7–S15.
31. Theodoratou E, Timofeeva M, Li X, Meng X, Ioannidis JPA. Nature, nurture, and cancer risks: genetic and nutritional contributions to cancer. Annu Rev Nutr. 2017;37:293–320.
32. Rock CL, Lampe JW, Patterson RE. Nutrition, genetics, and risks of cancer. Annu Rev Public Health. 2000;21:47–64.
33. Valle L. Genetic predisposition to colorectal cancer: where we stand and future perspectives. World J Gastroenterol. 2014;20(29):9828–49.
34. Huang Q, He X, Qin H, Fan X, Xie M, Triple LL. primary malignancies in a patient with colorectal adenocarcinoma: a case report. Int J Surg Case Rep. 2017;42:34–7.
35. Yang L, Huang XE, Xu L, Zhou JN, Yu DS, Zhou X, Li DZ, Guan X. Role of MYH polymorphisms in sporadic colorectal cancer in China: a case-control, population-based study. Asian Pac J Cancer Prev. 2013;14(11):6403–9.

Healthy Dietary Pattern for the Primary Prevention of Colorectal Cancer

Reema F. Tayyem

1 Introduction

In colorectal cancer (CRC) disease, several well-known dietary and non-dietary risk factors have been involved in its development. Some of those factors are high consumption of red meat and processed meat; low fiber intake; alcohol drinking; obesity; and a sedentary lifestyle [1]. Additionally, genetic susceptibility [2], tobacco smoking [3], and exposure to environmental carcinogens were found to promote proliferation and malignant transformation of CRC cells [4]. Several studies have focused on the effects of a single food item or a nutrient on lowering risk of CRC incidence [5]. However, the association of a single food item or food group with the risk of developing CRC may not be valid because of the presumption that each single food item or nutrient has an isolated effect [6]. A dietary pattern in food choice is defined as a combination of the dietary components (food items, food groups, nutrients, or both) used to summarize elements of the total diet or the major features of the food choices for the population under study [7]. The descriptive summary of the dietary pattern has been used in nutritional epidemiology to explain and assess the overall dietary experience, by suggesting that the synergistic effects of the variety of dietary and non-dietary factors can be used to explain the relationship between diet and health [8]. In general, there are two dietary patterns: "Healthy" and "Western." The healthy dietary pattern is largely characterized by a greater intake of fruits, vegetables, and grains, and a lower intake of sweets, red meat, and processed meat; this dietary pattern is considered to be associated with lowering the risk of developing CRC. Alternatively, the Western dietary pattern, reported to

R. F. Tayyem (✉)
Faculty of Agriculture, Department of Nutrition and Food Technology,
University of Jordan, Amman, Jordan

© Springer International Publishing AG, part of Springer Nature 2018
M. I. Waly, M. S. Rahman (eds.), *Bioactive Components, Diet and Medical Treatment in Cancer Prevention*, https://doi.org/10.1007/978-3-319-75693-6_11

contain more meat, highly processed food, potatoes, refined carbohydrates, and much lower in vegetables and dietary fiber, has been reported to increase the risk of developing CRC [7, 9].

2 Western Dietary Pattern and CRC

Recent studies that analyzed dietary patterns indicate that adoption of a "Western dietary pattern" (high intake of red meat and/or processed meat, high-fat dairy products, fast food, refined grains, and sweet foods and drinks) increases CRC risk. Recently, global publicity was generated by the World Health Organization International Agency for Research on Cancer consensus statement regarding the increased risk of CRC with consumption of processed or red meat [4]. The 2015 statement notes that processed meat is carcinogenic to humans and lists processed meat as a group 1 substance. Processed meats result from salting, smoking, fermenting, or curing the meat, and common examples include ham, bacon, and sausage [3]. Furthermore, red meat was declared as probably carcinogenic to humans, and red meat was listed as a group 2A substance [4]. Red and processed meats are considered significant components of a "Western" diet. Studies using factor analysis from both "Western" and other "developed" countries have linked the Western dietary pattern to the risk of developing CRC [10–13]. For example, Chen et al. [10] reported a positive association between "meat dietary pattern" and CRC risk (OR = 1.84; 95% CI = 1.19–2.86) in a Canadian population study involving 506 CRC cases and 673 controls. In another cohort study of African American women [11], the Western dietary pattern was found to be associated with a 42% higher risk of colorectal adenoma [11]. Similarly, a case-control study from Iran, conducted by Safari et al. [12], also reported that a Western dietary pattern was associated with an increased risk of CRC development (OR = 2.616; 95% CI = 1.361–5.030) [12]. Additionally, De Stefani et al. [13] also reported an increased risk of CRC development for colon cancer in Uruguayan men whose diet is similar to the western dietary pattern, OR of 2.62 (95% CI = 1.36–5.08).

Combined studies involved 137,217 participants who were followed for up to 32 years, with a total of 3,646,068 person-years of follow-up were analyzed. During the time of the study, 3260 incident CRCs were documented and they revealed that those in the highest quartile for Western dietary pattern consumption had a 31% increased CRC risk (relative risk [RR], 1.31; 95%, CI 1.15–1.48; $P < .0001$) compared with those in the lowest quartile [2]. On the other hand, in the prudent dietary pattern, those in the highest quartile had a 14% reduced risk of CRC (RR, 0.86; 95% CI, 0.77–0.95; $P < .01$) compared with those in the lowest quartile. In addition, of the 2800 tumors with location information available (1264 proximal colon, 866 distal colon, and 670 rectal tumors), the association of Western dietary pattern with CRC incidence was statistically significant for tumors of the distal colon (RR, 1.55; 95% CI, 1.22–1.96; $P < .0004$) and rectum (RR, 1.35; 95% CI, 1.03–1.77; $P < .01$), but not for the proximal colon (RR, 1.11; 95% CI, 0.91–1.35;

$P < .51$). There were no differences by anatomic location for prudent dietary pattern scores [2].

Total grains, sweets, and desserts are also components of the Western dietary pattern, and the increased risk of CRC with consumption of grains and sweets and deserts may be due to the high glycemic index of these foods. Foods that induce hyperinsulinemia have been implicated in the etiology of CRC [14].

3 Healthy Dietary Pattern and CRC

A dietary pattern that is rich in whole grains, vegetables, fruit, fish, legumes, and nuts and low in red and processed meat and alcohol has been linked to a substantial reduction in the risk of CRC [15–19]. This type of dietary pattern is either called healthy or prudent pattern. The WHO recommends improving dietary quality by increasing consumption of fruit and vegetables, as well as legumes, whole grains, and nuts [20]. These recommendations are similar to those studied in the Dietary Approaches to Stop Hypertension trial and are also similar to recommendations found in the Mediterranean Diet examined in the Seven Countries Study [21, 22].

Fung et al. [23] reported a significant protective association between the healthy dietary pattern and CRC. Nevertheless, healthy dietary patterns were mostly loaded with fruits and vegetables. Fruits and vegetables are good source of components of fiber and folic acid, reported to have anti-carcinogenic effects [24]. Previously Tayyem et al. [25] investigated and reported the lack of association of total fruit and vegetable intake with risk of CRC. Van Duijnhoven et al. [26] suggested that the association of fruit and vegetables with CRC risk may be a reflection of increased intake of other food groups. The healthy dietary pattern identified here also contained potatoes that earlier were identified in a report associated with increased risk of CRC in another study [6]. On the other hand, Chen et al. [10] identified that plant-based diet pattern which is loaded mostly with different kinds of fruits and vegetables, fish and whole grains decreases the risk of rectum cancer but not colon with a corresponding OR of 0.55 (95% CI: 0.35–0.87).

Other case-control studies have reported an inverse association between healthy, prudent, or plant-based dietary patterns and the risk of CRC. For example, Azizi et al. [27] found that a healthy eating pattern was protective against CRC in Iranians (OR = 0.18; 95% CI = 0.091–0.47). The healthy dietary pattern in the study by Azizi et al. [27] consisted mainly of fruits and vegetables, low fat dairy, fish, liquid oils, carrots, and nuts. Additionally, Satia et al. [28] reported that a fruit-vegetable pattern was inversely and significantly (OR = 0.4, 95% CI = 0.3–0.6) associated with the risk of having colon cancer in Whites, while another study showed that the prudent dietary pattern was significantly protective, with odds of 0.63 for men (95% CI 0.43–0.92) and 0.58 for women (95% CI 0.38–0.87) [29]. Adherence to the Mediterranean diet pattern was associated with lower risk of CRC (OR = 0.46, 95% CI = 0.28–0.75) [30]. A plant-based pattern mostly of fruits and vegetables as well as fish, was found to be protective against CRC in Uruguayan men (OR = 0.60, 95%

CI = 0.45–0.81) [13]. In a more recent review of 11 case-control and cohort studies, mostly involving Caucasian populations, the conclusion was that dietary patterns characterized by limited intakes of red and processed meat, moderate intakes of dairy products, and plenty fruits and vegetables reduce the risk of CRC [31].

4 Other Dietary Patterns and CRC

4.1 Alcohol Consumption Pattern

The "alcohol-consumption" pattern is characterized by high consumption of alcohol-containing beers, wines, and white spirits. Many articles reported the evidence of an increased risk of CRC in the highest compared with the lowest category of "alcohol-consumption" pattern [32–35]. Alcohol is initially metabolized into an intermediate metabolite, acetaldehyde, followed by further metabolism and then elimination from the body. Hence, the possible mechanism is that ethanol and its major metabolites (e.g., acetaldehyde) have been shown to be carcinogenic to the colon and rectum in animals [35]. In addition, alcohol and acetaldehyde may inhibit folate-mediated methionine synthesis and may thus impair DNA methylation, which is linked to carcinogenesis [34]. Furthermore, acetaldehyde increases the risk of CRC by inducing DNA lesions, generating free radicals, and damaging enzymes involved in DNA repair and antioxidant protection [35].

4.2 High Sugar Drinks Pattern

High-sugar drinks pattern loaded with sugar should be limited. A high risk of CRC cancer was evident for increasing tertiles of High-sugar drinks pattern [29]. The increased risk of CRC was documented in many studies [10, 15] and it was evidenced that low levels of deglycating enzymes are present in colorectal cancer patients [36] The increased risk of CRC with sugar consumption was documented in many studies [10, 15]. It was evidenced that low levels of deglycating enzymes are present in colorectal cancer patients [36]. Additionally, the risk of colorectal adenoma associated with the level of fructosamine, which is consdired as an indicator of the level of glucose in the blood and it is more sensitive to foods with a high glycemic index [37]. and the increased risk of colorectal adenoma with the level of fructosamine, an indicator of the level of glucose in the blood and it is more sensitive to foods with a high glycemic index [36]. Tayyem et al. [38] identified three dietary patterns, the first one is the "Healthy Pattern," and the second was identified as "High Sugar/High Tea Pattern," and the third as "Western Pattern." In the Healthy Pattern group, they found a 10.54% variation in food intake, while the intake variation was 11.64% in the Western Pattern [38]. After adjusting for confounding factors, the Western Pattern food choice was found to be significantly associated

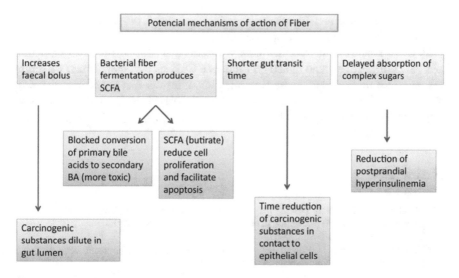

Fig. 1 Scheme of potential mechanisms of protection of fiber in colorectal cancer. SCFA, short-chain fatty acids (adapted from [40])

with an increased risk of developing CRC (OR = 1.88; 95% CI = 1.12–3.16). The results for the Healthy and High-Sugar/High Tea Patterns showed a decrease, but the statistic was not significant for the risk of CRC development [38].

5 Possible Mechanisms of Diet and CRC

The potential mechanisms related to the consumption of food and the development of CRC is not clear, however, it is possible that more than one metabolic pathway, dietary compounds or biochemical reactions are involved. However, there are different proposed physiological mechanisms through which diet may be associated with a reduced risk of CRC and through which this association may differ for men and for women. For example, studies focused on individual nutrients suggest that olive oil may exert a reduced risk of CRC by influencing secondary bile acid patterns in the colon. This may in turn affect polyamine metabolism in colonic enterocytes, reducing progression from normal mucosa to adenoma and carcinoma [39].

Fiber intake may reduce the contact between carcinogens and the lining of the colon/rectum and increase stool bulk, which dilutes fecal carcinogens and decreases transit time [15, 19]. In addition, bacterial fermentation of fiber produces short-chain fatty acids (SCFA) which reduce cancer cell proliferation and facilitate apoptosis (Fig. 1). SCFA may also help in preventing cancer development through blocking the conversion of primary bile acids to secondary toxic ones [41].

Red and processed meat may exert a carcinogenic effect due to heme iron, N-nitro compounds, polycyclic aromatic hydrocarbons (PAHs), malondialdehyde, nitrites and nitrates and heterocyclic amines generated during cooking at high temperatures as well as a proneoplastic effect due to increased adiposity and insulin [42]. Other studies suggested that dietary patterns that include a high consumption of high saturated fatty acid intake may increase CRC risk via their effects on serum insulin concentrations and on the bioavailability of insulin-like growth factor-I [43]. Whole grain intake has been associated with decreased fasting insulin level and improved insulin sensitivity [44].

References

1. World Cancer Research Fund/American Institute for Cancer Research. Food, nutrition, physical activity and the prevention of cancer: a global perspective. Washington, DC: American Institute for Cancer Research; 2007.
2. Heavy PM, McKenna D, Rowland IR. Colorectal cancer and the relationship between genes and the environment. Nutr Cancer. 2004;48:124–41.
3. Ulrich CM, Bigler J, Whitton JA, Bostick R, Fosdick L, Potter JD. Epoxide hydrolase Tyr113His polymorphism is associated with elevated risk of colorectal polyps in the presence of smoking and high meat intake. Cancer Epidemiol Biomarkers Prev. 2001;10:875–82.
4. Irigaray P, Newby JA, Clapp R, Hardell L, Howard V, et al. Lifestyle-related factors and environmental agents causing cancer: an overview. Biomed Pharmacother. 2007;61:640–58.
5. Sun Z, Zhu Y, Wang PP, Roebothan B, Zhao J, Dicks E, et al. Reported intake of selected micronutrients and risk of colorectal cancer: results from a large population-based case-control study in Newfoundland, Labrador and Ontario, Canada. Anticancer Res. 2012;32:687–96.
6. Flood A, Rastogi T, Wirfalt E, Mitrou PN, Reedy J, Subar AF, et al. Dietary patterns as identified by factor analysis and colorectal cancer among middle-aged Americans. Am J Clin Nutr. 2008;88:176–84.
7. Randi G, Edefonti V, Ferraroni M, La Vecchia C, Decarli A. Dietary patterns and the risk of colorectal cancer and adenomas. Nutr Rev. 2010;68:389–408.
8. Magalhaes B, Bastos J, Lunet N. Dietary patterns and colorectal cancer: a case-control study from Portugal. Eur J Cancer Prev. 2011;20:389–95.
9. Magalhaes B, Peleteiro B, Lunet N. Dietary patterns and colorectal cancer: systematic review and meta-analysis. Eur J Cancer Prev. 2012;21:15–23.
10. Chen Z, Wang PP, Woodrow J, Zhu Y, Roebothan B, Mclaughlin JR, Parfrey PS. Dietary patterns and colorectal cancer: results from a Canadian population-based study. Nutr J. 2015;15:14–8.
11. Makambi KH, Agurs-Collins T, Bright-Gbebry M, Rosenberg L, Palmer JR, Adams-Campbell LL. Dietary patterns and the risk of colorectal adenomas: the Black Women's Health Study. Cancer Epidemiol Biomarkers Prev. 2011;20(5):818–25.
12. Safari A, Shariff ZM, Kandiah M, Rashidkhani B, Fereidooni F. Dietary patterns and risk of colorectal cancer in Tehran Province: a case-control study. BMC Public Health. 2013;13:222.
13. Stefani ED, Deneo-Pellegrini H, Ronco AL, Correa P, Boffetta P, Aune D, Acosta G, Mendilaharsu M, Luaces ME, Lando G, Silva C. Dietary patterns and risk of colorectal cancer: a factor analysis in Uruguay. Asian Pac J Cancer Prev. 2011;12(3):753–9.
14. Giovannucci E. Insulin, insulin-like growth factors and colon cancer: a review of the evidence. J Nutr. 2001;131:3109S–20S.
15. Aune D, Chan DS, Lau R, et al. Dietary fibre, whole grains, and risk of colorectal cancer: systematic review and dose-response metaanalysis of prospective studies. BMJ. 2011;343:d6617.
16. Bamia C, Lagiou P, Buckland G, et al. Mediterranean diet and colorectal cancer risk: results from a European cohort. Eur J Epidemiol. 2013;28:317–28.

17. Bouvard V, Loomis D, Guyton KZ, et al. International Agency for Research on Cancer Monograph Working G. Carcinogenicity of consumption of red and processed meat. Lancet Oncol. 2015;16:1599–600.
18. Chan DS, Lau R, Aune D, et al. Red and processed meat and colorectal cancer incidence: meta-analysis of prospective studies. PLoS One. 2011;6:e20456.
19. Mehta RS, Song M, Nishihara R, et al. Dietary patterns and risk of colorectal cancer: analysis by tumor location and molecular subtypes. Gastroenterology. 2017;152:1944–53.
20. Amine E, Baba N, Belhadj M, et al. Diet, nutrition and the prevention of chronic diseases: report of a Joint WHO/FAO Expert Consultation: World Health Organization. 2002.
21. Knoops KT, de Groot LC, Kromhout D, et al. Mediterranean diet, lifestyle factors, and 10-year mortality in elderly european men and women: the HALE project. JAMA. 2004;292:1433–9.
22. Reedy J, Mitrou PN, Krebs-Smith SM, et al. Index-based dietary patterns and risk of colorectal cancer: the NIH-AARP Diet and Health Study. Am J Epidemiol. 2008;168:38–48.
23. Fung T, Hu FB, Fuchs C, Giovannucci E, Hunter DJ, Stampfer MJ, Colditz GA, Willett WC. Major dietary patterns and the risk ofcolorectal cancer in women. Arch Intern Med. 2003;163(3):309–11.
24. Harshman MR, Aldoori W. Diet and colorectal cancer: review of the evidence. Can Fam Physician. 2007;53:1913–20.
25. Tayyem RF, Shehadeh I, Abu-Mweis SS, Bawadi H, Bani-Hani K, Al-Jaberi T, Majed Alnusair HD. Fruit and vegetable intake among Jordanians: results from a case-control study of colorectal cancer. Cancer Control: Journal of the Moffitt Cancer Center. 2014;21(4):350–6.
26. Van Duijnhoven FJ, Bueno-De-Mesquita HB, Ferrari P, Jenab M, Boshuizen HC, Ros MM, et al. Fruit, vegetables, and colorectal cancer risk: the European Prospective Investigation into Cancer and Nutrition. Am J Clin Nutr. 2009;89:1441–52.
27. Azizi H, Asadollahi K, DavtalabEsmaeili E, Mirzapoor M. Iranian dietary patterns and risk of colorectal cancer. Health Promot Perspect. 2015;5(1):72–80.
28. Satia JA, Tseng M, Galanko JA, Martin C, Sandler RS. Dietary patterns and colon cancer risk in Whites and African Americans in the North Carolina Colon Cancer Study. Nutr Cancer. 2009;61(2):179–93.
29. Slattery ML, Boucher KM, Caan BJ, Potter JD, Ma KN. Eating patterns and risk of colon cancer. Am J Epidemiol. 1998;148(1):4–16.
30. Grosso G, Biondi A, Galvano F, et al. Factors associated with colorectal cancer in the context of the Mediterranean diet: a case-control study. Nutr Cancer. 2014;66(4):558–65.
31. Fung TT, Brown LS. Dietary patterns and the risk of colorectal cancer. Curr Nutr Rep. 2013;2(1):48–55.
32. Ben Q, Wang L, Liu J, et al. Alcohol drinking and the risk of colorectal adenoma: a dose-response meta-analysis. Eur J Cancer Prev. 2015;24:286–95.
33. Feng YL, Shu L, Zheng PF, et al. Dietary patterns and colorectal cancer risk: a meta-analysis. Eur J Cancer Prev. 2017;26(3):201–11.
34. Park JY, Dahm CC, Keogh RH, et al. Alcohol intake and risk of colorectal cancer: results from the UK Dietary Cohort Consortium. Br J Cancer. 2010;103:747–56.
35. Seitz HK, Stickel F. Molecular mechanisms of alcohol-mediated carcinogenesis. Nat Rev Cancer. 2007;7:599–612.
36. Notarnicola M, Caruso MG, Tutino V, et al. Low red blood cell levels of deglycating enzymes in colorectal cancer patients. World J Gastroenterol. 2011;17(3):329–33.
37. Misciagna G, De Michele G, Guerra V, et al. Serum fructosamine and colorectal adenomas. Eur J Epidemiol. 2004;19(5):425–32.
38. Tayyem RF, Bawadi H, Shehadeh I, et al. Dietary patterns and colorectal cancer. Clin Nutr. 2017;36:848–52.
39. Stoneham M, Goldacre M, Seagroatt V, et al. Olive oil, diet and colorectal cancer: an ecological study and a hypothesis. J Epidemiol Commun Health. 2000;54:756–60.
40. Romaneiro S, Parekh N. Dietary fiber intake and colorectal cancer risk. Top Clin Nutr. 2012;27(1):41–7.

41. Plotnikoff G. Three measurable and modifiable enteric microbial biotransformations relevant to cancer prevention and treatment. Glob Adv Health Med. 2014;3(3):33–43.
42. Santarelli R, Pierre F, Corpet D. Processed meat and colorectal cancer: a review of epidemiologic and experimental evidence. Nutr Cancer. 2008;60(2):131–44.
43. Sandhu MS, Dunger DB, Insulin GEL, et al. IGF-I, IGF binding proteins, their biologic interactions, and colorectal cancer. J Natl Cancer Inst. 2002;94:972–80.
44. Pereira MA, Jacobs DR, Van Horn L, et al. Dairy consumption, obesity, and the insulin resistance syndrome in young adults: the CARDIA Study. JAMA. 2002;287:2081–9.

Lifestyle Modification in Long-Term Management of Chronic Diseases

Haleama Al Sabbah

1 Introduction

Nowadays, unfortunately, obesity has been viewed as a cosmetic issue rather than a chronic disease; furthermore, health insurance systems do not include the costs of obesity treatment except if it is associated with a chronic disease such as hypertension and diabetes [1]. Obesity could be defined as an excess amount of energy intake and fat storage through overnutrition and adopting sedentary lifestyle [2, 3]. It can be caused by a combination of several factors including cultural and environmental factors, such as elevated energy diet, low levels of physical activity, eating disorders, and increased portion size. These factors can cause a fundamental change in the structure of adipose tissue leading to "hypertrophy and hyperplasia of adipocytes, inflammation" as well as it causes a change in the secretion of adipokines, which is a biologically active protein that can cause severe impact on the metabolism of glucose and lipids [3, 4]. A study found in UAE indicated that factors that may attribute to low levels of activities are mainly due to the hot climate that can reach up to 45° C in the summer, in addition to the cultural norms that can restrict female outdoor physical activities [5].

2 Obesity and Chronic Diseases

Obesity considers being the main cause of morbidity and mortality [6–8]. With increased duration of obesity, many forms of cancer may develop, as strong relationship is found between the increased duration of obesity and the incidence of

H. Al Sabbah (✉)
Health Sciences Department, Zayed University, Dubai, UAE
e-mail: haleama@hotmail.com

© Springer International Publishing AG, part of Springer Nature 2018
M. I. Waly, M. S. Rahman (eds.), *Bioactive Components, Diet and Medical Treatment in Cancer Prevention*, https://doi.org/10.1007/978-3-319-75693-6_12

developing other forms of cancer including postmenopausal breast cancer, colon, endometrial, and kidney cancer. In fact, obesity duration can be an indicator or an independent factor of type 2 diabetes and cardiovascular diseases, since obesity can cause a change in biological mechanisms which poses individual in a higher risk of developing hypertension and insulin resistance [2, 9, 10]. Hypertension is defined as having blood pressure exceeding 140/90 mmHg. In this case, hypertension can result in severe health outcomes, and it is called silent killer since it is not accompanied by symptoms; thus if it is untreated it can prompt heart attack and kidney and heart failure. Moreover, diabetic patients are more prone to develop nervous system diseases, dental problems, and loss of vision [6].

Obesity can lead to osteoarthritis which is a chronic disease responsible for the breaking down of the joint's cartilage causing pain and stiffness and hence difficulty in the movement of the joint. This happens because high body weight causes more stress in the joints [6, 11]. Another study showed that people who were obese in their childhood exhibit greater risk of developing cardiovascular diseases, which is associated with hypertension and dyslipidemia in their adulthood, unlike people who had normal weights as a child [12]. Obesity is a chronic disease and it affects all people regardless of their age. Childhood obesity can show early signs of cardiovascular dysfunction, arterial stiffness, and alter the myocardial structure as a result of excess adiposity [12]. In fact, fat distribution is found to be the main factor to predict cardiovascular disease as studies revealed. People with higher central obesity (also called upper body obesity measured by waist circumference) are more prone to develop cardiovascular diseases and metabolic syndrome [1, 3, 13].

As a consequence, obese people tend to have lower life expectancy and higher drug expenditure because of obesity-related diseases, meaning that the effect of obesity is not only limited to affect human health, but it also extends to higher costs in the healthcare sector. It is estimated in Europe that approximately 7% of total healthcare costs account for obesity-related diseases [3, 10]. Studies showed that obese people may face some discrimination in terms of employment, as they are seen to be less productive and less motivated in the workplace [14]. Several studies stated that obese people tend to have higher rate of absence because of sick leaves, as a result they receive discrimination because of the missing days which lead to low performance in the workplace. Moreover, employers often prevent employing obese people to avoid health insurance and other health-related expenses [14, 15]. In fact, most of the health insurance companies ignore the fact that including bariatric surgery in the insurance is economically sustainable, because of the increased number of obese people and the growing demand for surgical intervention and after-care [16].

3   Obesity Management and Prevention

Management of obesity should start from childhood since childhood obesity is the main sign of adult obesity [5, 8, 9]. Long-term follow-up and frequent measurements of weight and height are important to detect any dramatic changes in the body weight and to quantify the exposure level of obesity and overweight.

These parameters would also help in measuring the corresponding health effects of obesity-related diseases [9]. The application of effective strategies may help in reducing obesity-related diseases and help to sustain finance of the healthcare sector through lowering medical expenses [10]. For example, 10% reduction in total body weight resulted in decreasing the risk of developing diabetes and help to maintain blood pressure and reduce the insulin resistance [1, 7]. In addition, diabetes prevention program claimed that lifestyle modification and intervention can produce weight loss with an average of 7% at 6 months and 4.9% at 3 years; this moderate weight loss was successful enough to reduce the risk of developing diabetes by 58%. Another study with five thousand people with type 2 diabetes showed significant improvements in sleep apnea, urinary incontinence, and kidney disease. Moreover, weight loss can lead to psychological improvements as obese patients experience more depression, stress, and poor self-esteem than people with normal weight; however, the effects of these symptoms can be reduced with weight loss particularly through improved body image and reduced anxiety [2, 17].

As it is mentioned earlier, childhood obesity is a major predictor of adulthood obesity, so it is cost-effective to control obesity in early ages [5, 8, 9]. In childhood obesity management, the involvement of the parents is very important as they are considered as a risk factor for childhood obesity, but it is a challenge because some parents may be aware of their child's overweight but they are not aware enough about health consequences to be involved in the obesity management program [18, 19]. Parent's socioeconomic status (SES) can be an example of risk factors that contribute to obesity development. SES is measured by the level of education, income, and occupation. Several studies have shown that higher education level results in lower childhood obesity. Moreover, inverse relationship between the occupation and obesity was found, as the average BMI for professional workers were 25.9 and 27.2 for unskilled manual occupational workers, similar relationships were found with income, as obesity was inversely related to the income [19]. Another study sought to determine factors that may influence parent's decision in joining obesity management programs. Their results showed that parents were largely influenced by their failed attempts to control their children's weight and their children's emotions. Enhancing parent's awareness must be the first step in addressing the issue of childhood obesity in order to encourage them to join obesity management programs. However, this step might not be sufficient by itself, as health professionals must include activities and strategies for long-term follow-up. Finally, parent's awareness could not directly push parents to join obesity program but it can help the parent to take action toward this issue [18].

4 Obesity Treatment

4.1 Lifestyle Modification Programs

There is a growing body of literature that recognizes the importance of obesity treatment with a combination of several approaches rather than a single approach [7, 8]. The words lifestyle modification programs (LMP), behavioral treatment, or weight control always used alternately [20]. Those terms incorporate three main principles which are diet, exercise, and behavioral therapy (i.e., basically set of standers and strategies to modify eating behavior and exercise) [8, 17]. Often LMPs intended to enable patients to lose 1–2 lb/week bringing about 5–10% weight reduction by a half year, through controlled energy intake (500–1000 kcal/day) and this aim could be obtained by reducing portion size and sugar, eradicating fat, and increasing body energy consumption by physical activity [17, 20, 21].

In addition, the program emphasizes practices such as record keeping of physical activity and food intake, self-monitoring, stress control, and social support to achieve weight reduction [20, 22]. It has been suggested that school-based lifestyle intervention program is effective for obesity prevention. A study done in China to assess the effectiveness of school-based lifestyle intervention program further support the idea of obesity prevention on early onset, especially children who were involved in the program exhibit healthy behaviors as well as knowledge about obesity and its health outcomes, in contrast to the control group, the intervention group were able to lose weight more than 0.5 kg/m^2 BMI [23]. Obtaining family support can be facilitated through school-based intervention programs. It is important to get participant's family engagement in which parents or guardians enrolled in classes on how to adopt healthy lifestyle and behavioral changes at the level of the household. In addition, they are assigned to specific tasks and activities which needs to be done by the parents and children regarding healthy lifestyle and obesity prevention. Moreover, including fun events in the curriculum can also help to gain children's attraction as well as help to increase awareness, for example, arranging short writing, painting, and stage drama competition regarding the risk associated with obesity can help to increase awareness among school children [23, 24].

4.2   Three Main Components of Lifestyle Modification Programs

4.2.1   Diet Intervention

This component focuses on energy or calorie deficiency made basically through restricted food intake, where patients were assigned to a specific calorie objective in order to achieve 500–1000 kcal deficiency from their baseline of food calorie intake, hence they are likely to produce a weight loss of a 1–2 lb/week [17]. The assigned caloric intake is different from person to another, depending on their weights. For instance, patients with more than 200 lb are encouraged to consume 1500–1800 kcal/day, while patients under 200 are recommended to 1000–1500 kcal/day [17].

Despite the fact that there are many studies to prove that weight reduction is fundamentally related to controlled caloric intake rather than micronutrient composition of the eating routine, behavioral programs recommend patients to reduce fat intake (i.e., less than 30% of calories from fat) to accomplish caloric objectives [17]. Unfortunately, commercial diets such as ad-libitum, very low calorie, low glycemic index, protein and meal replacement diets are becoming more common, the main problem of these diets lies on its short-term effect on weight loss and sometimes these diets might be harmful without proper monitoring. The most critical thing in weight management programs is the adherence to a healthy lifestyle for weight loss maintenance, which cannot be accomplished with the commercial diets [22]. In fact, a moderate caloric restriction can be more effective in weight maintenance as it is easier for obese patients to adhere [22]. However, energy restriction alone can be an effective method in weight loss but its effect in weight loss maintenance is short-term; a number of studies showed that less than 5% of individuals were able to lose weight by only energy restriction for 2 years [2].

4.2.2   Physical Activity

Physical activity can enhance the effect of diet interventions in weight loss management because it increases the energy expenditure causing a reduction in energy consumption of the body [22]. It has a major role in weight maintenance and adherence to weight loss strategies, because exercise can reduce individual's stress and depression, thus it makes some improvements in the mood [2]. The program supports gradual increments in physical activity by using moderate force exercises, for example, quick walking. The duration of the exercise is important to achieve the desired weight loss. In order to sense the impact of physical activity on body weight, it is recommended to start with 50 min/week, with a gradual increase to 150/week. In addition, longer duration of physical activity (200–250 min/week) can contribute to the maintenance of the weight loss [17]. Researchers have found that the problem of being inactive started from childhood, a longitudinal study of 5 years follow-up from childhood to adolescence, the study found that physically active children were active as adults, while inactive children exhibit low physical activity as adults [19]. Physical activity can be assessed and measured based on four dimensions, which include type, intensity, frequency, and duration.

Each of those measurements requires direct observation, surveys reported from self or proxy, accelerometer, and monitoring heart rate. For instance, a questionnaire can provide enough information to assess all measures of physical activity while accelerometer can measure only intensity, duration, and frequency [19]. Moderate intensity of physical activity like walking as 30 min/day can reduce cardiovascular risk factors by 30–50%, in another simple form daily 5–10 min of stair climbing which can be equivalent to 30 min walking [25].

4.2.3   Behavioral Changes

Most of the behavioral changes programs help to make patients adhere to the healthy behaviors through specific strategies. Self-monitoring, record keeping of weight, and physical activity are the main components of behavioral weight loss programs; additional strategies include stimulus control, which is a way of keeping high-calorie food out of reach and making sure that healthy option and low-calorie foods are available [17]. The cornerstones of behavioral change program are self-monitoring and record keeping help individuals to understand better about the relationship between their eating behavior and weight loss, thus allowing them to adjust their eating and physical activity behaviors [17, 26]. Adherence to controlled caloric intake can be facilitated through frequent and consistent self-monitoring, investigated the effectiveness of frequent and consistent self-monitoring, the study found that individuals who self-monitored were able to maintain their weight changes better than those with less frequent and consistent self-monitoring [26]. Understanding the motives behind joining weight loss programs is important because poor adherence to weight loss programs is associated with a lack of self-motivation which has been viewed as a predictor of successful treatment, this can help healthcare professionals to relate the associated psychological needs with obesity intervention programs [15]. In academic medical centers, behavioral programs are usually performed in a group of 10–20 participants or individually, participants are enrolled in 60–90 min sessions often 16–24 weeks, which is arranged by a dietician, psychologist, or exercise specialist. Although individual treatment is expensive, it has been shown that it is less effective in terms achieving weight loss, because group care treatment provides the suitable environment that provides empathy, motivation, and social support which can promote a competitive environment between the participants [17, 20].

4.2.4 Pharmacotherapy

Weight loss cannot be obtained with only anti-obesity drugs, which is viewed as a "rescue strategy." Anti-obesity drugs, in fact, can enhance weight loss when it is used in a combination with behavioral change [17, 22]. Pharmacotherapy is recommended to an obese patient with body mass index (BMI) above 30 kg/m^2 and overweight people who suffer from obesity-related diseases such as hypertension and type 2 diabetes [7, 27]. An example of an anti-obesity drug which has been widely used and approved by FDA in 2003 is Orlistat, which restricts intestinal and pancreatic lipase and thus it prevents about 30% of triglycerides absorption by gastrointestinal [8, 22]. Orlistat can have a mild to moderate side effects on the intestinal (i.e., frequent stools due to unabsorbed fats) and abdominal pain and diarrhea. However, these side effects can be reduced by decreasing dietary fat intake and increasing the portion of natural dietary fibers [8]. Based on clinical trials, many studies have concluded that Orlistat can help in weight reduction in a combination with diet, exercise, and behavioral change. McDiffie, the first who studied Orlistat in American obese adolescence, observed a significant weight loss and decrease in cholesterol, lipoprotein, and fasting blood glucose in 3–6 months, compared with the baseline weight; Orlistat group lost 6.3–5.4 kg with a decrease in BMI approximately 4.1–2.9 kg/m^2 in contrast to the controlled group who gained weight (4.2–6.5 kg) with increase in BMI by 0.1 kg/m^2. Since the level of plasma fat-soluble vitamin is noticed to be decreased with Orlistat group, which is of particular concern affecting child growth, FDA suggested Orlistat must be accompanied with multivitamins and it is only recommended for adolescent [8].

4.2.5 Surgical Intervention

Typically, surgical interventions are used when obese patients fail to achieve weight loss with traditional methods of weight management. Surgical interventions have been viewed as the best option to treat very obese patients with greater risk [22, 28]. According to the National Institute for Health and Clinical excellence, surgical intervention is recommended when the BMI of an individual exceeds 50 and sometimes when it is more than 35 if the individual is suffering from serious comorbidities.

Bariatric surgery is classified into two basic categories depending on its mechanism of weight loss such as malabsorptive (which has a higher risk of mortality) and restrictive procedures [22]. Although malabsorptive procedure exposes obese patients to risk, it can cause a significant and rapid health improvement in serious metabolic comorbidities which are associated with very obese patients; therefore, the malabsorptive procedure seems to outweigh the effect of severe obesity that causes serious comorbidities [11, 22]. Bariatric surgery is not a long-term method for weight loss unless it is used in a combination with a long-term behavioral change; it requires weight loss maintenance, long-term follow-up, and adopting a healthy lifestyle. It is important to remember that the aim of the surgery must not only be weight loss and reducing the risk of comorbidities, but also improving psychological function which is an important step to ensure the adherence to a healthy lifestyle in long-term [11, 17].

Bioenterics intragastric balloon (BIB) is considered as a safe, nonsurgical and non-pharmacological option for obesity treatment, it is reversible and can be done several times. The main function of this method is to induce satiety through slowing down gastric emptiness and partially filling the stomach. An average of 12–13 kg of weight loss can be achieved by BIB treatment within 6 months. However, the short-term effect of this method must be considered, it must be remembered that after the removal of the BIB the probability of weight regain is high and it is a critical issue to consider, it has been reported that most of the patients who lose weight during the treatment have regained it after its removal [7, 8]. Therefore, many studies support the idea that one single treatment or step toward obesity management is not sufficient to address such a complex chronic disease [7, 28, 29]. Thus, a combination of long-term behavioral modification is recommended after the BIB removal in order to support the long-term weight maintenance and to avoid weight regain [7, 29].

References

1. Vega GL. Cardiovascular outcomes for obesity and metabolic syndrome. Obes Res. 2002;10:S27–32.
2. Rippe JM, Hess S. The role of physical activity in the prevention and management of obesity. J Am Diet Assoc. 1998:S31–8.
3. Tsigos C, Hainer V, Basdevant A, Finer N, Fried M, Mathus-Vliegen E, Micic D, Maislos M, Roman G, Schutz Y, Toplak H, Zahorska-Markiewicz B, Obesity Management Task Force of the European Association for the Study of Obesity. Management of obesity in adults: European clinical practice guidelines. Obes Facts. 2008;1(2):106–16.
4. Kondo T, Kobayashi I, Murakami M. Effect of exercise on circulating adipokine levels in obese young women. Endocr J. 2006;53(2):189–95.

5. Al Junaibi A, Abdulle A, Sabri S, Hagali M, Nagelkerke N. The prevalence and potential determinants of obesity among school children and adolescents in Abu-Dhabi, United Arab Emirates. Int J Obes (Lond). 2013;37(1):68–74.
6. Debraganza N. Self-monitoring in the long-term management of obesity (Order No. 3467696). 2010. Available from ProQuest Dissertations & Theses Global. (880861957). https://search. proquest.com/docview/880861957?accountid=15192.
7. Farina MG, Baratta R, Nigro A, Vinciguerra F, Puglisi C, Schembri R, Frittitta L. Intragastric balloon in association with lifestyle and/or pharmacotherapy in the long-term management of obesity. Obes Surg. 2012;22(4):565–71.
8. Rogovik AL, Chanoine J, Goldman RD. Pharmacotherapy and weight-loss supplements for treatment of pediatric obesity. Drugs. 2010;70(3):335–46.
9. Arnold M, Jiang L, Stefanick ML, Johnson KC, Lane DS, LeBlanc ES, Anton-Culver H. Duration of adulthood overweight, obesity, and cancer risk in the women's health initiative: a longitudinal study from the United States. PLoS Med. 2016;13(8):1–16.
10. Rappange DR, Brouwer WBF, Hoogenveen RT, Van Baal PHM. Healthcare costs and obesity prevention. Pharmacoeconomics. 2009;27(12):1031–44.
11. Cobbold A, Lord S. Treatment and management of obesity: is surgical intervention the answer? J Perioper Pract. 2012;22(4):114–21.
12. Russu G, Frasinariu O, Trandafir L. Cardiovascular suffering in childhood obesity. Romanian. J Pediatr. 2016;65(4):366–71.
13. Sharma AM. The value of current interventions for obesity. Nat Clin Pract Cardiovasc Med. 2008;5(Suppl 1):S3–9.
14. Tekle AT. Examination of factors associated with obesity, physical activity and income in metropolitan areas of the United States (Order No. 3576341). 2013. Available from ProQuest Dissertations & Theses Global. (1465413156). https://search.proquest.com/docview/1465413 156?accountid=15192.
15. Teixeira PJ, Silva MN, Mata J, Palmeira AL, Markland D. Motivation, self-determination, and long-term weight control. Int J Behav Nutr Phys Act. 2012;9:22–8.
16. Sidorov JE, Fitzner K. Obesity disease management opportunities and barriers. Obesity. 2006;14(4):645–9.
17. Olson K, Bond D, Wing RR. Behavioral approaches to the treatment of obesity. R I Med J. 2017;100(3):21–4.
18. Davidson K, Vidgen H. Why do parents enroll in a childhood obesity, management program: a qualitative study with parents of overweight and obese children? BMC Public Health. 2017;17(1):1–10.
19. Park H. Longitudinal relationships between physical activity, sedentary behaviors, and obesity in children and adolescents (Order No. 3289070). 2007. Available from ProQuest Central; ProQuest Dissertations & Theses Global. (304842292). https://search.proquest.com/docview/ 304842292?accountid=15192.
20. Wadden TA, Butryn ML, Byrne KJ. Efficacy of lifestyle modification for long-term weight control. Obes Res. 2004;12:S151–62.
21. U.S. Department of Health and Human services. Managing overweight and obesity in adults: systematic evidence review from the obesity expert panel. 2013. National institutes of Health website https://www.nhlbi.nih.gov.
22. Aditya BS, Wilding JPH. Modern management of obesity. Clin Med. 2009;9(6):617–21.
23. Xu F, Ware RS, Leslie E, Tse LA, Wang Z, Li J, Wang Y. Effectiveness of a randomized controlled lifestyle intervention to prevent obesity among Chinese primary school students: CLICK-Obesity Study. PLoS One. 2015;10(10):1–12.
24. Neumark-Sztainer D. Eating disorders prevention: looking backward, moving forward; looking inward, moving outward. Eat Disord. 2016;24(1):29–38.
25. Kouris-Blazos A, Wahlqvist ML. Health economics of weight management: evidence and cost. Asia Pac J Clin Nutr. 2007;16:329–38.
26. Peterson ND, Middleton KR, Nackers LM, Medina KE, Milsom VA, Perri MG. Dietary self-monitoring and long-term success with weight management. Obesity. 2014;22(9):1962–7.

27. Abyad A. Obesity management in primary health care. Middle East J Intern Med. 2016;9(3):26–8.
28. Dixon JB, Straznicky NE, Lambert EA, Schlaich MP, Lambert GW. Surgical approaches to the treatment of obesity. Nat Rev. 2011;8(8):429–37.
29. Dixon JB, Dixon ME. Combined strategies in the management of obesity. Asia Pac J Clin Nutr. 2006;15:63–9.

Early Detection and Screening of Cancer

Preeja Prabhakar and Sivaprasad Punnaveetil

1 Introduction

Cancer is one of the leading causes of morbidity and mortality worldwide, with approximately 14 million new cases in 2012 [1]. Cancer refers to a large group of diseases resulting from uncontrolled proliferation of tissues and its spread that can affect any part of the body. Malignancy, carcinoma, tumours and neoplasms are the other terms referring to different aspects of this medical condition. A defining feature of cancer is the accumulation of mutations resulting in an uncontrolled proliferation of abnormal cells that grow beyond their usual boundaries, and can even invade adjoining structures, spread to other organs, the latter process referred to as metastasis. Metastases or simply spread of cancer is one of the common causes of death in patients with cancer. Cancer being the second leading cause of death in the world is predicted to affect the future mankind in higher numbers. Half of men and one-third of women in the United States are considered to develop cancer during their lifetimes [2]. Today, millions of cancer patients extend their life due to early identification, timely intervention and treatment.

Cancer is not a new disease and has affected people throughout the world at all times. In the current era of modern medicine, antibiotics and novel therapeutics helped us tackle many morbidities and prevent mortalities to an extent. A decline in the infant and maternal mortalities and infectious diseases has occurred due to the improved sanitation, oral rehydration salts, vaccines and antibiotics and these have

P. Prabhakar (✉)
Department of Food Science and Nutrition, College of Agricultural and Marine Sciences,
Sultan Qaboos University, Muscat, Oman
e-mail: drpreeja@squ.edu.om

S. Punnaveetil
Department of Gastroenterology, Starcare Hospital LLC, Muscat, Oman

© Springer International Publishing AG, part of Springer Nature 2018
M. I. Waly, M. S. Rahman (eds.), *Bioactive Components, Diet and Medical Treatment in Cancer Prevention*, https://doi.org/10.1007/978-3-319-75693-6_13

reduced the medical cost burden. But, cancer still remains as a threat to the present and future worlds. In fact, Cancer deaths as documented by WHO in 2015 accounted to around 8.8 million.

2 History

Humans, animals and even trees have had cancer throughout history as recorded. So it is not a surprise that since the dawn of history itself people have known and have written about cancer. The word cancer (*carcinos* and *carcinoma*) originated from a Greek word 'karkinos' meaning crab to describe the invasive nature of the condition. It was first used by the Father of Medicine, Greek physician Hippocrates (460–370 BC) to describe non-ulcer forming and ulcer-forming tumours. But yet he may not be considered as the first to discover this disease. Oldest description of cancer (although the word cancer was not used) was discovered in Egypt and dates back to about 3000 BC. It's called the 'Edwin Smith Papyrus' and is a copy of part of an ancient Egyptian textbook on trauma surgery and it describes eight cases of tumours or ulcers of the breast that were removed by cauterization with a tool called the fire drill. The writing says about the disease, 'There is no treatment' [3].

Some of the earliest evidence of human bone cancer have been found in mummies in ancient Egypt and in ancient manuscripts that dates around 1600 B.C. The world's oldest recorded case of breast cancer hails from ancient Egypt in 1500 BC and it was even recorded that there was no treatment for the cancer, only supportive therapy. Growths suggested that the bone cancer called osteosarcoma have been seen in mummies. Bony skull destruction as seen in invasive malignancies of the head and neck has been found too [4].

The Roman physician, Celsus (28–50 BC), later translated the Greek term into *cancer*, the Latin word for crab. Galen (130–200 AD), another Greek physician, used the word *oncos* (Greek for swelling) to describe tumours. Although the crab analogy of Hippocrates and Celsus is still used to describe malignant tumours, Galen's term is now used as a part of the name for cancer speciality and specialists—Oncology and oncologists, respectively [3].

2.1 Facts and Figures

Cancer is a leading cause of death worldwide. It is estimated that nearly 1 in 6 deaths worldwide occurring is due to cancer. Prevention and early detection must be our aim to lead the fight for a world without much cancer burden. Much of the suffering and death from cancer could be prevented by systematic efforts in reducing tobacco use and alcohol binge and to improve dietary habits, increased physical activity, obesity and the use of established screening tests [5]. In 2017 about 190,500 cancer deaths in the USA is predicted to be caused by cigarette smoking alone [6].

An estimated 20% of all cancers diagnosed in the USA are caused by a combination of excess body weight, physical inactivity, excess alcohol consumption, and poor nutrition, and thus could also be prevented [7]. Cancer screening tests can also prevent thousands of additional cancer deaths through early detection of cancers at an early stage when timely treatment is more effective and interventions like removal of premalignant lesions (colorectal and cervical).

2.2 What Causes Cancer?

Cancer arises from the transformation of normal cells into tumour cells in a multi-stage process that generally progresses from a precancerous lesion to a malignant tumour. These changes are the result of the interaction between a person's genetic factors and external agents including [5, 8]:

(a) Physical carcinogens (ultraviolet and ionizing radiation).
(b) Chemical carcinogens (components of tobacco smoke, alcohol, aflatoxin, food contaminant and arsenic-containing water).
(c) Tobacco use is the most important risk factor for cancer and is responsible for approximately 22% of cancer deaths.
(d) Biological carcinogens, such as infections from certain viruses, bacteria or parasites.
(e) Chronic infections are risk factors for cancer and have major relevance in low- and middle-income countries. Approximately 15% of cancers diagnosed in 2012 were attributed to carcinogenic chronic inflammation associated with infections like *Helicobacter pylori*, human papillomavirus (HPV), hepatitis B virus, hepatitis C virus, HIV and Epstein-Barr virus. Ageing is another factor for the development of cancer. The incidence of cancer rises dramatically with age, most likely due to a build-up of risks for specific cancers that increase with age. The overall risk accumulation is combined with the less effective cell repair mechanisms.
(f) Genetic Factors: Knudson hypothesis, also known as the two-hit hypothesis or multiple-hit hypothesis, explained that cancer is the result of accumulated mutations to a cell's DNA. It was first proposed by Carl O. Nordling in 1953, and later formulated by Alfred G. Knudson in 1971, led indirectly to the identification of cancer-related genes [9–11]. Two hundred ninety-one cancer genes have been reported so far, i.e. more than 1% of all the genes in the human genome. The development of cancer, carcinogenesis depends both on the activation of proto-oncogenes and on the deactivation of tumour suppressor genes. Proto-oncogenes are genes that stimulate cell proliferation, and tumour suppressor genes are responsible for keeping proliferation in check. Ninety percent of cancer genes show somatic mutations in cancer, whereas 20% show germline mutations and 10% show both. The most common class of mutation among the known cancer genes is a chromosomal translocation that creates a chimeric gene or opposes a gene to the regulatory elements of another gene [12].

3 Reducing the Cancer Burden

According to World Health Organization (WHO), 30–50% of cancers could be prevented. This can be accomplished by avoiding risk factors and implementing existing evidence-based prevention strategies. The cancer burden can also be reduced through early detection of cancer and timely management of patients who develop cancer. Many cancers have a high chance of cure if diagnosed early and treated timely and adequately.

3.1 Modifiable Risk Factors

Modifying or avoiding key risk factors can significantly reduce the risk and burden of cancer cost. These risk factors include [13]: use of tobacco including cigarettes and smokeless tobacco, over eating that leads on to overweight or obese, unhealthy diet lacking fibre, fruits and vegetables, consumption of smoked foods, sedentary lifestyle and lack of physical activity, alcohol, prolonged sun exposure, ionizing and ultraviolet radiation, air pollution, indoor smoke from household use of solid fuels, occupational hazards involved with ship industry, infection by *H. pylori*, HPV, Hepatitis B and C or other carcinogenic infections, and human immunodeficiency virus (HIV) associated cancers.

To prevent cancer, people may increase avoidance of the risk factors listed above and have healthy life style and dietary habits vaccinate against HPV and hepatitis B virus control occupational hazards reduce exposure to ultraviolet radiation reduce exposure to ionizing radiation (occupational or medical diagnostic imaging). Early detection of *H.pylori* infection and adopting *H.pylori* eradication. Vaccination against these HPV and Hepatitis B viruses alone could prevent up to 1 million cancer cases each year.

3.2 Early Detection

Cancer mortality can be reduced if incident cases are detected and treated timely. There are two components of early detection and diagnosis. When identified early, cancer is more likely to respond to effective treatment and can result in a greater probability of surviving, lesser morbidity, and lesser expensive treatment. Early diagnosis consists of integration of these strategies in a timely manner: awareness and access to treatment and quality cancer care and clinical evaluation, diagnosis and staging of cancer. The early accurate diagnosis is relevant in all settings and the majority of cancers. In the absence of early diagnosis, patients are diagnosed at late stages when curative treatment may no longer be effective and supportive therapy and palliation may be the only option. Programmes can be designed to reduce delays in, and barriers to, care, allowing patients to access treatment in a timely manner.

Early detection of cancer greatly increases the chances for successful treatment. There are two major components of early detection of cancer: education to promote early diagnosis and screening. Recognizing possible warning signs of cancer and taking prompt action leads to early diagnosis. Increased awareness of possible warning signs of cancer, among physicians, nurses and other health care providers as well as among the general public, can have a great impact on the disease. Some early signs of cancer include lumps, sores that fail to heal, abnormal bleeding, persistent indigestion and chronic hoarseness. Early diagnosis is particularly relevant for cancers of the breast, cervix, mouth, larynx, colon and rectum, and skin.

3.3   Screening

Screening aims to identify individuals with abnormalities suggestive of a specific cancer or precancer who have not developed any symptoms and refer them promptly for diagnosis and treatment. Screening programmes can be effective for certain cancer types when appropriate tests are used, implemented effectively, linked to other steps in the screening process and when quality is assured. In general, a screening programme is a far more complex public health intervention compared to early diagnosis. Examples of screening methods are: visual inspection with acetic acid (VIA) for cervical cancer in low-income settings, HPV and PAP cytology test testing for cervical cancer, and mammogram screening for breast cancer in settings with strong or relatively strong health systems.

Screening refers to the use of simple tests across a healthy population in order to identify individuals who have disease, but do not yet have symptoms. Examples include breast cancer screening using mammography and cervical cancer screening using cytology screening methods, including Pap smears. Screening programmes should be undertaken only when their effectiveness has been demonstrated, when resources (personnel, equipment, etc.) are sufficient to cover nearly all of the target group, when facilities exist for confirming diagnoses and for treatment and follow-up of those with abnormal results, and when prevalence of the disease is high enough to justify the effort and costs of screening [14].

Screening is the presumptive identification of unrecognized disease or defects by means of tests, examinations, or other procedures that can be applied rapidly. In advocating screening programmes as part of early detection of cancer, it is important for national cancer control programmes to avoid imposing the 'high technology' of the developed world on third world countries that lack the infrastructure and resources to use the technology appropriately or to achieve adequate coverage of the population. The success of screening depends on having sufficient numbers of personnel to perform the screening tests and on the availability of facilities that can undertake subsequent diagnosis, treatment and follow-up.

Sensitivity, specificity, positive predictive value, negative predictive value and acceptability of the testing methods should be taken into account when the adoption of any screening technique is being considered. A screening test aims to be sure that as few as possible with the disease get through undetected (high sensitivity) and as few as possible without the disease are subject to further diagnostic tests (high specificity). Given high sensitivity and specificity, the likelihood that a positive screening test will give a correct result (positive predictive value) strongly depends on the prevalence of the disease within the population. If the prevalence of the disease is very low, even the best screening test will not be an effective public health programme.

Policies on early cancer detection differ markedly between countries. An industrialized country may conduct screening programmes for cervical and breast cancer. Such programmes are not, however, recommended in the least developed countries in which there is a low prevalence of cancer and a weak health care infrastructure. Further, only organized screening programmes are likely to be fully successful as a means of reaching a high proportion of the at-risk population.

Countries that favour early cancer detection as part of health care strategies should adopt screening measures based on the following principles: The target disease should be a common form of cancer, with high associated morbidity or mortality; effective treatment, capable of reducing morbidity and mortality, should be available and easily accessible to the screened population; test procedures should be acceptable, safe, and relatively inexpensive. An information system that can: (1) send out invitations for initial screening; (2) recall individuals for repeat screening; (3) follow those with identified abnormalities. (4) monitor and evaluate the programme.

For many reasons, patients fail to adhere to recommended cancer screening activities. While in many cases both the patients and the health care providers understand the concept of early detection, they fail to comply with recommendations. This is Non-compliance. Non-compliance is a general health problem and one that should be addressed in a comprehensive manner to improve outcome and reduce the waste of resources. Screening that concentrates solely on a high-risk group is rarely justifiable, as identified risk groups usually represent only a small proportion of the cancer burden in a country. In planning the coverage of screening programmes, however, steps must be taken to ensure that all those at high risk are included. This requirement may be difficult to fulfil. In screening for cancer of the cervix, for example, those at high risk are often difficult to recruit into screening.

3.4   Treatment

A correct cancer diagnosis is essential for adequate and effective treatment because every cancer type requires a specific treatment regimen that encompasses one or more modalities such as surgery, radiotherapy and chemotherapy. Determining the goals of treatment and palliative care is an important first step, and health services should be integrated and people-centred. The primary goal is generally to cure cancer or to considerably prolong life. Improving the patient's quality of life is also an important goal. This can be achieved by supportive or palliative care and psychosocial support.

Potential for cure among early detectable cancers; some of the most common cancer types, such as breast cancer, cervical cancer, oral cancer and colorectal cancer, have high cure rates when detected early and treated according to best practices. Potential for cure of some other cancers; Some cancer types, even when cancerous cells have metastasized to other areas of the body, such as testicular seminoma and leukaemia and lymphoma in children, can have high cure rates if appropriate treatment is provided.

3.5 Palliative Care

Palliative care aims to relieve, rather than cure, symptoms caused by cancer and improve the quality of life of patients and their families. It can help people live more comfortably. It is an urgent humanitarian need for people worldwide with cancer and other chronic fatal diseases and particularly needed in places with a high proportion of patients in advanced stages of cancer where there is little chance of cure. Relief from physical, psychosocial and spiritual problems can be achieved in over 90% of advanced cancer patients through palliative care.

Palliative care strategies; effective public health strategies comprising of community- and home-based care are essential to provide pain relief and palliative care for patients and their families in low-resource settings. Improved access to oral morphine is mandatory for the treatment of moderate to severe cancer pain, suffered by over 80% of cancer patients in terminal phase.

4   Selected Cancer Prevention and Control

4.1   Breast Cancer

Breast cancer is the cancer among females with highest prevalence both in the developed and in the developing world. The incidence of breast cancer is increasing in the developing world due to increased life expectancy, increased urbanization and adoption of western lifestyles. Although some risk reduction might be achieved with prevention, these strategies cannot eliminate the majority of breast cancers that develop in low- and middle-income countries where breast cancer is diagnosed in very late stages. Therefore, early detection in order to improve breast cancer outcome and survival remains the cornerstone of breast cancer control. Population-based cancer screening is a much more complex public health undertaking than early diagnosis and is usually cost-effective when done in the context of high-standard programmes that target all the population at risk in a given geographical area with high specific cancer burden, with everyone who takes part being offered the same level of screening, diagnosis and treatment services [15].

So far the only breast cancer screening method that has proved to be effective is mammography screening. Mammography screening is very costly and is cost-effective and feasible in countries with good health infrastructure that can afford a long-term organized population-based screening programmes. Low-cost screening approaches, such as clinical breast examination, could be implemented in limited resource settings when the necessary evidence from ongoing studies becomes available. Many low- and middle-income countries that face the double burden of cervical and breast cancer need to implement combined cost-effective and affordable interventions to tackle these highly preventable diseases. Early detection in order to improve breast cancer outcome and survival remains the cornerstone of breast cancer control. WHO promotes breast cancer control within the context of national cancer control programmes and integrated to non-communicable disease prevention and control.

The 2015 guidelines by American Cancer Society states that [16]: women aged 40–49 with average risk: Women aged 40–44 years should have the choice to start annual breast cancer screening with mammograms if they wish to do so and considering the risks of screening as well as the potential benefits. Women aged 45–49 years should get mammograms every year. Women aged 50–74 with average risk: women aged 50–54 years should get mammograms every year, women aged 55 years and older should switch to mammograms every 2 years, or have the choice to continue yearly screening. Women aged 75 or older with average risk: screening should continue as long as a woman is in good health and is expected to live 10 more years or longer. Women at higher than average risk: women who are at high risk for breast cancer based on certain factors (such as having a parent, sibling or child with a BRCA 1 or BRCA2 gene mutation) should get an MRI and a mammogram every year. Women should be familiar with the known benefits, limitations and potential harms associated with breast cancer screening. They should also be familiar with how their breasts normally look and feel and report any changes to a health care provider right away.

4.2   Cervical Cancer

Screening is testing of all women at risk of cervical cancer, most of whom will be without symptoms. Screening aims to detect precancerous changes, which, if not treated, may lead to cancer. It is only effective if there is a well-organized system for follow-up and treatment. Women who are found to have abnormalities on screening need follow-up, diagnosis and possibly treatment, in order to prevent the development of cancer or to treat cancer at an early stage.

Several tests can be used in screening for cervical cancer. The Pap smear (cytology) is the only test that has been used in large populations and that has been shown to reduce cervical cancer incidence and mortality. Regardless of the test used, the key to an effective programme is to reach the largest proportion of women at risk with quality screening and treatment. Organized screening programmes designed and managed at the central level to reach most women at risk are preferable to opportunistic screening.

The guidelines by American Cancer Society (ACS), American Society for Colposcopy and Cervical Pathology (ASCCP), and American Society for Clinical Pathology (ASCP) recommend to start screening: age 21. Women aged <21 years should not be screened regardless of sex initialization or other risk factors. Frequency of cervical cancer screening: cytology (conventional or liquid based) testing 21–29 years of age (Every 3 years), 30–65 years of age (Every 3 years), HPV co-test (cytology + hr HPV test administered together); in women 30–65 years of age (Every 5 years), HPV co-testing should not be used for women aged <30 years.

When to stop screening: Aged >65 years with adequate negative prior screening and no history of CIN 2 (Cervical Intraepithelial Neoplasia) or higher within the last 20 years. When to screen after age 65 years: Aged >65 years with a history of CIN2 CIN2, CIN3, or adenocarcinoma in situ, routine screening should continue for at least 20 years. Screening among those immunized against HPV 16/18: Women at any age in spite of HPV vaccination should be screened according to the age-specific recommendations for the general population [17].

4.3   Colorectal Cancer

Colorectal cancer is one of the malignancies where premalignant conditions can be detected easily and removed efficiently which directly results in an improved prognosis and longevity. Multiple modalities of screening have been suggested by various organizations. Scientific evidence suggests that sigmoidoscopy alone may be effective for colorectal cancer screening, with benefits lasting for up to 10 years. Several trials have evaluated the effect of the faecal occult blood test (FOBT). Even though, there seems to be a lack in sensitivity for detecting adenomas.

In 2015, the American College of Physicians (ACP) recommended that average-risk adults aged 50–75 years should be screened for colorectal cancer by one of the following strategies: Annual high-sensitivity FOBT or FIT, flexible sigmoidoscopy every 5 years, high-sensitivity FOBT or FIT every 3 years plus flexible sigmoidoscopy every 5 years, and colonoscopy every 10 years. Interval screening with faecal testing or flexible sigmoidoscopy in adults having 10-year screening colonoscopy is not recommended. Average-risk adults younger than 50 years, older than 75 years, or with an estimated life expectancy of less than 10 years should not be screened. For screening purposes, patients with one first-degree relative diagnosed with colorectal cancer or advanced adenoma at age 60 years or older are considered at average risk. For patients with a single first-degree relative diagnosed with colorectal cancer or advanced adenoma before age 60 years, or those with two first-degree relatives with colorectal cancer or advanced adenomas, the guideline recommends colonoscopy every 5 years, beginning at age 40 years or at 10 years younger than the age at diagnosis of the youngest affected relative. A new, simple, blood test called Septin 9 (Epi procolon) has been evaluated as a screening technique for Colorectal malignancy with 48% sensitivity. However, it's not efficient in detecting colonic polyps. Yearly Septin 9 testing has recently been US FDA approved and may replace FOBT and come into vogue in the future as the simplest screening test for CRC.

4.4   Oral Cancer

Early detection (as distinct from organized screening) of oral cancer using visual inspection of the mouth is being considered in countries where incidence is high, such as Bangladesh, India, Pakistan and Sri Lanka. The oral cavity is easily accessible for routine examination, and nonmedical personnel can readily detect lesions that are the precursors of carcinoma. Precursor lesions may regress if tobacco use ceases and that surgical treatment of early oral cancer is very effective. Some programmes have also encouraged early detection of oral cancer by self-examination using a mirror. However, so far it has not been shown that detection of precancerous lesions or early cancers can reduce mortality from the disease.

5   Challenges in Cancer Screening and Early Detection Research

Patients whose cancers are detected and treated early may have better long-term survival than patients whose cancers are not found until symptoms appear. Unfortunately, effective screening tests for early detection do not exist for many cancers. Considering cancers for which there are widely used screening tests, many of the tests have not proven effective in reducing cancer mortality. But, there have been some important successes in screening and early detection. Deaths from cervical cancer in the United States, for example, declined substantially after annual screening with the Pap test became common practice, and screening for colorectal and breast cancer have also been shown to reduce mortality from these cancers. Although research on cancer screening and early detection can be challenging, the potential results in terms of cancer deaths avoided. A greater understanding of the underlying biology of many cancers, as well as technological advances in areas such as imaging, are creating new avenues for advances in screening and early detection. Importantly, studies performed over the last decade have strongly suggested that, in addition to benefits, screening has downsides. In particular, there is the risk of over-diagnosis and overtreatment—the diagnosis and treatment of cancers that would not threaten life or cause symptoms.

Overdiagnosis and overtreatment expose patients unnecessarily to the potential physical harms of unneeded and often invasive diagnostic tests and treatment, as well as to the psychological stresses associated with a cancer diagnosis. This understanding has led to intensive study of ways to identify and distinguish those screen-detected cancers that are truly life threatening and require immediate treatment from those for which treatment is unnecessary or can be safely delayed. Based on research, investigators are pursuing key opportunities, including: developing 'liquid biopsy' technologies that can noninvasively identify the presence of genetic material from cancer cells in the blood or molecular markers in urine or saliva that can identify precursor lesions or cancer at its earliest stages, identifying and validating biomarkers that may distinguish aggressive, life-threatening cancers from non-life-threatening tumours, identifying genetic changes that point to potential avenues for more effectively monitoring people at increased risk of cancer, testing interventions, such as the use of health navigators and tailored outreach and education programmes, to increase the use of approved, effective screening tests among certain population groups, and better quantifying the benefits and harms of screening tests, as well as the relative contributions of cancer screening and improvements in treatment on mortality rates.

6 Conclusion

As with research on cancer prevention, time is a challenge when developing and testing new interventions for screening and early detection. Years or decades are often needed to determine whether an intervention, such as a new screening test or a patient risk assessment, reduces the number of people diagnosed with advanced cancer or who die from cancer. And these studies can be expensive and logistically challenging to conduct. Discovering and validating biomarkers that can accurately identify people at increased risk of cancer or who have potentially lethal cancers has also proven to be very difficult. Many biomarkers that have shown promise in early studies have not been validated subsequently in more advanced testing. In addition, screening and early detection on their own are often not enough. Ensuring that individuals receive the appropriate follow-up and treatment after a cancer diagnosis is essential but has proven to be difficult, particularly for those from low socioeconomic settings and certain racial or ethnic groups, resulting in delayed treatment and worse outcomes.

References

1. Ferlay J, Soerjomataram I, Ervik M, Dikshit R, Eser S, Mathers C, et al. Cancer incidence and mortality worldwide. Lyon, France: IARC, International Agency for Research on Cancer; 2013.
2. National Cancer Institute. Surveillance research program. http://surveillance.cancer.gov/devcan/.
3. American Cancer Society. The history of cancer. https://www.cancer.org/cancer/cancer-basics/history-of-cancer.html.

4. Sudhakar A. History of cancer, ancient and modern treatment methods. J Cancer Sci Ther. 2009;1(2):1–4.
5. World Cancer Research Fund and American Institute for Cancer Research. Continuous update project. http://www.wcrf.org/int/research-we-fund/continuous-update-project-cup.
6. Kohler LN, Garcia DO, Harris RB, Oren E, Roe DJ, Jacobs ET. Adherence to diet and physical activity cancer prevention guidelines and cancer outcomes: a systematic review. Cancer Epidemiol Biomarkers Prev. 2016;25:1018–28.
7. Kushi LH, Doyle C, McCullough M, et al. American Cancer Society Guidelines on Nutrition and Physical Activity for cancer prevention: reducing the risk of cancer with healthy food choices and physical activity. CA Cancer J Clin. 2012;62(1):30–67.
8. GBD 2015 Risk Factors Collaborators. Global, regional, and national comparative risk assessment of 79 behavioural, environmental and occupational, and metabolic risks or clusters of risks, 1990–2015: a systematic analysis for the Global Burden of Disease Study 2015. Lancet. 2016;388(10053):1659–724.
9. Nordling C. A new theory on cancer-inducing mechanism. Br J Cancer. 1953;7(1):68–72.
10. Marte B, Eccleston A, Nath D. Molecular cancer diagnostics. Nature. 2008;452(7187):547.
11. Knudson A. Mutation and cancer: statistical study of retinoblastoma. Proc Natl Acad Sci U S A. 1971;68(4):820–3.
12. Futreal PA, Coin L, Marshall M, Down T, Hubbard T, Wooster R, Stratton MR. A census of human cancer genes. Nat Rev Cancer. 2004;4(3):177–83.
13. Plummer M, de Martel C, Vignat J, Ferlay J, Bray F, Franceschi S. Global burden of cancers attributable to infections in 2012: a synthetic analysis. Lancet Glob Health. 2016;4(9):e609–16.
14. Stewart BW, Wild CP, editors. World cancer report. Lyon, France: International Agency for Research on Cancer; 2014.
15. White JD, Lin H, Jia L, Wu RS, Lam S, Li J, Dou J, Kumar N, Lin L, Lao L. Proceedings of the strategy meeting for the development of an International Consortium for Chinese Medicine and Cancer. J Glob Oncol. 2017;3(6):814–22.
16. Oeffinger KC, Fontham ET, Etzioni R, Herzig A, Michaelson JS, Shih YC, et al. American Cancer Society. Breast cancer screening for women at average risk: 2015 guideline update from the American Cancer Society. JAMA. 2015;314(15):1599–614.
17. Saslow D, Solomon D, Lawson HW, Killackey M, Kulasingam SL, Cain J, et al. American Cancer Society; American Society for Colposcopy and Cervical Pathology; American Society for Clinical Pathology. American Cancer Society, American Society for Colposcopy and Cervical Pathology, and American Society for Clinical Pathology screening guidelines for the prevention and early detection of cervical cancer. Am J Clin Pathol. 2012;137(4):516–42.

Prevention of Common Cancers of the Female Genital Tract

Ikram Ali Burney

1 Introduction

The world has seen incremental success in the outcomes of patients with cancer over the past 60 years. Ever-growing surgical expertise, improvements in radiation techniques, combination chemotherapy, supportive care, improved diagnostics, and more recently targeted therapy, all have led a changed landscape. A significant number of cancer patients, previously deemed incurable, is now cured. What cannot be cured does not have to be endured. Several incurable cancers are now managed like a chronic disease. However, despite the success in treatment of cancer, total number of patients who die as a result of cancer continue to increase, and this is a direct reflection of the rising incidence. According to the Globocan, 12.7 million patients were diagnosed with cancer in 2008, and the number is likely to increase almost twofold to 22.2 million by 2030. Similarly, 7.6 million people died of cancer in 2008, and the number is likely to increase to 17 million by 2030 [1]. Despite all the excitement and success in accurate diagnosis and refined treatment of cancer, clearly a lot more needs to be achieved in research and implementation of effective policies to reduce the incidence of cancer, in order to decrease the overall burden of the disease and the attendant mortality. Cancer should be treated across the continuum, if meaningful gain in survival is the goal (Fig. 1).

In this chapter, developments in the field of prevention of gynecological cancers are reviewed. Together, gynecological cancers rank among the top five cancers worldwide (Table 1). Female genital tract consists of ovaries and the fallopian tubes, uterus, cervix, vagina, and the vulva. Cancers of the vulva and vagina are uncommon. Furthermore, throughout the female genital tract, cancers may arise from the epithelium (carcinoma), mesothelium (sarcoma), connective tissue, or the germ cells

I. A. Burney (✉)
Department of Medicine, Sultan Qaboos University Hospital, Sultan Qaboos University, Muscat, Oman
e-mail: ikram@squ.edu.om

© Springer International Publishing AG, part of Springer Nature 2018
M. I. Waly, M. S. Rahman (eds.), *Bioactive Components, Diet and Medical Treatment in Cancer Prevention*, https://doi.org/10.1007/978-3-319-75693-6_14

161

Fig. 1 The cancer continuum

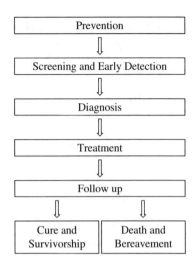

Prevention

⇓

Screening and Early Detection

⇓

Diagnosis

⇓

Treatment

⇓

Follow up

⇓   ⇓

| Cure and Survivorship | Death and Bereavement |

Table 1 Cancer prevalence

Cancer	No. in millions
Cancer of lung	1825
Cancer of breast	1677
Colorectal cancers	1361
Prostate cancer	1112
Gynecological cancers	1087

of the ovary, or may even be secondary from other organs, or because of infiltration of leukemic cells. Cancers of epithelial origin are by far the commonest, and account for 80–90% of all gynecological cancers. In this chapter, preventive strategies for epithelial cancers arising from ovary and the fallopian tubes, uterus, and the cervix are discussed.

The description would include the histological subtypes, incidence, risk factors, and prevention strategies. For the purposes of this chapter, discussion on prevention strategies would be restricted to published guidelines, phase III studies, meta-analyses, and systematic reviews. It would be simply out of scope of the chapter to deal with the individual studies and expert opinions. Before dealing with prevention strategies for the three cancers separately, it would be prudent to define "risk factors" and different types of preventive strategies of cancer in the clinical context.

1.1 Risk Factors of Cancers of the Female Genital Tract

A risk factor is an attribute, a characteristic, or an exposure which could increase the incidence of getting a certain disease, including cancer. It is important to note that a risk factor may increase the incidence, but may not necessarily be causal. The risk is estimated through correlation. Since the correlation of an attribute or a characteristic may increase the risk of developing cancer, it is plausible to use the risk factors to devise strategies for prevention. Common risk factors for cancer include age, smoking, infectious agents, diet, obesity, environmental carcinogens such as radiation and chemicals, and genetic factors. It is evident that some risk factors are modifiable and others are not. In the sections below, risk factors would be described as definitive (may be even causal), probable (unequivocal association), equivocal (no convincing evidence), or preventive.

1.2 Prevention Strategies of Cancers of the Female Genital Tract

Prevention strategies include a range of activities or interventions aimed at reducing the risks. Interventions to alter the modifiable risk factors can be employed in reducing the incidence of cancer. Generally, interventions include lifestyle modifications, pharmacological interventions, and sometimes even surgical interventions. The preventive strategies would be defined as either primary, secondary, or tertiary [1, 2].

1.2.1 Primary Prevention

Primary prevention aims to prevent cancer before it occurs. Usually, primary preventive strategies apply to all individuals at risk. This is done by either preventing or reducing the exposure through education and awareness, such as lifestyle factors and smoking cessation, or by immunization against the infective agent, such as HBV vaccination for hepatocellular cancer and HPV vaccination for cervical cancer.

1.2.2 Secondary Prevention

Secondary prevention aims to reduce the impact, especially in those who are predisposed. Examples include screening and early detection of cancers of the breast, cervix, prostate or colon, chemoprevention of colon cancers in those genetically predisposed, and surgical prevention in those who are at an exceedingly high risk of developing the cancer.

1.2.3 Tertiary Prevention

Tertiary prevention aims to reduce recurrences of cancer in those who have already been diagnosed to have cancer and are in remission after successful treatment.

Although targeted risk reduction in the form of secondary and tertiary prevention may seem cost-effective for the specific type of cancer, primary prevention remains the ultimate aim to reduce the burden of disease. A plethora of data has been published on the issue of primary prevention, and it would be out of scope of this chapter to review it here. More recently, the World Cancer Research Fund

Table 2 WCRF/AICR recommendations

Be as lean as is possible, maintaining BMI close to 25
Regular physical activity, at least 30 min per day
Restrict red meat consumption, five portions per week
Increase fruit and vegetable consumption 5/15 portions per day
Stop smoking
Restrict the intake of alcohol
Limit the use of high energy drinks
Avoid processed meat
Avoid dietary supplements
For women, breast-feeding for at least 6 months

(WCRF) published evidence-based guidelines for primary prevention of cancer (Table 2). Several lifestyle and dietary modifications were suggested.

Over the next few years, it became apparent that people who adhered to guidelines had a significant reduction in the incidence of and mortality from different types of cancers, including gynecological cancers. For example, the EPIC investigators reported that a greater concordance with the WCRF recommendations was significantly associated with a decreased risk of cancer [2].

One-point increment was associated with a 5% risk reduction for all cancers, 12% for colorectal cancers and 16% for the stomach cancer [3]. Furthermore, the investigators showed that participants with maximum adherence to the WCRF recommendations had a 34% reduced risk of death compared with those who had least adherence to the recommendations [4]. Similarly, the data from the VITAL study revealed that the breast cancer risk reduced by 60% in women who met at least five recommendations, and the incidence of hematologic malignancies reduced by 34% in cohort of people who carried out regular physical activity [5].

Having defined "risk factors" and "prevention strategies," and the WCRF recommendations for primary prevention, applicable to all cancers, we now describe the data on prevention of the three common cancers of the female genital tract.

2 Ovarian Cancer

2.1 Epidemiology

Ovarian cancer is one of the most common gynecological cancers, and predominantly affects postmenopausal women. According to the Globocan data, ovarian cancer is the 18th most common cancer in both genders, and the 7th most common cancer in women. Ovarian cancer is the leading cause of death among the gynecological cancers in the developed countries. There are several types, including epithelial ovarian cancer (EOC), germ cell tumors, sex cord-stromal tumors, metastatic tumors, and infiltration with leukemia and lymphoma. Epithelial ovarian cancer (EOC) is by far the commonest and account for 80–90% of all ovarian cancers. Pathological and molecular advances have revealed that most pelvic high-grade serous cancers, previously attributed to an ovarian origin, are probably implants from cancer originating in the fimbria of the fallopian tube. Epithelial cancers arising from the fallopian tube and the peritoneum share the natural course, response to treatment, outcome, and prognosis. Hence, for the purposes of diagnosis and treatment, tumors of the ovary, fallopian tubes, and peritoneum are considered together.

EOC can be divided into several histological subtypes: high-grade serous, endometrioid, and clear cell, mucinous and low-grade serous. These subtypes represent distinct disease entities, both clinically and at the molecular level. The vast majority of patients (60–80%) with high-grade serous epithelial cancer present with stage III and IV disease. Despite the currently available evidence-based management, the 5-year survival rates are 30–50% for stage IIIa–IIIc tumors, and 13% for stage IV tumors, while the median survival is 36 and 24 months, respectively. The standard care treatment includes debulking surgery and adjuvant combination chemotherapy. For the past two decades, the combination of paclitaxel and carboplatin has remained the standard of care. The two most important prognostic factors for a better outcome are the completeness of surgery (debulking surgery leading to minimal residual disease defined as tumor less than 5 mm in any given place), and sensitivity to platinum-based chemotherapy. Despite a high initial response rate to platinum and taxane treatment, the effectiveness of the treatments diminishes over time, and most patients experience disease relapse. Clearly, there is an unmet need to either prevent or detect the disease early.

2.2 Risk Factors

Although the etiology of ovarian cancer is not clear, certain factors are implicated in the etiology of this disease, such as ovulation, gonadotropic and steroid hormones, germ cell depletion, oncogenes and tumor suppressor genes, growth factors, cytokines, and environmental agents [6]. Family history of breast or ovarian cancer, or a personal history of breast cancer is a prominent risk factor for ovarian cancer, with 5–15% of ovarian cancers due to heritable risk. Hormone replacement therapy is known to cause a modest increase in risk. Obesity and diet may affect ovarian cancer risk. Reproductive factors such as age at menopause and infertility contribute to greater risk of ovarian cancer. Exposure to environmental agents such as talc may increase risk of ovarian cancer. Hormonal factors such as oral contraceptive (OC), pregnancy, tubal ligation, and hysterectomy reduce risk.

2.2.1 Definitive Risk Factors

Family/Personal History of Breast/Ovarian Cancer and Inherited Cancer
Genetic Syndromes

The strongest risk factor for EOC is the genetic predisposition. (For comprehensive review see [7]). Women with a family history of ovarian cancer, especially in a first-degree relative, and those with an inherited predisposition to ovarian cancer, such as a *BRCA1* or *BRCA2* mutation, have an increased risk of developing ovarian cancer. *BRCA1* or *BRCA2* genes are tumor suppressor genes, and mutations in either of these genes increase the susceptibility. Mutations in *BRCA1* and *BRCA2* are very high in certain kindreds, such as the Ashkenazi Jews. The lifetime ovarian cancer risk for women with a *BRCA1* mutation is estimated to be up to 45%, and between 10% and 30% for women with *BRCA2* mutations, compared to less than 2% for general population.

Other inherited cancer genetic syndromes in which the risk of ovarian cancer is significantly higher than the general population are the PTEN tumor hamartoma syndrome also known as Cowden disease (due to inherited mutations in the *PTEN* gene); hereditary nonpolyposis coli cancer syndrome (due to mutations in *MLH1*, *MSH2*, *MSH6*, *PMS1*, and *PMS2* genes); and Peutz-Jeghers syndrome due to mutations in the *STK11* gene. More recently, germline mutations in BRIP1, RAD51D, and RAD51C have been associated with increased risk of developing EOC over lifetime [8].

Hormone Replacement Therapy (HRT)

Is strongly associated with a moderate increase in the risk of developing epithelial ovarian cancer. A meta-analysis of 52 studies including more than 21,000 patients found an increased risk of ovarian cancer with current or recent use of HRT, especially for the serous and endometrioid subtypes. Recent use was more strongly related to the risk, even among women who had used HRT for less than 5 years, whereas the risk declined among women after discontinuation for longer periods of cessation.

2.2.2   Probable Risk Factors

Obesity

The association between obesity and ovarian cancer risk has been extensively investigated, but studies have yielded inconsistent findings. Based on an overview analysis of 25,157 women with ovarian cancer and 81,211 women without ovarian cancer from 47 epidemiological studies, there was a limited, inconsistent evidence of a positive association between obesity and ovarian cancer risk. Out of the 43 studies, 14 studies found a statistically significant positive association, 26 studies found no significant association, and 3 studies found a negative association between ovarian cancer risk and higher body mass index. However, a further analysis revealed the interplay between obesity and the use of hormone therapy. The RR of ovarian cancer per 5 kg/m^2 increase in body mass index (BMI) was 1.10 (95% CI, 1.07–1.13) among never-users of hormone therapy and 0.95 (95% CI, 0.92–0.99) among ever-users of hormone therapy [9, 10].

Dietary Factors

No consistent association has been observed between a variety of dietary factors and the risk of ovarian cancer [10, 11]. An analysis from the Women's Health Initiative (WHI) prospective, low fat dietary modification trial of 48,835 postmenopausal women suggested that long-term adoption of a low fat diet was associated with a 40% reduction in ovarian cancer risk [12]. A systematic review suggested that total, animal, and dairy fat were consistently associated with a higher risk [13]. The role of physical activity in ovarian cancer is not clearly understood. A randomized, controlled trial, the Lifestyle Intervention for Ovarian Cancer Enhanced Survival (LIVES) is prospectively assessing the effect of diet in combination with physical activity on increasing progression-free survival (PFS) in women previously treated for ovarian cancer. When completed, LIVES will be the largest behavior-based lifestyle intervention trial conducted among ovarian cancer survivors [11–14].

2.2.3   Equivocal Risk Factors

Alcohol

A systematic review and meta-analysis including 23 case-control studies and 3 cohort studies found no evidence of an association between alcohol use and EOC [15, 16].

Aspirin and Nonsteroidal Anti-Inflammatory Drugs

A systematic review and meta-analysis of 21 observational studies found a decreased risk of invasive ovarian cancer with aspirin use, but no statistically significant association with nonsteroidal anti-inflammatory drugs (NSAIDs). A population-based case-control study of 902 incident cases and 1802 population controls observed a decreased risk of ovarian cancer associated with continual use.

Perineal Talc Exposure

There is no consistent association between talc exposure and an increased risk of ovarian cancer. A meta-analysis of 16 studies observed an increased risk with the use of talc, whereas a pooled analysis from the Ovarian Cancer Association Consortium including 8525 cases and 9859 controls found a modest increased risk of EOC with genital powder use. On the other hand, a cohort study among nurses did not observe a risk of ovarian cancer associated with perineal talc use, and in the WHI study, no association of ovarian cancer with talc powder use was found.

Ovarian Hyperstimulation Due to Infertility Treatment

Controversy persists concerning the association between ovarian hyperstimulation and ovarian cancer. Results of a systematic review and meta-analysis of nine cohort studies comprising 109,969 women provided inconclusive evidence for an association. A Cochrane systematic review including 11 case-control studies and 14 cohort studies, for a total of 186,972 women, was also indeterminate for an association.

2.2.4 Preventive Factors

Oral Contraceptives

OCs reduce the risk of developing EOC. The degree of risk reduction varies by duration of OC use, and the time since last use. For example, for 1–4 years of OC use, the risk reduction is 22%, and for 15 or more years of use, the risk reduction is 56%. The reduction in risk persists for more than 30 years after discontinuing the use. On the other hand, use of combined estrogen-progestin OC is associated with an increased risk of venous thromboembolism, particularly among smokers. A meta-analysis of 24 case-control and cohort studies reported risk reduction by duration of use. The risk reduction among women using OC for more than 1 year but less than 5 years was 0.77; and for more than 10 years, 0.43. Based on an estimated lifetime risk of 1.38% and prevalence of ever-use of oral contraceptives of 83%, the estimated lifetime reduction of ovarian cancer attributable to oral contraceptives was 0.54%.

Tubal Ligation

Tubal ligation provides a relative reduction in the odds of developing ovarian cancer of about 30%. A meta-analysis of 16 case-control studies, three retrospective studies, and two prospective cohort studies observed a decreased risk of ovarian cancer associated with tubal ligation. The reduced risk was observed up to 14 years after tubal ligation. The risk reduction is more for the serous subtype as compared to clear cell, endometroid, and the mucinous subtypes.

Multiparity

Parous women have appropriately 30% lower ovarian cancer risk than nulliparous women.

Salpingectomy

Data relating salpingectomy to risk of ovarian/tubal cancer are limited, but consistent. A meta-analysis of three studies found an OR of 0.51 for risk of these cancers among women who had undergone salpingectomy, compared with women who had intact fallopian tubes. Protection for bilateral salpingectomy was approximately twice that for unilateral salpingectomy.

Breast-Feeding

Breast-feeding reduces the risk of EOC. A meta-analysis including 5 prospective studies and 30 case-control studies examined the association between breast-feeding and the risk of ovarian cancer. Any breast-feeding was associated with a decreased risk of ovarian cancer. The risk decreased by 8% for every 5-month increase in duration of breast-feeding. Another meta-analysis including 5 prospective and 35 case-control studies also found that breast-feeding was associated with a decreased risk of ovarian cancer. Yet another meta-analysis of 19 studies, including 4 cohort and 15 case-control studies, also found an overall decreased risk of ovarian cancer.

2.3   Screening for Early Detection

Almost 75% of patients with high-grade EOC are diagnosed with stage IIIc/IV disease. There are no appropriate screening tests to detect EOC early. This observation provides the rationale to look for screening tests to diagnose the disease early. The most commonly used tests are serum tumor marker CA125 and pelvic ultrasound. However, because of suboptimal sensitivity, and a poor predictive value, there are concerns about the use of these tests. Data to show improved survival with screening for ovarian cancer in any population are lacking. Whereas, four large trials demonstrated that screening may detect the disease early, they failed to show a survival benefit. The US Preventive Services Task Force (USPSTF) recommends against screening for ovarian cancer in asymptomatic women of average risk, however, the UK Collaborative Trial of Ovarian Cancer Screening (UKCTOCS) has shown encouraging early data; the final results are awaited [17, 18]. Also, for the high-risk group, such as those with hereditary breast ovarian cancer syndrome, or a strong family history of ovarian cancer, the NCCN does not consider screening for ovarian cancer to be a reasonable substitute for salpingo-oophorectomy. However, a woman who declines salpingo-oophorectomy may undergo screening with serum measurement of CA-125 and transvaginal ultrasonography every 6–12 months, starting at age 30–35 years or 5–10 years before the earliest diagnosis of ovarian cancer in the family.

2.4   Prevention of Ovarian Cancer

There are several ways to reduce the risk of developing EOC. It is important to realize that some of these strategies reduce the risk only slightly, while others decrease it much more [19].

2.4.1 Primary Prevention

The World Cancer Research Fund (WCRF) recommends eating a variety of healthy foods, with an emphasis on plant sources. Eat at least 2 ½ cups of fruits and vegetables every day, as well as several servings of whole grain foods from plant sources such as breads, cereals, grain products, rice, pasta, or beans. Limit the amount of red meat and processed meats you eat. Even though the effect of these dietary recommendations on ovarian cancer risk remains uncertain, following them can help prevent several other diseases, including some other types of cancer [2, 3].

Oral contraceptives reduce the risk of developing ovarian cancer, especially for long-term users. Women who use oral contraceptives for more than 5 years have about a more than 50% reduction in the risk of developing ovarian cancer [6]. Tubal ligation and hysterectomy may reduce the chance of developing ovarian cancer; these surgeries should be done for valid medical reasons. Even if there were no increased risk of ovarian cancer, some authorities recommend bilateral salpingo-oophorectomy if there were a need for hysterectomy, if the woman had already gone through menopause or is close to menopause [19].

2.4.2 Secondary Prevention

Risk-Reducing Salpingo-Oophorectomy

Based on solid evidence, risk-reducing bilateral salpingo-oophorectomy is associated with a decreased risk of ovarian cancer. Risk-reducing surgery is generally reserved for women at high risk of developing ovarian cancer, such as women who have an inherited susceptibility to ovarian cancer. A 90% reduction in risk of ovarian cancer was observed among women with a *BRCA1* or *BRCA2* mutation [20]. Seven efficacy studies of risk-reducing salpingo-oophorectomy for prevention of ovarian cancer and one meta-analysis showed a significant risk reduction of approximately 80% among BRCA1 and BRCA2 carriers. Beyond its use for the prevention of ovarian cancer, salpingo-oophorectomy also reduces the risk of breast cancer significantly in the mutation carriers. In the Prevention and Observation of Surgical Endpoints (PROSE) multicenter prospective cohort study, involving 2482 BRCA1 and BRCA2 carriers, the surgical group had lower all-cause mortality after risk-reducing salpingo-oophorectomy [21]. Current guidelines recommend risk-reducing salpingo-oophorectomy for both BRCA1 and BRCA2 carriers between the ages of 35 and 40 years who have completed their childbearing. For premenopausal women who have *BRCA* gene mutations and undergo bilateral salpingo-oophorectomy, the risk of ovarian cancer is reduced by 85–95%, and the risk of breast cancer by 50%.

The discovery that many pelvic serous cancers originate in the fallopian tubes raises the question of whether bilateral salpingectomy with delayed oophorectomy may be an option for premenopausal women who want to delay surgical menopause. Anecdotal reports indicate that this option is being used occasionally. However, data regarding the efficacy of this investigational approach are lacking.

Non-surgical Approaches

Data from randomized, controlled trials of oral contraceptives for the prevention of ovarian cancer are lacking. Observational studies have shown associations between the use of oral contraceptives and a reduced risk of ovarian cancer among BRCA1 and BRCA2 carriers, with odds ratios suggesting a 40–50% reduction in risk. However, in this group of patients, there was a concern about a possible increased risk of breast cancer.

3 Uterine Cancer

3.1 Epidemiology

Uterine cancer is one of the most common gynecological cancers, and predominantly affects postmenopausal women [1]. According to the Globocan data, uterine cancer is the 14th most common cancer in both genders, and the 5th most common cancer in women. In developed countries, uterine cancer is the most common gynecological cancer. The vast majority of uterine cancers are adenocarcinomas, arising from the endometrium. Hence, the term endometrial carcinoma is used synonymously with uterine carcinoma, and the term would be used throughout this chapter. Sarcoma is much less common and accounts for 2% of all uterine cancers. The most common form is leimyosarcoma, and the tumor could be either low or high grade. Occasionally, tumors may metastasize to the uterus. Throughout this chapter, the discussion about prevention of uterine cancer would be limited to endometrial cancer.

More than 90% of cases of endometrial cancer occur in women older than 50 years of age, with a median age at diagnosis of 63 years. However, around 5% of women with endometrial cancer are younger than 40 years of age at the time of diagnosis. The majority of endometrial cancers are diagnosed early (80% in stage I); however, mortality rates are high if regional or distant disease is present at the time of diagnosis.

Endometrial cancer can be classified into two main clinic-pathological subtypes: Type I or endometrioid adenocarcinoma (80–90%) is much more common and usually presents at an early stage, and has a favorable prognosis. Type I carcinomas are associated with genetic alterations in PTEN, KRAS genes, and MLH1 promoter hypermethylation. Type II comprises serous, clear cell, undifferentiated carcinomas, and carcinosarcoma. These tumors are aggressive, often present with advanced stage disease and the prognosis is stage dependent. Serous carcinomas are associated with TP53 mutations [22].

More recently, The Cancer Genome Atlas (TCGA) research network has classified the endometrial cancers into four molecular subtypes: POLE (ultramutated) tumors, Microsatellite unstable tumors, copy-number high tumors with mostly TP53 mutations, and the remaining group without these alterations. Microsatellite unstable tumors are mostly seen in families with hereditary nonpolyposis colon cancer (HNPCC) syndrome, and the majority are type I cancers; however, mutations in the genes can also occur sporadically [23].

3.2   Risk Factors

Several factors increase the risk of developing endometrial cancer. These include obesity, high estrogen levels, estrogen-producing ovarian tumors, polycystic ovarian syndrome, increasing age, diabetes mellitus, family history of endometrial or colorectal cancer, past medical history of breast or ovarian cancer, endometrial hyperplasia, or treatment with radiotherapy to the pelvis. On the other hand, pregnancy, OCPs, and the use of intrauterine contraceptive devices are linked with a reduced risk [24].

3.2.1   Defintive Risk Factors

Obesity

Endometrial cancer is strongly associated with obesity [25]. Most patients with endometrial cancer have a high body mass index (BMI), and several other components of metabolic syndrome (e.g., hypertension, diabetes). There is convincing evidence that overweight and obesity are a cause of endometrial cancer. A recent meta-analysis involving six studies and 3132 cancer cases revealed a relative risk (RR) of 1.89 for developing endometrial cancer in women with metabolic syndrome. Obesity was associated with the greatest increase in RR of 2.21. The strength of association between obesity and cancer risk increased with increasing BMI; RR for overweight was 1.32 and for obesity was 2.54. Compared with normal-weight women, women who have class-3 obesity (BMI ≥ 40 kg/m^2) were seven times more likely to develop endometrial cancer.

Weight cycling is also known to be associated with obesity-related cancers in postmenopausal women. In the Women's Health Initiative (WHI) observational study, almost 81,000 postmenopausal women, aged 63.4 ± 7.4 years, were categorized by self-reported weight change (weight-stable; weight-gain; lost weight weight-cycled) groups during early to mid-adulthood (18–50 years). A total of 7464 (breast = 5564; endometrial = 788; colorectal = 1290) cancers were diagnosed. Compared with weight-stable group, the weight-gain group had significantly increased risk of breast cancer and endometrial cancer. Weight cycling "4–6 times" was consistently associated with a 38% increased risk for endometrial cancer compared to weight-stable women. The data suggested that both weight-cycling and weight-gain increase the risk of endometrial and breast cancer in postmenopausal women. Further analysis revealed that the role of adult weight-change and weight-cycling tend to be stronger for the endometrioid subtype. The Australian National Endometrial Cancer study collected self-reported information on height and weight at three time points (age 20, maximum, and 1 year prior to diagnosis), intentional weight loss/regain (weight cycling) from 1398 women with endometrial cancer and 1538 controls. Relative to women who maintained a stable weight during adulthood, greater weight-gain after the age of 20 was associated with an increased risk of endometrial cancer, 5.3-fold for all types, and 6.5-fold for endometroid subtype. Interestingly, women who had lost weight intentionally and subsequently maintained that weight were not at an increased risk.

The mechanism of obesity as a cause of cancer has been adequately described. Obesity promotes endometrial carcinogenesis by conversion of androgens to estrogen. Increased adiposity in postmenopausal women leads to increased estrogen production, stimulating endometrial proliferation, hyperplasia, and cancer. The increasing rate of obesity corresponds with increasing incidence of endometrial cancer in developed countries. This represents a major public health challenge. Fortunately, high BMI correlates with good prognostic features of endometrial cancer, such as low tumor grade, endometrioid histology, and presentation at an early stage; however, prevention or treatment of obesity can reduce the overall burden of disease. The link between obesity and endometrial cancer is under-recognized among women. For example, one report suggested that as many as 58% women interviewed were not aware of obesity as a risk factor for endometrial cancer.

Family History of Endometrial or Colorectal Cancer

Endometrial cancer tends to run in some families, who have an inherited tendency to develop colon cancer. The disorder is called *hereditary nonpolyposis colon cancer* (HNPCC). HNPCC is an autosomal dominant disorder caused by germline mutations in DNA mismatch repair genes. Women with mutations in MLH1, MSH2, MSH6, or PMS2 have up to a 40–60% lifetime risk of developing both endometrial and colorectal cancers, as well as a 9–12% lifetime risk of developing ovarian cancer. Some families have a high rate of only endometrial cancer [24]. Tumors associated with mismatch repair abnormalities appear to have adverse prognostic factors and clinical outcome.

Endometrial Hyperplasia

Endometrial hyperplasia increases the risk of malignant transformation; however, the risk depends on the degree of complexity. Simple hyperplasia has a very small risk of becoming malignant. Simple atypical hyperplasia has about 5% risk of malignant transformation and complex atypical hyperplasia (CAH) has 30% chance of transformation, if left untreated. The risk of having an undetected endometrial cancer is even higher. Radiation used to treat some other cancers can damage the DNA, increasing the risk of endometrial cancer [25].

Treatment with Radiotherapy to the Pelvis

Radiation used to treat some other cancers can damage the DNA, increasing the risk of endometrial cancer.

Excess Estrogen Levels

Hormone balance plays an important part in the development of most endometrial cancers. Many of the risk factors for endometrial cancer affect estrogen levels. Before menopause, the ovaries are the major source of estrogen and progesterone. A shift in the balance toward more estrogen increases the risk. Even after menopause, estrogen is produced in the adipose tissue. Estrogen from the adipose tissue has a bigger impact after menopause than it does before menopause [24].

Treating menopausal symptoms using estrogen alone can lead to type I endometrial cancer, and the risk is 10- to 30-fold higher than the general population, if the treatment continues for 5 years or more. In case treatment is required for menopausal symptoms, combination hormone therapy is commonly employed, where progestin is given along with estrogen. Despite the use of combination therapy, yearly follow-up with pelvic exams, and a low threshold for abnormal bleeding or discharge from the vagina should be maintained.

Nulliparity and infertility are classical risk factors for endometrial cancer. Infertility secondary to polycystic ovarian syndrome (PCOS) seems to be the most important with an almost threefold increase in the risk. Women with PCOS have higher androgen and estrogen levels and lower levels of progesterone.

Estrogen-producing granulose-theca cell tumors carry an increased risk, with up to 20% of women with these tumors reported as having a simultaneous endometrial cancer. Both early menarche and late menopause are associated with a twofold increased risk.

Administration of tamoxifen increases the risk by 2.5-fold. Tamoxifen acts as an anti-estrogen in breast tissue, but it acts like an estrogen in the uterus. The risk differs depending on the menopausal status. Premenopausal women treated with tamoxifen have no increased risk, whereas, in postmenopausal women the risk is fourfold higher.

3.2.2   Probable

Diabetes Mellitus

Diabetes mellitus, particularly type II DM, is an independent risk factor for endometrial cancer, with an approximate doubling of risk. A recent meta-analysis consisting of 21 cohort studies involving 12,195 incident cases and 575 deaths caused by EC revealed that DM was associated with an increased incidence of endometrial carcinoma compared with individuals without diabetes or the general population. However, the risk of mortality was not increased. Moreover, the fact that people with type II diabetes mellitus tend to be obese is a confounding factor. A recent epidemiological study from the United States questioned the independent role of type II DM as a risk factor for endometrial cancer.

3.2.3 Equivocal

Past Medical History of Breast or Ovarian Cancer

Women who have had breast cancer or ovarian cancer may have an increased risk of developing endometrial cancer, too. Some of the dietary, hormonal, and reproductive risk factors for breast and ovarian cancer also increase the risk of endometrial cancer.

3.2.4 Preventive Factors

Pregnancy, OCPs and the use of intrauterine contraceptive devices are linked with a reduced risk.

3.3 Screening for Early Detection

There is no evidence that population-based screening could help in the early detection of endometrial cancer in asymptomatic women who are at average risk of developing endometrial cancer. There is also no standard or routine screening test for endometrial cancer. Furthermore, there is no evidence that screening reduces mortality from endometrial cancer. To the contrary, screening asymptomatic women may result in anxiety and complications due to unnecessary biopsies because of false-positive test results. The current recommendations are that at the time of menopause, women should be strongly encouraged to report any vaginal bleeding, discharge, or spotting to ensure appropriate investigations and treatment. Similarly, women with an increased risk for endometrial cancer due to a history of unopposed estrogen therapy, late menopause, nulliparity, infertility or failure to ovulate, diabetes or hypertension should be informed of the risks and symptoms of endometrial cancer and strongly encouraged to report any unexpected bleeding or spotting. There are no recommendations for screening in this group as well [22, 23].

Women who are at significantly increased risk, such as those with endometrial thickening over 11 mm, taking tamoxifen, and history of adult granulosa cell tumor should be managed on a case-by-case basis. The potential benefits, risks, and limitations of testing for early endometrial cancer should be explained to ensure informed decision-making.

Women with a substantial likelihood of developing endometrial cancer, such as those having an HNPCC-associated mutation, should be informed of the potential benefits, risks, and limitations of testing for early endometrial cancer; but they should also be informed that the recommendation for screening is based on expert opinion in the absence of definitive scientific evidence. Surveillance of the endometrium by gynecological examination, transvaginal ultrasound, and aspiration biopsy starting from the age of 35 years should be offered to all mutation carriers of HNPCC.

3.4   Prevention of Endometrial Cancer

Strategies to reduce mortality as a result of endometrial cancer have relied largely on early detection through patient and physician awareness. Most women with endometrial cancer present with vaginal bleeding, which should trigger evaluation. Fortunately, the vast majority of patients have type I endometrial cancers, where they are diagnosed with early-stage tumors associated with a high cure rates. However, despite these efforts, the incidence of endometrial cancer is increasing, and so is the mortality. There is an urgent need to reduce the burden of disease.

3.4.1   Primary Prevention

It is clear that reducing risk factors and introducing protective factors may lower the risk of developing endometrial cancer. All women should follow the WCRF guidelines for primary prevention of cancer. They should be strongly encouraged to engage in regular physical activity to attain and maintain a healthy weight. The use of OCPs is significantly associated with a decrease in endometrial cancer, the benefit being greater with increasing duration of use; however, this intervention needs to be balanced with the side effects, and needs a discussion.

Weight Loss

Intentional weight loss has been positively associated with decreasing the risk of endometrial cancer and mortality. The association between intentional weight loss and endometrial cancer risk in postmenopausal women by using data from the WHI study. More than 36,000 postmenopausal women, aged 50–79 years, had their body weights measured and body mass indices calculated at baseline and at year 3. Intentional weight loss was assessed by self-report at year 3. Compared with women who had stable weight, women who had a 5% or greater loss of body weight had a nearly 30% reduction in the risk of endometrial cancer. Furthermore, among obese women, an intentional weight loss of 5% or greater lowered the risk of endometrial cancer by 66%. Not unexpectedly, the reduction in endometrial cancer risk was due in large part to a reduction in type I, estrogen-dependent tumors. In addition, the risk reduction was most pronounced in those women who received hormone replacement therapy with combination of estrogen and progesterone. These data suggest that even a modest amount of weight loss can lead to a significant reduction in endometrial cancer risk in the long-term [28].

The effect of fluctuations in weight loss was studied in the Iowa Women's Health study. More than 21,000 postmenopausal women, free of cancer completed a questionnaire about intentional and unintentional weight loss episodes of 20 pounds or more during adulthood. Compared with women who never had the desired degree of weight loss, in women who had a more than 20 pounds intentional weight loss, the incidence rates of developing any cancer were 11% lower, more marked for breast cancer, followed by colon and the endometrial cancer. Furthermore, women who were not overweight at the time of analysis also had an incidence of cancer similar to non-overweight women [29].

Since, chronic hyperinsulinemia is linked both to obesity and metabolic syndrome which influences endometrial proliferation through direct and indirect actions, hence weight loss, calorie restriction, and physical activity have been known to reduce the risk of endometrial pathology. For these reasons, lifestyle modifications, and the oral hypoglycemic agent, metformin have been proposed as preventive factors. Metformin reduces the metabolic syndrome, lowers insulin and testosterone levels in postmenopausal women, and has been shown to be a potent inhibitor of endometrial cancer cell proliferation [30].

Oral Contraceptive Pill

Combination hormone therapy can reduce the risk. The risk is lowest in women who take the pill for a long time, and this protection continues for at least 10 years after stopping the OCP. Despite the use of combination therapy, yearly follow-up with pelvic exams, and a low threshold for abnormal bleeding or discharge from the vagina should be maintained.

3.4.2 Secondary Prevention

Bariatric Surgery

Given the difficulty of weight loss, other, more aggressive preventive strategies also may be beneficial in high-risk women. A meta-analysis to examine the impact of bariatric surgery on the development of endometrial cancer noted a 60% reduction in cancer risk in women who underwent the procedure compared with women in a control group [31, 32].

Intrauterine Contraceptive Device and Progestational Agents

Although findings from a meta-analysis verified the efficacy of the levonorgestrel intrauterine device (LNG-IUD) in preventing uterine polyps in breast cancer patients treated with tamoxifen, there was insufficient evidence to ascertain whether the LNG-IUD was associated with any benefit in reducing the incidence of precancerous or cancerous lesions. A cost-effectiveness analysis of the prophylactic use of LNG-IUD for the prevention of endometrial cancer in obese women found that such a strategy was potentially cost-effective to prevent deaths as a result of endometrial cancer. Among patients who had a body mass index of 40 kg/m^2 or greater, the LNG-IUD was more effective than usual care, and the incremental cost-effectiveness rate was just less than $75,000 [24].

Hysterectomy

Women with a very high risk (60%) for endometrial cancer include: carriers of
HNPCC-associated genetic mutations, those who have a substantial likelihood of
being a mutation carrier, women without genetic testing results but who are from
families with a suspected autosomal dominant predisposition to colon cancer.

In women with HNPCC, the following options are available: annual screening
beginning at age 35 years, regular hysteroscopy and endometrial biopsies or hysterectomy (current options), the application of local progesterone, treatment of
premalignant disease.

Hysterectomy and Bilateral Salpingo-oophorectomy

Prophylactic surgery (hysterectomy and bilateral salpingo-oophorectomy), prefer-
ably using a minimally invasive approach, should be discussed at the age of 40 as an
option for HNPCC mutation carriers to prevent endometrial and ovarian cancer.
Findings from a prospective observational cohort study of women with HNPCC
opting for endometrial cancer screening and who underwent annual outpatient hysteroscopy and endometrial sampling suggested that in women with HNPCC, annual
endometrial sampling is acceptable and has high diagnostic accuracy in screening
for endometrial cancer and atypical endometrial hyperplasia. However, larger multi-
institutional studies are needed for confirmation [23].

4 Cervical Cancer

4.1 Epidemiology

Cervical cancer is one of the most preventable cancers. Cervical cancer is the most
common gynecological cancer, and predominantly affects women in the fourth and
the fifth decades of life. According to the Globocan data, cervical cancer is the seventh most common cancer in both genders, and the fourth most common cancer in
women. It is one of the most common cancers among women in more than 40 countries in the world. Despite the possibility of prevention, it is one of the leading
causes of death worldwide, and is the most common cause of cancer-related death
in more than 50 countries [1].

The vast majority of deaths secondary to cervical cancer occur in low- and
middle-income countries (LMICs). Out of half-a-million cases diagnosed worldwide, 85% occur in LMICs. Almost quarter-of-a-million women die of cervical
cancer, and it is the leading cause of cancer deaths in eastern and central Africa and
some central and South American countries. Cervical cancer is of two main
histological subtypes. More than 90% of cervical cancers are squamous cell carcinoma, beginning in the transformation zone between exo-cervix and the endo-cervix. The rest are adenocarcinomas, arising from the mucus-producing cells off the
endo-cervix. The incidence of adenocarcinoma is increasing over the last

20–30 years. Less commonly there are mixed tumors, adeno-squamous carcinoma. In addition, melanoma, sarcoma, or lymphoma may involve the cervix, like any other part of the body. The discussion in the ensuing paragraphs would be about squamous cell carcinoma and adenocarcinoma.

4.2   Risk Factors

The primary cause of cervical cancer is a persistent or chronic infection with human papilloma virus (HPV) [33]. There are several strains. Cancer of the cervix is caused by one or the several of "high-risk" strains. More than 70% of all the cervical cancers are caused by two types of HPV, 16 and 18. A small percentage of cervical cancer is caused by strains 31, 33, 45, and 58. The low risk groups of HPV, 6 and 11, cause genital warts or condylomas, and do not cause cancer.

HPV is acquired during sexual intercourse, usually early during the sexual life. Whereas, infection with HPV is the underlying cause of almost all cases of cervical cancer, all infections do not cause cancer. For the vast majority of men and women, who become infected with HPV, the infection resolves spontaneously. However, only in a small percentage of people, the infection persists, and lead to a process of carcinogenesis through the stages of precancer, cancer in situ, invasive cancer, and in some cases to metastasis at the time of presentation. The process of carcinogenesis may take 10–20 years. The slow progression of changes due to persistent HPV infection provides ample opportunity to detect lesions early and offer treatment either at precancer stage, or earlier in the course of invasive cancer. Women who are coinfected with human immunodeficiency virus (HIV) may develop the invasive cervical cancer earlier than those who do not have HIV infection.

Besides HPV, other etiological/risk factors include: immunocompromised individuals are more likely to have persistent HPV infection and faster progression to cancer, individuals who have concomitant infection with herpes simplex, chlamydia, and gonorrhea are at a higher risk, multiparity and younger age of the first birth may increase the risk, tobacco smoking is associated with an increased risk.

4.3   Screening for Early Detection

Because of the slow progression of changes due to persistent HPV infection, there is an ample opportunity to detect the precancerous lesions early through screening and follow-up. Two types of screening tests are widely available and recommended. Screening is recommended in women aged 21–65 years with cytology (papanicolaou smear—pap smear) every 3 years. For women who would like to have less frequent screening, a combination of pap smear and HPV DNA is recommended every 5 years. Although the pap test has been more successful than any other screening test in preventing a cancer, it has its limitations, such as false-positive, false-negative, and equivocal results. If the pap smear shows epithelial cell abnormalities, such as atypical squamous cells of uncertain significance (ASC-US) or atypical squamous cells where high-grade squamous intraepithelial lesion (HSIL) can't be excluded (ASC-H) or atypical glandular cells (AGC), more tests can be done [34].

Since the most important risk factor for developing cervical cancer is infection with HPV, the HPV DNA test is used in combination with the pap smear to screen for cervical cancer for women aged 30 and older. The HPV DNA test can also be used in women who have slightly abnormal pap test results. If the pap test result is normal, but the test is positive for HPV, the test is done specifically for HPV types 16 or 18. In case either pap test or HPV DNA is positive, then several other tests are carried out to identify the nature of lesion. These include colposcopy, cervical biopsy, endocervical curettage, or a cone biopsy.

4.4   Prevention of Cervical Cancer

One of the most significant advances in the fight against cervical cancer is the development of HPV vaccines. Early vaccination with regular screening is now the most effective way to prevent cervical cancer. In June 2006, the first vaccine was approved by the FDA for use in 9–26-year-old women and girls. In large clinical trials, the vaccine was found to be very effective in protecting women from developing precancerous lesions of the cervix, vulva, and vagina. More recently, this vaccine has been approved and recommended for boys. Vaccine is administered as an injection, in a 3-dose series. Ideally, girls and boys should be vaccinated before beginning sexual activity. Studies show that the vaccines are extremely safe. Three vaccines are approved by the FDA to prevent HPV infection: *Gardasil*, *Gardasil*, and *Cervarix*. All three vaccines prevent infections with HPV types 16 and 18, the two high-risk HPVs responsible for 70% of all cervical cancers. *Gardasil* also prevents infection with HPV types 6 and 11, which cause 90% of genital warts [35].

The incidence and mortality secondary to cervical cancer is related largely to socioeconomic factors, gender bias, and culture-dependent factors, which restrict access to programs related to primary and secondary prevention, early detection and treatment. To support the argument further, the incidence and mortality rates of cervical cancer has fallen in the last 30 years where social and economic status has improved, largely through the implementation of secondary prevention, screening and early detection, and evidence-based treatment programs.

In order to implement a robust program for prevention of cervical cancer, the World Health Organization (WHO) has suggested a framework consisting of six building blocks. These include service delivery, health workforce, information, medical products, vaccine technologies, finance, and leadership. WHO program recognizes the inequalities in access to effective screening and treatment programs across the globe, and is designed to decrease the incidence of cervical cancer, and morbidity and mortality associated with the cancer [36].

The premise of the comprehensive program is that it should include primary, secondary, and tertiary prevention, and that the screening programs should be linked to treatment, post-treatment follow-up, and access to palliative care. The recent progress in prevention programs is outlined as follows.

4.4.1   Primary Prevention

The goal of the primary prevention is to reduce the HPV infections, because some of those may lead to persistent infections and cause cancer. The strategies for primary prevention include vaccination for girls aged 9–13 years, healthy sexual education, condom promotion or provision, and male circumcision. Recently, the American Society of Clinical Oncology (ASCO) issued a clinical practice guideline on HPV vaccination for primary prevention of cervical cancer. The recommendations are based on four levels of resource settings, pertaining to financial resources of a country or region.

The key recommendations are: For all resource settings two doses of HPV vaccines should be administered to girls aged 9–14 years, with an interval of at least 6 months and up to 15 months, and girls who have a concomitant HIV infection should receive three doses. Boys may be vaccinated if there is an at least 50% coverage in priority female target population. For maximal and enhanced resource settings are: If girls are 15 years or older and have received their first dose before the age of 15, they may complete the two-dose course, and if they did not receive the first dose before age 15, they should receive three doses. The last dose could be given till age 26. For, Basic and limited resource settings: If resources are still available after vaccinating girls 9–14 years of age, then girls who received one dose may receive additional doses between ages 15 and 26 years.

4.4.2   Secondary Prevention

The goal of secondary prevention is to reduce the incidence and prevalence of cervical cancer and associated mortality, by intercepting the progress from pre-cancer to cancer. The evidence-based strategies for secondary prevention include: counseling and information sharing, screening for all women aged 30–49 years; and treatment of identified precancerous lesions.

In the recent past, ASCO issued a clinical practice guideline on HPV vaccination for secondary prevention of cervical cancer in the resource-stratified manner. The key recommendations are:

a. Screening: for all resource settings HPV DNA testing is recommended (visual inspection with acetic acid is acceptable in basic settings) for women between the ages 25 to 65 every 5 years; and between the ages 30 to 65, if two consecutive tests are negative at 5-year intervals, then every 10 years
b. Triage using either visual assessment (basic settings); or genotyping and/or cytology (all other settings).
c. Women who are HIV positive should be screened with HPV testing after diagnosis and screened twice as many times per lifetime as the general population.

Triage; basic (visual assessment), other settings (genotyping and/or cytology), treatment; basic (treatment if abnormal triage results are present), options include cryotherapy or loop electrosurgical excision procedure. Other settings (colposcopy for abnormal triage results, options include loop electrosurgical excision procedure or ablation). Follow-up: Twelve-month post-treatment follow-up in all settings, and women who are HIV positive should be screened with HPV testing after diagnosis and screened twice as many times per lifetime as the general population. In basic settings without mass screening, infrastructure for HPV testing, diagnosis, and treatment should be developed.

4.4.3 Tertiary Prevention

The goal of tertiary prevention is to decrease the number of deaths due to cervical cancer. The strategies for tertiary prevention include effective referral mechanisms to cancer centers, timely diagnosis, evidence-based, clinical stage-guided treatment and palliative care plan.

5 Conclusion

Gynecological cancers are the fifth most common cancer globally. Epithelial cancer of the ovary, uterus, and the cervix constitute almost 80–90% of all gynecological cancers. The risk factors for all three common cancers have been described (Table 3).

Table 3 Risk factors for common gynecological cancers

| | Risk factors | | |
	Definitive	Probable	Equivocal
Ovarian cancer	BRCA 1 or BRCA 2 related inherited genetic syndrome Family history of breast or ovarian cancer Past history of breast or ovarian cancer syndrome HNPCC Cowden's syndrome Peutz-Jeghers syndrome Hormone replacement therapy	Obesity	High total, animal and dairy fat Alcohol Aspirin NSAIDs Peritoneal talc Ovarian hyperstimulation
Uterine cancer	Obesity HNPCC Family history of endometrial or ovarian cancer Endometrial hyperplasia Radiotherapy to pelvis	Diabetes mellitus Estrogen therapy Nulliparity Infertility Estrogen-producing tumors Tamoxifen therapy	Past medical history of breast or ovarian cancer
Cervical cancer	HPV Immunosuppression	Immunosuppression Multiparity Tobacco smoking	

HNPCC Hereditary nonpolyposis coli cancer syndrome, *NSAIDs* Nonsteroidal anti-inflammatory drugs, *HPV* Human papilloma virus

Preventive strategies revolve around the risk factors. Evidence-based guidelines have been discussed in this chapter. Lifestyle changes as suggested by the WCRF have been shown to reduce the risk of uterine cancer, and may also help in reducing the risk of ovarian and the cervical cancer. Intentional weight loss reduces the risk of endometrial cancer in a dose-dependent manner. Vaccination has been shown to reduce the risk of cervical cancer, but the success has been modest, as only a small percentage of target population is aware of the intervention, and is available to even a smaller percentage of population. Risk-reducing salpingo-oophorectomy reduces the risk in high-risk patients with ovarian cancer, such as those with genetic mutations, and hysterectomy is increasingly being employed in those with genetic mutations predisposing to endometrial cancer (Table 4).

Table 4 Prevention of common gynecological cancers

	Preventive strategies		
	Primary	Secondary	Tertiary
Ovarian cancer	WCRF recommendations Oral contraceptive pills Tubal ligation and hysterectomy	Risk-reducing bilateral salpingo-oophorectomy Salpingectomy	WCRF recommendations Effective referral mechanisms to cancer centers Timely diagnosis Evidence-based, clinical stage-guided treatment
Uterine cancer	Weight loss Oral contraceptive pill	Bariatric surgery Intrauterine contraceptive devices Progestational agents Hysterectomy	
Cervical cancer	Vaccinations for girls aged 9–13 years Healthy sexual education Condom promotion or provision Male circumcision	Counseling and information sharing Screening for all women aged 30–49 years Treatment of identified precancerous lesions	

WCRF World Cancer Research Fund

References

1. Ferlay J, Soerjomataram I, Ervik M, Dikshit R, Eser S, Mathers C, Rebelo M, Parkin DM, Forman D, Bray F. GLOBOCAN 2012 v1.1, cancer incidence and mortality worldwide: IARC CancerBase No. 11 [Internet]. Lyon, France: International Agency for Research on Cancer; 2014. Available from: http://globocan.iarc.fr. Accessed 16 January 2015.
2. Romaguera D, Vergnaud AC, Peeters PH, van Gils CH, Chan DS, Ferrari P, et al. Is concordance with World Cancer Research Fund/American Institute for Cancer Research guidelines for cancer prevention related to subsequent risk of cancer? Results from the EPIC study. Am J Clin Nutr. 2012;96:150–63.
3. Vergnaud AC, Romaguera D, Peeters PH, van Gils CH, Chan DS, Romieu I, et al. Adherence to the World Cancer Research Fund/American Institute for Cancer Research guidelines and

risk of death in Europe: results from the European Prospective Investigation into Nutrition and Cancer cohort study1,4. Am J Clin Nutr. 2013;97:1107–20.

4. Hastert TA, Beresford SA, Patterson RE, Kristal AR, White E. Adherence to WCRF/AICR cancer prevention recommendations and risk of postmenopausal breast cancer. Cancer Epidemiol Biomarkers Prev. 2013;22:1498–508.

5. Walter RB, Buckley SA, White E. Regular recreational physical activity and risk of hematologic malignancies: Results from the prospective vitamins and lifestyle (VITAL) study. Ann Oncol. 2013;24:1370–7.

6. Sueblinvong T, Carney ME. Current understanding of risk factors for ovarian cancer. Curr Treat Options in Oncol. 2009;10:67–81.

7. Hartmann LC, Lindor NM. The role of risk-reducing surgery in hereditary breast and ovarian cancer. N Eng J Med. 2016;374:454–68.

8. Toss C, Tomasello E, Razzaboni G, et al. Hereditary ovarian cancer: not only BRCA 1 and 2 genes. BioMed Res Int. 2015:341–8.

9. Foong KW, Bolton H. Obestiy and ovarian cancer risk: a systematic review. Post Reprod Health. 2017;23(4):183–98. https://doi.org/10.1177/2053369117709225.

10. Crane TE, Khulpateea BR, Alberts DS, et al. Dietary intake and ovarian cancer risk: a systematic review. Cancer Epidemiol Biomark Prev. 2014;23(2):255–73.

11. Dolecek TA, McCarthy BJ, Joslin CE, et al. Prediagnosis food patterns are associated with length of survival from epithelial ovarian cancer. J Am Diet Assoc. 2010;110(3):369–82.

12. Thomson CA, Crane E, Wertheim BC, et al. Diet quality and survival after ovarian cancer: results from the Women's Health Initiative. J Natl Cancer Inst. 2014;106(11):pii: dju314.

13. Zhou Y, Chlebowski R, LaMonte MJ, et al. Body mass index, physical activity, and mortality in women diagnosed with ovarian cancer: Results from the Women's Health Initiative. Gynecol Oncol. 2014;133(1):4–10.

14. Thomson CA, Crane TE, Miller A, et al. A randomized trial of diet and physical activity in women treated for stage II–IV ovarian cancer: rationale and design of the Lifestyle Intervention for Ovarian Cancer Enhanced Survival (LIVES): an NRG Oncology/Gynecologic Oncology Group (GOG-225) Study. Contemp Clin Trials. 2016;49:181–9.

15. https://www.cancer.org/cancer/ovarian-cancer/causes-risks-prevention/risk-factors.html.

16. https://www.cancer.gov/types/ovarian/hp/ovarian-prevention-pdq.

17. Moyer VA, U.S. Preventive Services Task Force. Screening for ovarian cancer: U.S. Preventive Services Task Force reaffirmation recommendation statement. Ann Intern Med. 2012; 157(12):900–4. https://doi.org/10.7326/0003-4819-157-11-201212040-00539.

18. Menon U, McGuire AJ, Raikou M, et al. The cost-effectiveness of screening for ovarian cancer: results from the UK Collaborative Trial of Ovarian Cancer Screening (UKCTOCS). Br J Cancer. 2017 Aug 22;117(5):619–27. https://doi.org/10.1038/bjc.2017.222.

19. Tewari KS, Monk BJ. The 21st century handbook of clinical ovarian cancer. Switzerland: Springer International Publishing; 2015. https://doi.org/10.1007/978-3-319-08066-6_2.

20. Paluch-Shimon S, Cardoso F, Sessa C, et al. on behalf of the ESMO Guidelines Committee. Prevention and screening in BRCA mutation carriers and other breast/ovarian hereditary cancer syndromes: ESMO Clinical Practice Guidelines for cancer prevention and screening Ann of Oncol 27 (Suppl 5): v103–v110, 2016 doi:https://doi.org/10.1093/annonc/mdw327.

21. Olopade OI, Artioli G. Efficacy of risk-reducing salpingo-oophorectomy in women with BRCA-1 and BRCA-2 mutations. Breast J. 2004;10(Suppl 1):S5–9.

22. Colombo N, Preti E, Landoni F, et al. Endometrial cancer: ESMO clinical practice guidelines for diagnosis, treatment and follow up. Ann Oncol. 2011;22(Suppl 6):vi35–9.

23. Colombo N, Creutzberg C, Amant F, et al. ESMO-ESGO-ESTRO Endometrial Consensus Conference Working Group. ESMO-ESGO-ESTRO consensus conference on endometrial cancer: diagnosis, treatment and follow-up. Radiother Oncol. 2015;117(3):559–81. https://doi.org/10.1016/j.radonc.2015.11.013.

24. https://www.cancer.gov/types/uterine/hp/endometrial-prevention-pdq.

25. Anderson AS, Key TJ, Norat T, et al. European code against cancer 4th Edition: obesity, body fatness and cancer. Cancer Epidemiol. 2015;39(Suppl 1):S34–45. https://doi.org/10.1016/j.canep.2015.01.017.

26. Welti LM, Beavers DP, Caan BJ, et al. Weight fluctuation and cancer risk in post-menopausal women: The women's health initiative. Cancer Epidemiol Biomarkers Prev. 2017;26(5):779–86. pii: cebp.0611.2016.
27. Nagle CM, Marquart L, Bain CJ, et al. Australian National Endometrial Cancer Study Group. Impact of weight change and weight cycling on risk of different subtypes of endometrial cancer. Eur J Cancer. 2013;12:2717–26.
28. Luo J, Chlebowski RT, Hendryx M, et al. Intentional weight loss and endometrial cancer risk. J Clin Oncol. 2017;35(11):1189–93.
29. Parker ED, Folsom AR. Intentional weight loss and incidence of obesity-related cancers: the Iowa Women's Health Study. Int J Obes Relat Metab Disord. 2003;27(12):1447–52.
30. Campagnoli C, Abbà C, Ambroggio S, et al. Life-style and metformin for the prevention of endometrial pathology in postmenopausal women. Gynecol Endocrinol. 2013;29(2):119–24.
31. Ward KK, Roncancio AM, Shah NR, et al. Bariatric surgery decreases the risk of uterine malignancy. Gynecol Oncol. 2014;133(1):63–6. https://doi.org/10.1016/j.ygyno.2013.11.012.
32. Anveden Å, Taube M, Peltonen M, et al. Long-term incidence of female-specific cancer after bariatric surgery or usual care in the Swedish Obese Subjects Study. Gynecol Oncol. 2017;145(2):224–9. https://doi.org/10.1016/j.ygyno.2017.02.036.
33. https://www.cancer.gov/types/cervical/hp/cervical-prevention-pdq.
34. Jeronimo J, Castle PE, Temin S, et al. Secondary prevention of cervical cancer: ASCO resource-stratified clinical practice guideline. J Global Oncol. 2017;3(5):635–57. https://doi.org/10.1200/JGO.2016.006577.
35. Arrossi S, Temin S, Garland S, et al. Primary prevention of cervical cancer. *ASCO*. First Global Guidance for HPV Vaccination for Cervical Cancer Prevention. ASCO's website. Mar. 17, 2017. doi: https://doi.org/10.1200/JGO.2016.008151.
36. http://apps.who.int/iris/bitstream/10665/144785/1/9789241548953_eng.pdf.

Medical Aspects of Gastrointestinal Cancer Etiology, Therapy, and Survivorship

Sivaprasad Punnaveetil and Preeja Prabhakar

1 Introduction

Cancer is a major public health problem all over the world. It is a much bigger issue in the developing world where a lack of resources, public awareness, and lack of political encouragement exist in combating this dreaded illness, which contributes to its increased incidence, sustained prevalence, and poor medical and psychological outcomes. Increases in the number of individuals diagnosed with cancer each year, due in large part to aging and growth of the population, as well as improving detection and survival rates, have led to an ever-increasing number of cancer survivors.

Neoplasia in the gastrointestinal (GI) tract is one of the commonest illnesses that gastroenterologists confront. Advances in our understanding of the cellular and molecular basis of GI neoplasia have provided a foundation for the development of novel diagnostic and therapeutic approaches. Although some features are tissue site specific, depending on its anatomical and embryological origin, many mechanisms of tumorigenesis are common to the most structures throughout the GI tract. Neoplasia results from disruption of the regulatory mechanisms of normal cell growth and division. Growth is determined by the balance of cellular proliferation, differentiation, senescence, and programmed cell death. Apoptosis (or programmed cell death) is an important mechanism that counterbalances cell proliferation, and abnormalities involving downregulation of apoptosis play a critical role in oncogenesis.

S. Punnaveetil (✉)
Department of Gastroenterology, Starcare Hospital LLC, Muscat, Oman

P. Prabhakar
Department of Food Science and Nutrition, College of Agricultural and Marine Sciences, Sultan Qaboos University, Muscat, Oman
e-mail: drpreeja@squ.edu.om

© Springer International Publishing AG, part of Springer Nature 2018
M. I. Waly, M. S. Rahman (eds.), *Bioactive Components, Diet and Medical Treatment in Cancer Prevention*, https://doi.org/10.1007/978-3-319-75693-6_15

187

Replicative senescence plays a role in determining overall growth in cell populations. Most primary cells when grown in vitro have a limited replicative potential and eventually undergo senescence [2]. In contrast, malignant cells replicate indefinitely. Telomeres are repetitive DNA sequences at the ends of all chromosomes that regulate chromosomal stability. Telomeres shorten with each cell division, and when they have been reduced to a certain critical length, cellular senescence or aging occurs. Activation of the telomerase enzyme is essential to escape from replicative senescence. Cancer cells are able to maintain their telomere length despite multiple cell divisions through the reactivation of telomerase enzyme activity.

2   Factors for Cancer Development

2.1   Intestinal Tumor Development: Multistep Pathways

Multiple genetic alterations occur during the transformation of normal intestinal epithelium to malignancy. This multistep nature of neoplasia is illustrated by the changes accumulated that lead to the development of colonic neoplasia. In colonic malignancy, the accumulation of genetic alterations roughly parallel the progression from normal epithelium through adenomatous polyps (or, in the case of ulcerative colitis, flat dysplastic mucosa) to malignant neoplasia. Studies on the molecular pathogenesis of colon cancer have served as an ideal example for the elucidation of genetic alterations in other GI cancers. Similar progression is also seen in the transition from normal squamous epithelium to metaplastic mucosa (Barrett's esophagus) through dysplasia to adenocarcinoma of the esophagus. Gastric and pancreatic oncogenesis are each thought to proceed through their own similar multistep pathways [1–3].

A number of factors could promote the likelihood of malignant transformation by promoting stimuli for increased cell turnover, which increases opportunities for somatic mutations to accumulate [4]. In the GI tract, these promoting factors include dietary constituents as well as chronic inflammation, which are associated with increased cell proliferation. Thus, a number of chronic inflammatory conditions increase the tissue-specific risk of cancer, such as ulcerative colitis, chronic gastritis, chronic pancreatitis, Barrett's esophagus, and chronic hepatitis. Although the mechanisms by which inflammatory processes lead to tumor development are incompletely understood, cytokines produced by inflammatory cells can inhibit apoptosis, stimulate tumor cells, and stimulate proliferation [5].

Clonal expansion is essential to tumor development. Clonal expansion occurs when a specific gene mutation results in survival advantage for the cell. A second round of clonal expansion occurs when a cell within this population sustains still another genetic alteration, which further enhances its growth properties. After several mutations, a final genetic alteration eventually confers a property that, together with the preceding genetic alterations, makes a cell malignant [6]. A genetically unstable environment was thought to be necessary for the development of the multiple mutations that ultimately result in cancer. Genomic instability is observed in almost all cancers, regardless of organ site. Instability of the genome may result from several mechanisms. In colon cancer, there are at least two well-recognized forms of genetic instability, and they have been termed chromosomal instability and microsatellite instability [7].

2.2   Neoplasia-Associated Genes

The genes that collectively play an important role in oncogenesis generally lead to disruption of the regulated mechanisms of normal cell proliferation. All these genes that become altered appear to belong to one of three distinct groups: (a) oncogenes, which actively confer a growth-promoting property; (b) tumor suppressor genes, the products of which normally restrain growth or proliferation; (c) DNA repair genes, which contribute to transformation by fostering genomic instability and facilitating mutations in other genes. Activation of oncogenes or inactivation of tumor suppressor genes and DNA repair genes contributes to malignant transformation. A list of the various neoplasia-associated genes is provided in Table 1. This list is not comprehensive and covers only the most common neoplasia-associated genes in GI cancers.

2.3   Environmental Mutagenesis

Fundamentally, even though cancer is a genetic disorder, environmental factors play an important role in tumor formation. They ultimately lead to the expression of abnormal genes or inappropriate expression of normal genes, the products of which lead to the malignant phenotype. Mutations can result from any class of carcinogen, including chemical mutagens and ionizing and ultraviolet radiation. Dietary constituents and their metabolites may act as important environmental mutagens within the GI tract. Viral agents also can lead to disruption of normal genes by entry into the host genome in a position that disrupts normal gene sequences or through the introduction of aberrant genes present in the virus's own genetic material. Viral agents that appear to play a role in oncogenesis in the GI tract include human papillomavirus in squamous cell cancers of the esophagus and anus, Epstein-Barr virus in gastric lymphoepithelial malignancies, and hepatitis B virus in hepatocellular carcinoma. Infection and chronic inflammation in stomach due to *Helicobacter pylori* is also implicated as the predominant factor in the causation of gastric carcinoma and lymphoma.

Table 1 Neoplasia-associated genes

Gene	Esophagus	Stomach	Biliary tract	Pancreas	Colon	Liver	Gist
Oncogenes							
K-ras		+	+	+	+		
c-Myc	+	+		+	+	+	
EGFR	+				+		
ErbB2		+					
B-Raf			+		+		
c-Src					+		
c-Kit							+
β-catenin		+	+		+	+	
Tumor suppressor genes							
TP53	+	+	+	+	+	+	
p16^{INK4A}	+	+	+	+		+	
p14^{ARF}				+	+		
APC			+		+		
DPC4, SMAD4			+	+			
E-cadherin		+					
Rb						+	
BRCA2				+			
Axin						+	
LKB1				+			
DNA repair genes							
MSH2, MLH1, MSH6, PMS2		+		+	+		
MYH					+		

GIST Gastrointestinal stromal tumor
Adapted from Sleisenger and Fordtrans Gastrointestinal and Liver diseases [1]

2.4   *Chemical Carcinogenesis*

Metabolic activation by the host is a key determinant of the carcinogenic potential of many chemical compounds. The initial compound, the procarcinogen, is converted by host enzymes to an electrophilic derivative usually free radicals (reactive oxygen or nitrogen species), which then chemically modifies DNA. Mutations result from errors that occur during DNA replication. These mutations, along with other tumor-promoting factors, facilitate or cause malignancy.

These principles are exemplified by experimental colonic carcinomas that arise in rodents fed cycasin, a glucosylated compound present in the cycad nut. The glucose residue of cycasin is cleaved in the rat liver by β-glucosidase to form methylazoxymethanol (MAM), which is subsequently deformylated by enzymes in the liver and colon to give rise to methyldiazonium, a carcinogen. These same metabolites are formed through hepatic enzymatic modification of the compound dimethylhydrazine and result in colon cancer in rats [1].

2.5   Dietary Factors

The mucosal surfaces from which most primary cancers in the GI tract develop are exposed to a complex mixture of dietary constituents which are potential carcinogens or procarcinogens. The ability of dietary factors to act as mutagens in humans was demonstrated directly in 1995. The frequency of contamination of foodstuffs with aflatoxins, a fungal metabolite, parallels the incidence of hepatocellular carcinoma in various areas of the world [8]. Studies have demonstrated that aflatoxins cause mutations in the *TP53* gene in hepatocellular carcinoma and have provided a compelling link between genes and the environment [8].

Nitrates present in many foods, commonly smoked preparations, appear to be additional dietary constituents that may act as procarcinogens in the GI tract. Diet-derived nitrates can be converted by bacterial action in a hypochlorhydric stomach to nitrites and subsequently to nitrosamines which are carcinogenic [9]. These events may underlie the documented correlation between dietary intake of foods high in nitrates and the incidence of gastric cancer in different populations. Variations in the relative and absolute amounts of dietary fats may lead to alterations in the composition of the colonic microbiome and their metabolic characteristics, resulting in modulation of the production of enzymes that convert dietary constituents into potentially mutagenic compounds.

Changes in dietary fiber content can alter the transit time of luminal contents in the bowel, thereby changing the duration of exposure of the mucosa to potential mutagens. Bile salt content may be an additional luminal factor that can modulate the biological effect of procarcinogens. Deconjugated bile salts may promote carcinogenesis through mucosal injury and enhanced epithelial proliferation. Populations that have a high fiber intake and resulting fast colonic transit times generally exhibit a lower incidence of colon cancer than populations with low fiber intake and delayed transit. The incidence of colon cancer in Japanese immigrants to the United States who consume a Western diet is much higher than that of native Japanese who consume a traditional Japanese diet [10].

Alcohol consumption is a well-known association with an increased risk of cancers of the mouth, pharynx, larynx, esophagus, liver, colorectum, and breast. Though not a dietary constituent, smoking increases the risk of more than 15 different types of cancer and accounts for at least 30% of all cancer deaths. Smoking also interferes with some common cancer treatments.

3   Cancer Treatment and Survivorship

There are several definitions of cancer survivors; here, the term "cancer survivor" is used to describe any person who has been diagnosed with cancer, from the time of diagnosis through the rest of his/her life. There are at least three distinct phases associated with cancer survival, including the time from diagnosis to the end of initial treatment, the transition from treatment to extended survival, and long-term survival [11]. The goal of treatment is to "cure" the cancer, or prolong survival in patients with advanced disease, while preserving the highest possible quality of life in both the long and short term. Many survivors, even among those who are cancer free, must cope with the long-term effects of treatment, as well as psychological concerns, such as fear of recurrence.

3.1 Staging of Cancer

A number of different staging systems are used to classify cancers. The TNM staging system is most commonly used and assesses cancer in three ways: the size and extension of the tumor (T), regional lymph node involvement (N), and the presence of distant metastases (M). Once the T, N, and M classifications are determined, a stage of 0, I, II, III, or IV is assigned. The TNM staging system is commonly used in clinical settings and is used for the description of treatment patterns.

3.2 Treatment of Bowel Cancer

Treatment of cancers depends on its stage at the time of diagnosis. Once cancer of the GIT is diagnosed, the only curative treatment is surgery. Other modes of therapy exist like chemotherapy and radiotherapy. A lengthy discourse on GI cancer treatment is beyond the scope of this chapter. After diagnosis, a multidisciplinary team consisting of the treating physician, oncologist, gastroenterologist, surgeon, cancer psychologist, and dietician sits together with the patient and discusses the viable options, which include curative options, induction of remission, and treatment of cancer-related symptoms like pain, bowel obstruction, jaundice, and psychological issues. Together a plan of action is chalked out, which attends not only to control cancer but a holistic approach is used wherein the patients' physical, mental, and psychological well-being is aimed rather than just cure of physical disease [12].

In most instances, by the time the cancer is diagnosed, it would have reached a stage where treatment with surgery alone may not be curative. Hence surgery followed by chemotherapy and radiotherapy may need to be employed. Sometimes, radiotherapy and chemotherapy are given in advance to a patient before surgery so as to downstage the cancer and thereby facilitate a curative surgery. This methodology is called the use of neoadjuvant chemo/radiotherapy.

In this age of technology, molecule-specific cancer therapies have become the vogue. The use of medications that target minute molecules like cytokines and growth factors which are indispensable to cancer progression have been developed which are better than the use of broad spectrum anticancer drugs that are fraught with side effects. In some cancers, which are very advanced, no benefit is expected from the curative modes of treatment and hence only palliative care in the form of analgesia, medication for symptom relief, and hospice is provided. The aim of palliative care is to provide the patient with comfort and dignity during his last days of life.

3.3   Common Effects of Cancer and Its Treatment

The management of symptoms related to cancer and toxicities from its treatment are an important part of cancer care, affecting the completion of treatment and both short-term and long-term quality of life and physical and psychological functioning. The vast majority of cancer patients experience one or more symptoms or side effects during active treatment [12]. Commonly reported symptoms are pain, fatigue, and emotional distress [13].

3.3.1   Fatigue

Fatigue is the most common side effect of active cancer treatment, reported in 28–90% of cancer patients [14]. It is more common in patients with advanced cancers and those who undergo treatment with radio/chemotherapy. Compared with fatigue experienced by healthy individuals, cancer-related fatigue is more severe and less likely to be relieved with rest. For many patients, chronic fatigue persists long after treatment has ended. Cancer-related fatigue is commonly associated with sleep disturbance, emotional distress, and pain. Cancer patients may experience fatigue due to anemia, which can be treated with a variety of medications or blood transfusion. Causes of cancer-related fatigue are multifactorial, and may include depression, chronic inflammatory processes with elevated cytokines, and alterations in muscular energy systems activity. A variety of interventions are recommended for cancer patients experiencing fatigue. Exercise, especially moderate-intensity resistance exercise reduces cancer-related fatigue.

3.3.2   Pain

A recent meta-analysis estimated the prevalence of pain to be 59% among patients in active treatment, 33% among survivors after treatment, and 64% among those with advanced/metastatic/terminal disease [15]. Both surgery and radiation therapy can cause nerve damage, resulting in chronic pain. Chemotherapy drugs, especially vincristine and the taxanes, can damage sensory nerve cells, causing peripheral neuropathy. Cancer-related pain reduces quality of life and is associated with depression and poor functioning. Although studies suggest that pain control can be achieved for 80% of cancer patients experiencing pain, it is frequently underassessed, underreported, and undertreated. Clinical practice guidelines from both the World

Health Organization and the National Comprehensive Cancer Network recommend pain assessment throughout the course of treatment and continuing care [16, 17].

3.3.3 Bone Mineral Density

Many cancer therapies cause a reduction in bone density. Osteopenia and osteoporosis are common side effects in breast cancer patients with chemotherapy-induced ovarian failure and those treated with aromatase inhibitors. Osteoporosis increases the risk of fractures, which are associated with a reduced quality of life, particularly among older survivors [18].

3.3.4 Cardiotoxicity

A number of cytotoxic drugs used in cancer therapy, particularly anthracyclines (e.g., doxorubicin) but also cyclophosphamide, cisplatin, fluorouracil, and taxanes, can result in cardiomyopathy, ischemia, and dysrhythmias [19]. Cardiovascular toxicity from radiotherapy can present in a number of ways, including as accelerated atherosclerosis of coronary arteries in the irradiated areas, dysrhythmia, and valvular disease. A large, long-term study of excess cardiovascular mortality in survivors of childhood cancer reported a fourfold increased risk for chemotherapy recipients and a fivefold increased risk for patients treated with radiotherapy [20].

3.3.5 Cognitive Deficits

Cognitive deficits from cancer treatment, often referred to as "chemo brain," may include problems with attention, concentration, memory, and mental processing speed. Although only a subgroup of survivors suffers long-term cognitive dysfunction, these deficits can be debilitating [21]. Any study that aims to look at the brain dysfunction in these patients is complicated by chemotherapy-related fatigue, depression, and anxiety, which can also contribute to poor cognitive performance.

3.3.6 Distress

Cancer-related distress has been defined as a multifactorial, unpleasant emotional experience of a psychosocial nature that may interfere with the ability to cope effectively with cancer and its treatment. Almost all cancer patients experience some level of distress, ranging from mild, which may be addressed by discussions with the treatment team, to more severe, which should be referred to appropriate supportive services (mental health, social work, and counseling). A recent meta-analysis found that 30–40% of cancer patients had diagnosable mood disorders.

Early detection and treatment of distress can improve treatment adherence and patient-provider communication and decrease the risk of severe depression or anxiety [22].

3.3.7   Infertility

Infertility can result from surgery, radiation therapy, or chemotherapy. Chemotherapy has a highly toxic effect on the ovaries that increases with dose and duration. Risk of ovarian failure is highest among women closest to natural menopause, who have smaller follicular reserves. Uterine radiation is associated with infertility, miscarriage, preterm labor, and low-birth weight infants. Male infertility from cancer surgery or radiation therapy can result from anatomic changes, hormonal imbalances, or lower production and quality of sperm.

3.3.8   Sexual Dysfunction

Although sexual dysfunction is typically associated with males treated for prostate cancer, a large percentage of female survivors of gynecologic and breast cancers also experience sexual dysfunction. In female survivors, painful sex is the most prevalent symptom, while the most common symptom for men is erectile dysfunction. For both sexes, a diminished interest in sex is frequently reported and is often persistent [23].

3.4   Recovery Phase

Regular medical care following primary treatment is particularly important for cancer survivors because of the potential persistent and delayed effects of treatment, as well as the risk of recurrence and additional primary malignancies. The patients and their primary care providers be given a treatment summary and comprehensive survivorship care plan developed by one or more members of the oncology team. The survivorship care plan may include a schedule of follow-up visits, symptoms of which to be aware, potential long-term treatment effects, health behaviors to enhance recovery, and community resources. The implementation of survivorship care plans could be facilitated by the development of consensus guidelines for survivor care to provide content for the plans and the use of electronic systems to reduce the time required of clinicians to individually tailor the plans.

3.5   Long-Term Survivorship

The last phase of the cancer continuum can be both stressful and hopeful. Survivors are relieved to have completed treatment, but may need to make physical, emotional, social, and spiritual adjustments to find a "new normal."

3.5.1   Quality of Life

The majority of long-term, disease-free cancer survivors (5 years or more) report a quality of life comparable to those with no history of cancer [24]. Rather than just physical improvement, it is desirable for the patients to have emotional, spiritual, and financial well-being all of which contributes to the holistic approach that must be encouraged for a well-rounded recovery. More invasive and aggressive treatment regimens tend to be associated with poorer functioning in the long term. Certain groups report greater difficulty regaining quality of life, including women; nonwhites; and those who are diagnosed at a younger age, have other chronic health conditions, have lower socioeconomic status, or are unemployed. Age is also an important predictor of quality of life; survivors diagnosed at a younger age tend to have poorer emotional functioning, whereas an older age at diagnosis is often associated with poorer physical functioning.

3.5.2   Physical Activity

Low physical activity can hasten recovery from the immediate side effects of treatment, prevent long-term effects, and may reduce the risk of recurrence and increase survival. Intervention studies have shown that exercise can improve fatigue, anxiety, depression, self-esteem, happiness, and quality of life in cancer survivors [25]. Exercise for cancer survivors should be individualized and tailored according to the disease site and stage and the survivor's capabilities.

3.5.3   Nutrition and Maintaining a Healthy Body Weight

During treatment, though many patients become underweight due to treatment-related side effects, some patients gain weight. A diet that is plentiful in fruit, vegetables, and whole grains but contains limited amounts of fat, red and processed meat, and simple sugars may reduce both the risk of developing second cancers and the risk of chronic diseases. Alcohol consumption is associated with an increased risk of cancers of the mouth, pharynx, larynx, esophagus, liver, colorectal, and breast [26].

3.5.4 Smoking Cessation

A substantial number of cancer survivors continue to smoke after their diagnosis. Forty percent of cancer survivors aged 18–44 years are current smokers, compared with 24% of the general population [27]. Studies have shown that smoking cessation efforts are most successful when they are initiated soon after diagnosis.

3.5.5 Sun Exposure

Cancer survivors, particularly those diagnosed with skin cancers, should be encouraged to adopt skin care behaviors to decrease their risk of developing skin cancer, including wearing sunscreen and protective clothing and avoiding sunbathing and artificial tanning [28].

3.5.6 Care Givers

It is important to provide supports to the caregivers. Over time, caregivers may become increasingly vulnerable to psychological distress, depression, and anxiety, which can be exacerbated by feelings of social isolation [28]. Social support can help buffer the negative consequences of caregiver stress and serve to maintain, protect, or improve health. Numerous studies have shown that female caregivers experience more care-related distress and have a higher risk of poor physical and emotional health than their male counterparts [29]. Anxiety about the future and fear of cancer recurrence are lingering issues for caregivers. Caregivers can be apprehensive as they reintegrate into life after the patient's complete treatment. To ease this transition, caregivers may benefit from coping strategies, such as stress management or relaxation techniques. Recent studies show that both survivors and their caregivers often find benefit in the challenges associated with cancer [30]. Better adjustment and overall quality of life have been attributed to such positive growth. Ensuring that caregivers are healthy, both emotionally and physically, is imperative for optimal survivorship care.

4 Conclusion

In conclusion, the increase in the number of individuals diagnosed with cancer each year, due in large part to aging and growth of the population, as well as improving detection and survival rates, have led to an ever-increasing number of cancer survivors. Advances in our understanding of the cellular and molecular basis of the gastrointestinal (GI) neoplasia have provided a foundation for the development of novel diagnostic and therapeutic approaches. Although some features are tissue site specific, depending on its anatomical and embryological origin, many mechanisms of tumorigenesis are common to the most structures throughout the GI tract. Neoplasia results from disruption of the regulatory mechanisms of normal cell growth and division. Growth is determined by the balance of cellular proliferation, differentiation, senescence, and programmed cell death. Apoptosis (or programmed cell death) is an important mechanism that counterbalances cell proliferation, and abnormalities involving downregulation of apoptosis plays a critical role in oncogenesis.

References

1. Feldman M, Friedman LS, Brandt LJ. Sleisenger and Fordtrans gastrointestinal and liver diseases. 9th ed. Philadelphia: Saunders; 2010.
2. Hayflick L. Mortality and immortality at the cellular level. A review. Biochemistry. 1997;62:1180–90.
3. Cech TR. Beginning to understand the end of the chromosome. Cell. 2004;116:273–9.
4. Thompson TC, Southgate J, Kitchener G, Land H. Multistage carcinogenesis induced by ras and myc oncogenes in a reconstituted organ. Cell. 1989;56:917–30.
5. Lin WW, Karin M. A cytokine-mediated link between innate immunity, inflammation, and cancer. J Clin Invest. 2007;117:1175–83.
6. Nowell PC. The clonal evolution of tumor cell populations. Science. 1976;194:23–8.
7. Lengauer C, Kinzler KW, Vogelstein B. Genetic instabilities in human cancers. Nature. 1998;396:643–9.
8. Ozturk M. p53 mutations in nonmalignant human liver: fingerprints of aflatoxins? Hepatology. 1995;21:600–1.
9. Bortsch H. N-nitroso-compounds and human cancer: where do we stand? IARC Sci Publ. 1991;105:1–10.
10. Haenszel W, Kurihara M. Studies of Japanese migrants. I. Mortality from cancer and other diseases among Japanese in the United States. J Natl Cancer Inst. 1968;40:43–68.
11. Mullan F. Seasons of survival: reflections of a physician with cancer. N Engl J Med. 1985;313:270–3.
12. Barbera L, Seow H, Howell D, et al. Symptom burden and performance status in a population-based cohort of ambulatory cancer patients. Cancer. 2010;116:5767–76.
13. Patrick DL, Ferketich SL, Frame PS, et al. National Institutes of Health State-of-the Science Panel. National Institutes of Health State-of-the-Science Conference Statement: symptom management in cancer: pain, depression, and fatigue, July 15–17, 2002. J Natl CancerInst Monogr. 2004;32:9–16.
14. Hofman M, Ryan JL, Figueroa-Moseley CD, Jean-Pierre P, Morrow GR. Cancer related fatigue: the scale of the problem. Oncologist. 2007;12(1):4–10.
15. van den Beuken-van Everdingen MH, de Rijke JM, Kessels AG, Schouten HC, van Kleef M, Patijn J. Prevalence of pain in patients with cancer: a systematic review of the past 40 years. Ann Oncol. 2007;18:1437–49.
16. World Health Organization. Cancer pain relief: with a guide to opioid availability. 2nd ed. Geneva, Switzerland: World Health Organization; 1996.
17. National Comprehensive Cancer Network. NCCN clinical practice guidelines in oncology. Adult cancer pain. Version 2.2011. Fort Washington, PA: National Comprehensive Cancer Network; 2011.
18. Tipples K, Robinson A. Optimal management of cancer treatment-induced bone loss: considerations for elderly patients. Drugs Aging. 2011;28:867–83.

19. Steinherz LJ, Yahalom J. Cardiactoxicity. In: VT Jr DV, Hellman S, Rosenberg SA, editors. Cancer: principles and practice of oncology. 6th ed. Philadelphia, PA: Lippincott Williams&Wilkins; 2001. p. 2904–31.
20. Tukenova M, Guibout C, Oberlin O, et al. Role of cancer treatment in long-term overall and cardiovascular mortality after childhood cancer. J Clin Oncol. 2010;28:1308–15.
21. Ahles TA, Saykin A. Cognitive effects of standard-dose chemotherapy in patients withcancer. Cancer Investig. 2001;19:812–20.
22. Mitchell AJ, Chan M, Bhatti H, et al. Prevalence of depression, anxiety, and adjustment disorder in oncological, haematological, and palliative-care settings: a meta-analysis of 94 interview-based studies. Lancet Oncol. 2011;12:160–74.
23. Schover LR. Sexuality and fertility after cancer. Hematology Am Soc Hematol Educ Program. 2005:523–7. https://doi.org/10.1182/asheducation-2005.1.523.
24. Ganz PA, Desmond KA, Leedham B, Rowland JH, Meyerowitz BE, Belin TR. Quality of life in long-term, disease-free survivors of breast cancer: a follow-up study. J Natl Cancer Inst. 2002;94:39–49.
25. Courneya KS, Mackey JR, Bell GJ, Jones LW, Field CJ, Fairey AS. Randomized controlled trial of exercise training in postmenopausal breast cancer survivors: cardiopulmonary and quality of life outcomes. J Clin Oncol. 2003;21:1660–8.
26. Kushi LH, Byers T, Doyle C, et al. American Cancer Society 2006 Nutrition and Physical Activity Guidelines Advisory Committee. American Cancer Society Guidelines on Nutrition and Physical Activity for cancer prevention: reducing the risk of cancer with healthy food choices and physical activity. CA Cancer J Clin. 2006;56:254–81; quiz 313–314.
27. Burke L, Miller LA, Saad A, Abraham J. Smoking behaviors among cancer survivors: an observational clinical study. J Oncol Pract. 2009;5:6–9.
28. Yabroff KR, Kim Y. Time costs associated with informal caregiving for cancer survivors. Cancer. 2009;115(18):4362–73.
29. Hagedoorn M, Buunk BP, Kuijer RG, Wobbes T, Sanderman R. Couples dealing with cancer: role and gender differences regarding psychological distress and quality of life. Psychooncology. 2000;9:232–42.
30. Kim Y, Schulz R, Carver CS. Benefit-finding in the cancer caregiving experience. Psychosom Med. 2007;69:283–91.

Cholangiocarcinoma: Etiology, Pathogenesis, Diagnosis, and Management

Pushpendra Pratap, Syed Tasleem Raza, and Sanju Pratap

1 Introduction

Cholangiocarcinoma (CCA) is leading a neoplasm melanoma of the biliary duct system and accounting for 3% of gastrointestinal tumors [1]. It is the subordinate most extensive primary hepatic malignancy, representing 10–25% of primary hepatic malignancies worldwide [2]. CCA infrequently occurs earlier than the age of 40; the typical age at presentation is the seventh decade of life. Men have a higher incidence of CCA than women with ratios of 1:1.2–1.5. The incidence of CCA varies significantly by geographic area secondary to variations in risk factors. CCA is deadly due to its ability to recur, metastasize, late diagnosis, and drug-refractory nature. While the incidence of ICC is rising, the occurrence of ECC is trending down suggesting that different risk factors may be involved. The prognosis of CCA is poor; therefore, the mortality and prevalence rates are parallel. Even though there are recognized risk factors for the development of CCA, most patients do not have an identifiable risk aside from age [3].

The deprived prognosis of this sarcoma is furthermore explained from the fact that no helpful tools intended for early diagnosis for this neoplasia are still accessible. Because of the absence of particular symptoms combined with greater invasiveness and ordinary participation of critical anatomical organs [4], the patient typically presents with an unrespectable disease at the diagnostic way. These features advocate why a surgical restorative treatment is often impossible. Besides surgery, the other kinds of treatments for CCA are radiotherapy and chemotherapy [5]. However, CCA cells do not respond or weakly respond to these ways, which hence encompass often an analgesic role. Recent therapeutic options include brachytherapy and photodynamic therapy (PDT), with promising results. CCA develops from

P. Pratap (✉) · S. T. Raza · S. Pratap
Department of Biotechnology, ERA'S Lucknow Medical College & Hospital,
ERA University, Lucknow, India

© Springer International Publishing AG, part of Springer Nature 2018   201
M. I. Waly, M. S. Rahman (eds.), *Bioactive Components, Diet and Medical Treatment in Cancer Prevention*, https://doi.org/10.1007/978-3-319-75693-6_16

the accumulation of genetic and epigenetic alterations in regulatory genes of cholangiocyte cells that lead to the activation of oncogenes and the dysregulation of tumor suppressor genes (TSGs) [6]. The principal characteristics of malignant cholangiocytes can be summarized in (1) uncontrolled growth, (2) high capability of tissue invasiveness, and (3) capability to metastasize [7].

2   Classification of Cholangiocarcinoma

Anatomically cholangiocarcinoma (CCA) can be classified on the basis of location into intrahepatic or extrahepatic. Hilar CC (Klatskin tumors) is classically considered extrahepatic. Most common form is extrahepatic, accounting for 80–90% of CCAs. Further it is classified into proximal or perihilar concerning the bifurcation of the major ducts (50% of all CCA) and distal compartments depending on the locality of the tumor inside the extrahepatic biliary system. Perihilar disease is also frequently known as a Klatskin tumor. Three diverse expansion patterns of extrahepatic CCA can be observed: periductal penetrate, papillary or intraductal, as well as throng forming [8]. Intrahepatic CCA typically presents as an intrahepatic mass (Figs. 1 and 2).

The distinction between intrahepatic cholangiocarcinoma (ICCA) and extrahepatic cholangiocarcinoma (ECCA) has become progressively more significant, as the epidemiological aspect (i.e., incidence and risk factors) associated with each may be different. In the last several years there have been significant new insights into the molecular pathogenesis of CCA [9]. Innovative diagnostic and therapeutic modalities have also been developed, resulting in improved detection rates and outcomes. Further, we have currently entered the era of targeted therapies for human cancers. Therefore, it is timely and topical to evaluate these advances with a focus on hopeful targeted therapies intended for this disorder. An additional objective is to motivate further curiosity in this disease with the trust of improving conclusions for this still very much lethal malignancy.

3   Epidemiology of Cholangiocarcinoma (CCA)

Universally, occurrence of CCA varies, reflecting differentiations in genetic and environmental risk factors. The highest incidence is in northeast region of Thailand (by means of 80–90 cases/100,000 people), whereas Australia has the lowest incidence (with 0.4 cases per 100,000 people). Hepatobiliary malignancies account for 13% of the 7.6 million annual cancer-related deaths widespread and for 3% of the 560,000 every year cancer-related deaths in the United States. CCA accounts for 10–20% of the deaths from hepatobiliary malignancies [9]. The prevalence of CCA shows a wide geographic variability, with the highest rates in Asia and the lowest in Australia. In the United States, the incidence of CCA has been reported to be 0.82/100,000 for extrahepatic forms and 0.95/100,000 for intrahepatic forms of the

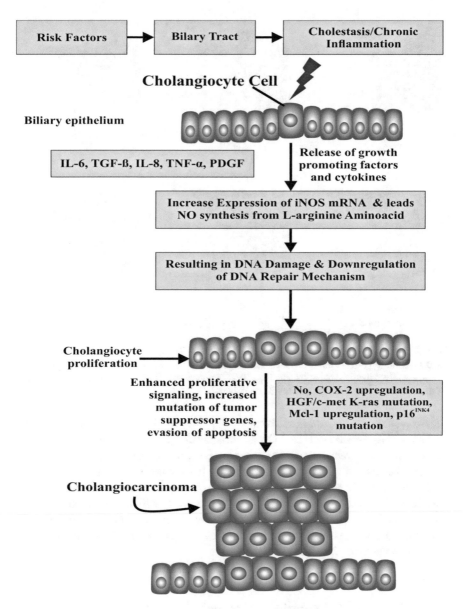

Fig. 1 Summary of key mechanisms regulating cholangiocarcinogenesis

disease. Its prevalence in diverse ethnic and cultural groups is heterogeneously distributed, with the highest age-adjusted prevalence in Hispanics (1.22/100,000) and the least in African Americans (0.17–0.5/100,000). In the last four decades, United States incidence rates of intrahepatic form of CCA have raised by 165%, while the extrahepatic CCA incidence has remained stable [4]. The significant enhance in

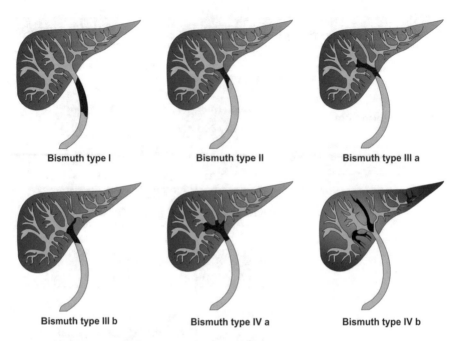

Fig. 2 Bismuth's classification of cholangiocarcinomas. Type I—Tumor involves the common hepatic duct, Type II—Tumor involves the bifurcation of the common hepatic duct, Type IIIa—Tumor involves the right hepatic duct, Type IIIb—Tumor involves the left hepatic duct, Type IV—Tumor involves both the right and left hepatic duct

age-adjusted occurrence of intrahepatic CCA was confirmed after correction for a prior misclassification of hilar CCA as intrahepatic CCA. Similarly, increasing incidence rates of intrahepatic CCA have also been reported in Western Europe and Japan. The cause for the increasing incidence has not been identified. We speculate that increased lipid conciliator such as oxysterols may provide the current increased incidence in Western societies [10]. In Western populations, the median age at appearance is >65 years, and it is only rarely diagnosed in patients <40 years of age excluding in patients with primary sclerosing cholangitis (PSC). There is a slight male predominance for CCA.

4 Etiology of Cholangiocarcinoma

In the Western planet, 80% of cholangiocarcinoma (CCA) cases are intermittent and have no identifiable risk factor. Smoking, alcohol consumption, obesity, and diabetes have not been consistently revealed to increase risk, although a small contribution cannot be ruled out [11]. Risk factors that have been identified are generally associated with chronic biliary inflammation. For example, primary sclerosing cholangitis is associated with 10% of CCA cases in the Western world [12]. In patients with PSC, the possibility of developing CCA is 1% per annum over 10 years, with a cumulative lifetime risk of 9–31%—1500-fold that of the general population [13]. In the management of this high-risk group, because of the often desmoplastic nature of cholangiocarcinoma (CCA) it is challenging to differentiate between malignancy and the benign strictures trait of PSC. Diverse etiology of liver cirrhosis conveys a tenfold relative risk. Uncommon abnormalities of biliary anatomy, for instance choledochal (bile duct) cysts, intrahepatic biliary cysts (Caroli's syndrome), biliary papillomatosis, and adenomata, are related with a high lifetime risk of CCA of 6–30%. This high rate of malignant transformation warrants prophylactic resection. Inborn or acquired irregularities of pancreatic biliary-duct junctions allow pancreatic reflux and resulting chronic cholangitis, increasing risk of CCA [14]. Chronic intraductal gallstones and hepatolithiasis are primarily allied to CCA in Asia (10% of patients with this trouble develop CCA), but are a much weaker risk factor in Western countries.

Several different infections are also associated with CCA. In areas of Southeast Asia, where the incidence of CCA is greater, biliary infestation with parasites (including Opisthorchis viverrini, Schistosomiasis japonica, and Clonorchis sinensis) is endemic. High fecal egg loads and high titers of fluke-specific antibodies are associated with a 14- and 27-fold boost in CCA risk, respectively, even though the mechanism of cholangiocarcinogenesis is unknown [15].

4.1 Primary Sclerosing Cholangitis

Primary sclerosing cholangitis (PSC) consequence in stricturing of extrahepatic and/or intrahepatic bile ducts is established risk factor for CCA. Chronic inflammation, proliferation of biliary epithelium, construction of endogenous bile mutagens, and bile stasis are hypothesized carcinogenic mechanisms [16]. The lifetime incidence of CCA among PSC patients ranges from 6 to 36%. Although PSC is known to be a strong risk factor for CCA, no more than 10% of CCA is attributed to PSC [14]. Data on the incidence of PSC suggest either no change or a small increase over time. A current study by Card et al. showed a nonsignificant growing tendency in the incidence of PSC, however the generally incidence estimates in this study were normally lesser than nearly all other reports [13]. An ensuing study by Lindkvist et al. [17] reported a considerably increased incidence of PSC. Given PSC is the most common known risk factor for CCA in the West, trending the occurrence of PSC is imperative for monitoring trends in CCA.

Heritable variations in the natural killer cell receptor G2D (NKG2D) are related with the expansion of cholangiocarcinoma (CCA) among primary sclerosing cholangitis (PSC) patients, while communication of natural killer cell receptor G2D (NKG2D) and major histocompatibility class I polypeptide-related sequence A is involved in defense against CCA in PSC [18]. Chronic inflammation due to stones or contagion is a risk factor in non-PSC patients, and the chronic gallbladder inflammation in PSC probably also leads to carcinogenesis. Primary sclerosing cholangitis (PSC) patients have an augmented incidence of gallbladder lesions with an expected prevalence of 3–14% versus 0.35% in the general inhabitants [19]. The well-built relationship among dysplasia/adenocarcinoma of gallbladder and bile duct dysplasia/cholangiocarcinoma (CCA) supports the concept of a neoplastic "field effect" along the extrahepatic/intrahepatic biliary tract in PSC. The existence of gallbladder epithelial cell dysplasia proposes a dysplasia-carcinoma progression in PSC similar to that observed in ulcerative colitis [20].

4.2 Parasitic Infection

The high occurrence of CCA is geologically interrelated with the parasite liver fluke, *Opisthorchis viverrini* [21]. The liver flukes parasite *O. viverrini* and *Clonorchis sinensis* are primary risk factors of CCA in Asia [22]. Liver fluke contagion outcomes in many pathological transformations, principally in the bile ducts where worms are found, and to the liver as well as gallbladder [23]. The importunate periductal fibrosis, however after praziquantel treatment, might be ultimately contributed to CCA carcinogenesis. Chronic inflammatory disease opisthorchiasis is mediated by interleukin-6 (IL-6), which is substantially allied with the expansion of advanced periductal fibrosis [12]. This unrelieved infection results in bile duct inflammation, which induces oxidative and/or nitrative tissue and DNA damage and may eventually lead to CCA [24].

4.3 Pancreaticobiliary Maljunction

Pancreaticobiliary maljunction (PBM) causes the integration and regurgitation of bile and pancreatic juices, which stagnate in the bile duct and the gallbladder, particularly in the dilated ordinary bile duct. This long-term pathophysiological situation may activate pancreatic enzymes, transform the bile acid fraction, and result in mutagenic and/or carcinogenic substances. A statement by Nagai et al. [25] showed 0% MSI in PBM patients with hyperplasia, 85.7% with dysplasia, and 80% with cancer, suggesting that MSI, similar to TP53 mutation, is a late incident in the PBM carcinogenic process.

4.4 Bile-Duct Cysts

It is a well-known risk factor for CCA. Class I (solitary, extrahepatic) and IV (extrahepatic and intrahepatic) bile-duct cysts have the greater prevalence of CCA. The lifespan prevalence of CCA in these patients varies from 6 to 30%. The incidence of bile-duct cysts is high in Asian as compared to the Western countries. The incidence of CCA is also higher in Asians with bile-duct cysts, virtually 18%, with the United State incidence closer to 6% [26]. There is an increase in incidence of CCA in patients with bile-duct cysts from 0.7% in the first decade of life to >14% after the age of 20. The normal age of malignancy identification has been reported to be 32 years, which is younger than the age at which CCA develop in the general inhabitants. The risk of malignancy turns down after entire choledochal cyst elimination, though these patients are still at increased risk of developing CCA compared with the general inhabitants [15]. Patients with bile-duct cysts are demonstrated to have at least 10- to 50-fold increased risk of developing CCA. In a Korean, hospital-based, case-control study by Lee et al., there was a strong relationship between choledochal cysts and ICC, with the OR at 10.7 (95% CI 1.8–63.9). In a large, SEER-Medicare study, there was a strong relationship between choledochal cysts and augmented risk of both ICCA and ECCA, with an OR of 36.9 (95% CI 22.7–59.7) and 47.1 (95% CI 30.4–73.2), respectively [27].

4.5   Chemical Exposure (Toxins)

Concern has been raised on the subject of the relationship among occupational chemical exposure and occurrence of CCA among employees in the offset color proof-printing part of a minute printing company in Osaka, Japan [28]. The report concluded that dichloromethane (DCM) and/or 1, 2-dichloropropane (1, 2-DCP) may cause CCA in human beings. Revelation to chemicals, counting chlorinated organic solvents, outcome in a high occurrence of CCA in relatively youthful employees of a printing corporation [29].

4.6   Genetics and Epigenetics

KRAS mutation is one of the most recurrent heritable alterations in CCA and other form of cancers. Alterations in PIK3CA, CDKN2A, PTEN, and TP53 have been established only in intrahepatic cases of CCA through normal liver [30]. BRAF and KRAS mutant of CCA cases have been linked with a worse long-term endurance, and hence screening of BRAF and KRAS could be precious in improving equally prognosis and outcome stratification [31]. KRAS mutation is an early molecular incident throughout the succession of biliary intraepithelial neoplasia to intrahepatic CCA in patients with hepatolithiasis, while p53 overexpression was acknowledged as a late molecular incident [32]. In response to inflammation cytokines produced play an imperative role in pathogenesis of cancer. Interleukin-6 (IL-6), transforming growth factor-β, tumor necrosis factor-α, and platelet-derived growth factor (PDGF) outlined the foundation of biliary epithelial cell and/or cholangiocyte proliferation [33]. Interleukin-6 (IL-6) plays a crucial role in CCA, inducing appearance of the forceful anti-apoptotic protein myeloid cell leukemia 1 (Mcl-1) in cholangiocarcinoma (CCA) cells using phosphorylation of signal transducers and activators of transcription 3 (STAT-3) [34]. Gankyrin is essential for cholangiocarcinoma (CCA) carcinogenesis and metastasis, activating IL-6/STAT3 signaling during the downregulation of Rb [35].

Epigenetic quietness of suppressor of cytokine signaling 3 (SOCS-3) controls the IL-6/STAT-3 signaling pathway through a typical feedback loop, and is accountable for sustained IL-6/STAT-3 signaling and improved Mcl-1 expression in cholangiocarcinoma (CCA) [36]. Epigenetic regulation by interleukin-6 (IL-6) can be implicated in tumor progression by changing promoter methylation as well as gene expression of growth regulatory pathways, such as those involving epidermal growth factor receptor (EGFR) [37].

4.7   Pathogenesis of Cholangiocarcinoma

Cholangiocarcinoma (CCA) likely outcomes from malignant transformation of cholangiocyte cells, however conversion of epithelial cells within biliary stem cells and/or peribiliary glands may also give rise to its development. There is also confirmation that subsets of CCA and mixed hepatocellular carcinoma (HCC)/CCA are derived from hepatic stem/progenitor cells [38]. Experimental and etiologic evidence implicates cholestasis and inflammation as key factors in the pathogenesis of cholangiocarcinoma (CCA). They produce an atmosphere that promotes injury in DNA mismatch repair genes and/or proteins, proto-oncogenes, and tumor suppressor genes (TSG) [39]. Growth factors, cytokines, and bile acids are found to be in elevated concentrations during cholestasis and inflammation, and contribute to these molecular alterations and enhance the growth and existence of altered cells. Cytokines motivate inducible nitric oxide synthase (iNOS) expression in epithelial cells, and upregulation of inducible nitric oxide synthase (iNOS) is present in inflammatory cholangiopathies and cholangiocarcinoma (CCA) [40]. Augmented inducible nitric oxide synthase (iNOS) activity outcomes in production of nitric oxide (NO) as well as reactive nitrogen oxide species (RNOS) recognized to communicate with cytoplasmic DNA and proteins. The interaction of reactive nitrogen oxide species (RNOS) and the cellular genome outcomes in transmutations and DNA strand breaks. Mutagenesis is additionally promoted by interaction of nitric oxide (NO) and RNOS with DNA repair enzymes like human 8-oxoguanine glycosylase, which is straightforwardly inactivated by S-nitrosylation of its active site cysteine residues [41].

A diversity of oncogenic mutations has been known in tissues of human cholangiocarcinoma (CCA). Their incidence depends on cancer stage, type of tumor, anatomical position, etiology, and ethnic population. Nevertheless dysregulation of the KRAS proto-oncogene and the p53 tumor suppressor gene (TSG) is frequently detected in malignancies; KRAS mutations have only been illustrated in 20–54% of intrahepatic cholangiocarcinoma (iCCA). This is in rapid distinction to pancreatic ductal adenocarcinoma (PADC), whereas mutations in KRAS are present in >90%

of tumors [42]. Hence, apart from communal developmental ontology among the pancreatic ducts and the biliary tree, their fully developed tumors are unlike. Nuclear accretion of p53 and upregulation of the allied protein WAF-1 and mdm-2 have been reported in 21.7–76% of cholangiocarcinoma (CCAs) [43]. Additional inactivated tumor suppressor genes (TSG) encompass p16INK4a, APC, and DPC4/Smad4. Interrelationship between these indicators (markers) and prognosis varies among studies. The majority of these heritable alterations were illustrated in intrahepatic cholangiocarcinoma (iCCA). specified the paucicellular, desmoplastic temperament of extrahepatic bile ducts, hereditary analysis of these cancers will necessitate attentive laser capture micro-dissection of the cholangiocarcinoma (CCA) cellular elements—a tedious procedure that has rarely been applied to this cancer [44].

5   Diagnosis of Cholangiocarcinoma

In majority of cases, cholangiocarcinoma (CCA) is clinically quiet, with indications merely rising at a higher stage. Once upon a time symptomatic, the clinical appearance depends on locality and escalation pattern of tumor. More than 90% patients with extrahepatic ductal cholangiocarcinoma (CCA) present with painless hyperbilirubinemia (jaundice), and 10% of patients with cholangitis [45]. Obstruction of unilobar biliary with ipsilateral vascular encasement results in atrophy of the pretentious lobe and hypertrophy of the unaltered lobe. Depending upon physical exploration, this "atrophy–hypertrophy complex" event presents as clear prominence of one hepatic lobe. Intrahepatic mass-forming cholangiocarcinoma (iCCA) presents with indications characteristic for hepatic masses, counting abdominal pain, night sweats, malaise, and cachexia. The serum cancer markers like carbonic anhydrase-125 (CA-125) and carcinoembryonic antigen (CEA) can be increased in cholangiocarcinoma (CCA), although they are non-specific and can be elevated in other malignancies like gastrointestinal or gynecologic and/or cholangiopathies [46]. Carbonic anhydrase (CA19-9) is the most frequently used tumor growth marker for cholangiocarcinoma (CCA). Sensitivity and specificity of these markers for detection of cholangiocarcinoma (CCA) in Primary Sclerosing Cholangitis (PSC) are 79% and 98%, respectively, at a cutoff value of 129 U/mL. Further investigators have acknowledged an elevated cutoff of >180 U/mL to accomplish this level of specificity [47]. An alteration from baseline of >63 U/L has a sensitivity of 90% and specificity of 98% for cholangiocarcinoma (CCA). In patients without PSC, sensitivity is 53% at a cutoff of >100 U/L and its negative prognostic value is 76–92% [48]. Carbonic Anhydrase (CA19-9) can also be increased in bacterial cholangitis (BC) and other gastrointestinal (GIT) and gynecologic neoplasias; patients missing the blood type Lewis antigen (10% of persons) do not produce this tumor marker [49]. Ultrasounds (USG) as well as computed tomography (CT) are only of limited significance for recognition of intra and extrahepatic cholangiocarcinoma (CCA) because of their low sensitivity as well as specificity, and low exactness in estimating tumor extent of intrahepatic and extrahepatic cholangiocarcinoma (CCA) [50].

Its main role in cholangiocarcinoma (CCA) is recognition of obstruction in bile duct, vascular compression/encasement, tumor staging, and preoperative planning.

For the assessment of tumor site and intraductal extent, cholangiography is the most significant diagnostic modality, principally for extrahepatic cholangiocarcinoma (eCCA) [51]. Magnetic resonance cholangiopancreatography (MRCP), percutaneous transhepatic cholangiography (PTC), and/or endoscopic retrograde cholangiopancreatography can be used for this objective. ERCP and PTC allow remedial interventions (for example, assignment of biliary stents) and compilation of tissue samples for pathological as well as cytological examination. MRCP/MRI (magnetic resonance imaging) provides instruction about site and tumor dimensions of intrahepatic CCA, ductal and periductal tumor extent of extrahepatic CCA, vascular involvement, and metastases. Its sensitivity and imaging excellence of tumor tissue can be elevated significantly with enhancement of ferumoxide [52]. The most sensitive method for assessment of provincial lymphadenopathy is endosonography. Biopsy of lymph nodes via fine needle aspiration (FNA) for further pathologic analysis can also be performed during the endosonographic procedure [53]. Nevertheless, biopsy of hilar lesions throughout endosonography is disheartened, because it can outcome in tumor seeding. In undefined cases, establishment of a diagnosis can be attempted with positron emission tomography (PET) with [18F]-2-deoxy-glucose. Sensitivity and specificity of integrated positron emission tomography (PET)/computed tomography (CT) in the recognition of primary lesions has been evaluated as 93% and 80% for intrahepatic CCA (iCCA) and 55% and 33% for extrahepatic CCA [54]. For provincial lymph node metastases, the sensitivity of positron emission tomography (PET)/computed tomography (CT) was 12% and the specificity was 96%. False positive PET scans have been reported in the setting of chronic inflammation [55].

6   Herbal Management of Cholangiocarcinoma

Throughout the past, traditionally herbal medication has afforded an affluent repository of remedies with diverse chemical structures and bioactivities in opposition to numerous health disorders. A frequent subject of herbal medicine is the constraint of information on their pharmacological activities and essential components. Traditionally, the use of herbal medicine has been dependent upon empirical management and passed on from generation to generation through information accessible simply in confined journals. This prevents various herbal medicines from creature developed to their complete prospective. The presentation will focus on research and expansion of *Atractylodes lancea* (Thunb) DC. (AL: family Asteraceae) as a probable chemotherapeutic treatment for cholangiocarcinoma (CCA). The desiccated rhizome of AL is a curative herb used in Japan, China, and Thai, intended for its various pharmacological properties including antitumor, contrary-inflammation and incompatible-microbial activities, activities on central nervous, cardiovascular, and gastrointestinal systems. The primary constituents in the necessary oils from AL rhizome are β-eudesmol, atractylon, and hinesol [56, 57].

7 Conclusion

Nonetheless, most cases of CCA are not related to recognized risk, in region endemic for liver flukes. The well-known risk factors for CCA consist of parasitic infections, biliary-duct cysts, primary sclerosing cholangitis (PSC), and hepatolithiasis. Less-established risk factors include IBD, HBV, HCV, cirrhosis, diabetes, obesity, smoking, alcohol, and genetic polymorphisms. The escalating universal occurrence of CCA collectively with the nonexistence of its valuable therapeutic tools explains the upward general curiosity for the study of this type cancer. The poor prognosis of patient affected by CCA is specified by the information that this sarcoma is frequently diagnosed when previously at an advanced stage. In spite of recent indicative advances, such as cytology techniques and imaging, additional investigations are essential to identify CCA at an early stage. Additional studies on novel diagnostic and therapeutic ways to influence the malignant behavior of CCA are required.

References

1. Gatto M, Bragazzi MC, Semeraro R, Napoli C, Gentile R, Torrice A, et al. Cholangiocarcinoma: update and future perspectives. Dig Liver Dis. 2010;42(4):253–60.
2. Sripa B, Pairojkul C. Cholangiocarcinoma: lessons from Thailand. Curr Opin Gastroenterol. 2008;24(3):349–56.
3. Blechacz BR, Gores GJ. Cholangiocarcinoma. Clin Liver Dis. 2008;12(1):131–50.
4. Khan SA, Thomas HC, Davidson BR, Taylor- Robinson SD. Cholangiocarcinoma. Lancet. 2005;366:1303–14.
5. Lazaridis KN, Gores GJ. Cholangiocarcinoma. Gastroenterology. 2005;128(6):1655–67.
6. Fava G, Marzioni M, Benedetti A, et al. Molecular pathology of biliary tract cancers. Cancer Lett. 2007;250(2):155–67.
7. Sandhu DS, Shire AM, Roberts LR. Epigenetic DNA hypermethylation in cholangiocarcinoma: potential roles in pathogenesis, diagnosis and identification of treatment targets. Liver Int. 2008;28(1):12–27.
8. Lim JH, Park CK. Pathology of cholangiocarcinoma. Abdom Imaging. 2004;29:540–7.
9. Khan SA, Emadossadat S, Ladep NG, Thomas HC, Elliott P, Taylor-Robinson SD, et al. Rising trends in cholangiocarcinoma: is the ICD classification system misleading us? J Hepatol. 2012;56:848–54.
10. Okuda K, Nakanuma Y, Miyazaki M. Cholangiocarcinoma: recent progress. Part 2: molecular pathology and treatment. J Gastroenterol Hepatol. 2002;17:1056–63.
11. Yoon JH, Canbay AE, Werneburg NW, Lee SP, Gores GJ. Oxysterols induce cyclooxygenase-2 expression in cholangiocytes: implications for biliary tract carcinogenesis. Hepatology. 2004;39:732–8.
12. Tyson GL, El-Serag HB. Risk factors for cholangiocarcinoma. Hepatology. 2011;54(1):173–84.
13. LaRusso NF, Shneider BL, Black D, Gores GJ, James SP, Doo E, Hoofnagle JH. Primary sclerosing cholangitis: summary of a workshop. Hepatology. 2006;44(3):746–64.
14. Claessen MM, Vleggaar FP, Tytgat KM, Siersema PD, van Buuren HR. High lifetime risk of cancer in primary sclerosing cholangitis. J Hepatol. 2009;50(1):158–64.
15. Söreide K, Körner H, Havnen J, Söreide JA. Bile duct cysts in adults. Br J Surg. 2004;91(12):1538–48.

16. Hughes NR, Pairojkul C, Royce SG, Clouston A, Bhathal PS. Liver fluke-associated and sporadic cholangiocarcinoma: an immunohistochemical study of bile duct, peribiliary gland and tumour cell phenotypes. J Clin Pathol. 2006;59:1073–8.
17. Card TR, Solaymani-Dodaran M, West J. Incidence and mortality of primary sclerosing cholangitis in the UK: a population-based cohort study. J Hepatol. 2008;48(6):939–44.
18. Lindkvist B, Benitod V, Gullberg B, Bjornsson E. Incidence and prevalence of primary sclerosing cholangitis in a defined adult population in Sweden. Hepatology. 2010;52(2):571–7.
19. Melum E, Karlsen TH, Schrumpf E, Bergquist A, Thorsby E, Boberg KM, et al. Cholangiocarcinoma in primary sclerosing cholangitis is associated with NKG2D polymorphisms. Hepatology. 2008;47:90–6.
20. Buckles DC, Lindor KD, Larusso NF, Petrovic LM, Gores GJ. In primary sclerosing cholangitis, gallbladder polyps are frequently malignant. Am J Gastroenterol. 2002;97:1138–42.
21. Lewis JT, Talwalkar JA, Rosen CB, Smyrk TC, Abraham SC. Prevalence and risk factors for gallbladder neoplasia in patients with primary sclerosing cholangitis: evidence for a metaplasiadysplasia-carcinoma sequence. Am J Surg Pathol. 2007;31:907–13.
22. Sibulesky L, Nguyen J, Patel T. Preneoplastic conditions underlying bile duct cancer. Langenbeck's Arch Surg. 2012;397:861–7.
23. Sithithaworn P, Yongvanit P, Duenngai K, Kiatsopit N, Pairojkul C. Roles of liver fluke infection as risk factor for cholangiocarcinoma. J Hepatobiliary Pancreat Sci. 2014;21:301–8.
24. Sripa B, Mairiang E, Thinkhamrop B, Laha T, Kaewkes S, Sithithaworn P, et al. Advanced periductal fibrosis from infection with the carcinogenic human liver fluke Opisthorchis viverrini correlates with elevated levels of interleukin-6. Hepatology. 2009;50:1273–81.
25. Yongvanit P, Pinlaor S, Loilome W. Risk biomarkers for assessment and chemoprevention of liver fluke-associated cholangiocarcinoma. J Hepatobiliary Pancreat Sci. 2014;21:309–15.
26. Beltrán MA. Pancreaticobiliary reflux in patients with a normal pancreaticobiliary junction: pathologic implications. World J Gastroenterol. 2011;17:953–62.
27. Lee TY, Lee SS, Jung SW, Jeon SH, Yun SC, Oh HC, et al. Hepatitis B virus infection and intrahepatic cholangiocarcinoma in Korea: a case-control study. Am J Gastroenterol. 2008;103(7):1716–20.
28. Welzel TM, Graubard BI, El-Serag HB, Shaib YH, Hsing AW, Davila JA, et al. Risk factors for intrahepatic and extrahepatic cholangiocarcinoma in the United States: a population-based casecontrol study. Clin Gastroenterol Hepatol. 2007;5(10):1221–8.
29. Kumagai S, Kurumatani N, Arimoto A, Ichihara G. Cholangiocarcinoma among offset colour proof-printing workers exposed to 1,2-dichloropropane and/or dichloromethane. Occup Environ Med. 2013;70:508–10.
30. Kubo S, Nakanuma Y, Takemura S, Sakata C, Urata Y, Nozawa A, et al. Case series of 17 patients with cholangiocarcinoma among young adult workers of a printing company in Japan. J Hepatobiliary Pancreat Sci. 2014;21:479–88.
31. Jang S, Chun SM, Hong SM, Sung CO, Park H, Kang HJ, et al. High throughput molecular profiling reveals differential mutation patterns in intrahepatic cholangiocarcinomas arising in chronic advanced liver diseases. Mod Pathol. 2014;27:731–9.
32. Robertson S, Hyder O, Dodson R, Nayar SK, Poling J, Beierl K, et al. The frequency of KRAS and BRAF mutations in intrahepatic cholangiocarcinomas and their correlation with clinical outcome. Hum Pathol. 2013;44:2768–73.
33. Hsu M, Sasaki M, Igarashi S, Sato Y, Nakanuma Y. KRAS and GNAS mutations and p53 overexpression in biliary intraepithelial neoplasia and intrahepatic cholangiocarcinomas. Cancer. 2013;119:1669–74.
34. Al-Bahrani R, Abuetabh Y, Zeitouni N, Sergi C. Cholangiocarcinoma: risk factors, environmental influences and oncogenesis. Ann Clin Lab Sci. 2013;43:195–210.
35. Kobayashi S, Werneburg NW, Bronk SF, Kaufmann SH, Gores GJ. Interleukin-6 contributes to Mcl-1 up-regulation and TRAIL resistance via an Akt-signaling pathway in cholangiocarcinoma cells. Gastroenterology. 2005;128:2054–65.
36. Zheng T, Hong X, Wang J, Pie T, Liang Y, Yin D, et al. Gankyrin promotes tumor growth and metastasis through activation of IL-6/STAT3 signaling in human cholangiocarcinoma. Hepatology. 2014;59:935–46.

37. Isomoto H, Mott JL, Kobayashi S, Warneburg NW, Bronk SF, Haan S, et al. Sustained IL-6/STAT-3 signaling in cholangiocarcinoma cells due to SOCS-3 epigenetic silencing. Gastroenterology. 2007;132:384–96.
38. Wehbe H, Henson R, Meng F, Mize-Berge J, Patel T. Interleukin-6 contributes to growth in cholangiocarcinoma cells by aberrant promoter methylation and gene expression. Cancer Res. 2006;66:10517–24.
39. Nomoto K, Tsuneyama K, Cheng C, Takahashi H, Hori R, Murai Y, et al. Intrahepatic cholangiocarcinoma arising in cirrhotic liver frequently expressed p63-positive basal/stem-cell phenotype. Pathol Res Pract. 2006;202:71–6.
40. Jaiswal M, LaRusso NF, Gores GJ. Nitric oxide in gastrointestinal epithelial cell carcinogenesis: linking inflammation to oncogenesis. Am J Physiol Gastrointest Liver Physiol. 2001;281:G626–34.
41. Jaiswal M, LaRusso NF, Burgart LJ, Gores GJ. Inflammatory cytokines induce DNA damage and inhibit DNA repair in cholangiocarcinoma cells by a nitric oxide-dependent mechanism. Cancer Res. 2000;60:184–90.
42. Jaiswal M, LaRusso NF, Nishioka N, Nakabeppu Y, Gores GJ. Human Ogg1, a protein involved in the repair of 8-oxoguanine, is inhibited by nitric oxide. Cancer Res. 2001;61:6388–93.
43. Z'Graggen K, Rivera JA, Compton CC, Pins M, Werner J, Fernandez-del Castillo C, et al. Prevalence of activating K-ras mutations in the evolutionary stages of neoplasia in intraductal papillary mucinous tumors of the pancreas. Ann Surg. 1997;226:491–8.
44. Boberg KM, Schrumpf E, Bergquist A, Broome U, Pares A, Remotti H, et al. Cholangiocarcinoma in primary sclerosing cholangitis: K-ras mutations and Tp53 dysfunction are implicated in the neoplastic development. J Hepatol. 2000;32:374–80.
45. Taniai M, Higuchi H, Burgart LJ, Gores GJ. p16INK4a promoter mutations are frequent in primary sclerosing cholangitis (PSC) and PSC-associated cholangiocarcinoma. Gastroenterology. 2002;123:1090–8.
46. Olnes MJ, Erlich R. A review and update on cholangiocarcinoma. Oncology. 2004;66:167–79.
47. Chen CY, Shiesh SC, Tsao HC, Lin XZ. The assessment of biliary CA 125, CA 19-9 and CEA in diagnosing cholangiocarcinoma—the influence of sampling time and hepatolithiasis. Hepato-Gastroenterology. 2002;49:616–20.
48. Nehls O, Gregor M, Klump B. Serum and bile markers for cholangiocarcinoma. Semin Liver Dis. 2004;24:139–54.
49. Levy C, Lymp J, Angulo P, Gores GJ, Larusso N, Lindor KD. The value of serum CA 19-9 in predicting cholangiocarcinomas in patients with primary sclerosing cholangitis. Dig Dis Sci. 2005;50:1734–40.
50. Akdogan M, Sasmaz N, Kayhan B, Biyikoglu I, Disibeyaz S, Sahin B. Extraordinarily elevated CA19-9 in benign conditions: a case report and review of the literature. Tumori. 2001;87:337–9.
51. Foley WD, Quiroz FA. The role of sonography in imaging of the biliary tract. Ultrasound Q. 2007;23:123–35.
52. Gores GJ. Early detection and treatment of cholangiocarcinoma. Liver Transpl. 2000;6:S30–4.
53. Braga HJ, Imam K, Bluemke DA. MR imaging of intrahepatic cholangiocarcinoma: use of ferumoxides for lesion localization and extension. AJR Am J Roentgenol. 2001;177:111–4.
54. Gleeson FC, Rajan E, Levy MJ, Clain JE, Topazian MD, Harewood GC, et al. EUS-guided FNA of regional lymph nodes in patients with unresectable hilar cholangiocarcinoma. Gastrointest Endosc. 2008;67:438–43.
55. Petrowsky H, Wildbrett P, Husarik DB, Hany TF, Tam S, Jochum W, et al. Impact of integrated positron emission tomography and computed tomography on staging and management of gallbladder cancer and cholangiocarcinoma. J Hepatol. 2006;45:43–50.
56. Fritscher-Ravens A, Bohuslavizki KH, Broering DC, Jenicke L, Schafer H, Buchert R, et al. FDG PET in the diagnosis of hilar cholangiocarcinoma. Nucl Med Commun. 2001;22:1277–85.
57. Na-Bangchang K, Karbwang J. Traditional herbal medicine for the control of tropical diseases. Trop Med Health. 2014;42(2):3–13.

Index

© Springer International Publishing AG, part of Springer Nature 2018
M. I. Waly, M. S. Rahman (eds.), *Bioactive Components, Diet and Medical Treatment in Cancer Prevention*, https://doi.org/10.1007/978-3-319-75693-6

Printed in the United States
By Bookmasters